PARASITOLOGY

Edited by **Mohammad Manjur Shah**

Parasitology
Edited by Mohammad Manjur Shah

Published by InTech

Janeza Trdine 9, 51000 Rijeka, Croatia

Publishing Process Manager Dragana Manestar

Technical Editor Teodora Smiljanic

Cover Designer InTech Design Team

Additional hard copies can be obtained from orders@intechopen.com

Parasitology, Edited by Mohammad Manjur Shah
p. cm.
ISBN 978-953-51-0149-9

For EU product safety concerns:
IN TECH d.o.o., Prolaz Marije Krucifikse Kozulić 3, 51000 Rijeka, Croatia,
info@intechopen.com or visit our website at intechopen.com.

Meet the editor

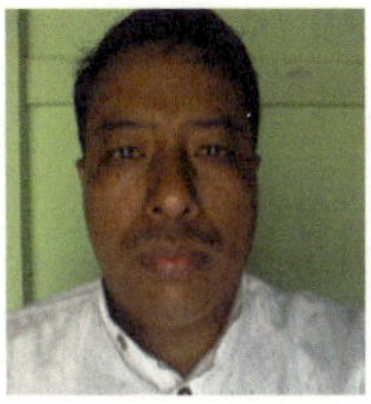

Dr Md. Mohammad Manjur Shah was born on August 01, 1972 at Hatta, Imphal East, Manipur, India. He obtained his Intermediate and BSc from Manipur University, and MSc and PhD from Aligarh Muslim University in the years 1991, 1995, 1997 and 2003. He worked as JRF and later Administrative Assistant in the Ministry of Environment, Government of India, New Delhi. As a Principal Investigator he has successfully completed the Fast Track Scheme of DST from 2006-2009 at Aligarh Muslim University, Aligarh, India. Currently he is working as a Post Doctoral Fellow at the Department of Biotechnology, Government of India, New Delhi and at the Life Sciences Department of Manipur University, Canchipur, Imphal, India. He has undertaken pioneering work on entomophilic nematodes from the entire north east region of India. He attended many conferences where he presented his findings and has published several papers in reputed, peer reviewed national and international journals. He has one monograph to his credit published in Zootaxa which is considered to be one of the world's best journals in taxonomy. In recognition of his academic credentials, he has been listed in several international biographies published in the UK and USA.

Contents

Preface

Parasitology can be defined as a discipline that deals with the study of parasites and their interactions with their hosts. Parasites may live in (as an intracellular/ intercellular parasite) or on the host (as an ectoparasite) without causing any discomfort or disease. Such parasites may be regarded as non-pathogenic parasites whereas those which cause disease or illness are pathogenic parasites. Pathogenic parasites pose numerous threats, not only to humans but also to domesticated animals everywhere. The various challenges imposed by these parasites have led to the subject attracting the interest of not only parasitologists but also other experts in biology and medicine.

The book is mainly intended for biologists in general, zoologists, nematologists, parasitologists, microbiologists, medical doctors, pathologists, as well as molecular biologists. The book addresses the role of parasitology in medicine and public health, while promoting a greater understanding of the intricate issues involving parasites and hosts. Recent advances in the basic and applied approaches (including research on the genetics of parasites) that are discussed in the book will assist in developing chemotherapeutic strategies. World population growth and its impact on agriculture and the emerging field of aquaculture also offers parasitologists an opportunity to contribute at many different levels of research, including the development of new diagnostic tools. Readers of this book can choose a topic of their interest among some of the challenging areas of research like physiological mechanisms underlying the process of locating intermediate/definitive hosts by larval helminth parasites, the physiology of the activation and excystation in many parasites, the complex and varied nature of site selection and pattern of migration seen within helminthes, the sensory biology of parasites, chemical communication between parasites, complex biology of helminth parasites regulated by conserved families of developmental hormones, defined media for helminth parasites, the excretory systems in acanthocephalans and nematodes, production of vaccines by employing recombinant technology, and finally the use of isoenzymes and DNA probes accompanied by PCR for diagnosis that could possibly bring more breakthroughs in parasitology in years to come.

The book was edited by collecting the expert opinions of the scientific community in the field of parasitology from different countries. It presents very interesting and important articles on some of the challenging areas of parasitology and its related human/animal diseases comprising epidemiology, evolution, and control approach involving vaccine development. The entire book contains up-to-date information in 8 chapters placed under two sections namely A. Medical Parasitology and B. Parasite ecology, evolution, morphology, epidemiology and biodiversity. The book is well illustrated with line diagrams, colored plates, and colored and black and white photomicrographs as graphical representations to help the reader easily understand the important information being discussed in the text.

The editor is very thankful to the Publishing Process Managers namely Ms Dragana Manestar, Ms Martina Blecic and Ms Natalia Reinic and also to Aleksandar Lazinica, CEO for believing me to carry on the task and also giving me co-operation throughout the process. Without their initiative and help this book would never have come to light. I also wish to thank all the technical staff associated with publication of the book (both online and in print edition) for making the task a reality. Numerous suggestions from various quarters for improving the book are highly appreciated. I hope this book will be useful to a wide range of readers by giving them a better understanding of the subject.

Lastly, I would like to thank my wife Ruhana who always supported me whenever I got an assignment.

Mohammad Manjur Shah, PhD
DBT-Research Associate
Department of Life Sciences
Manipur University, Canchipur
Imphal,
India

Part 1

Medical Parasitology

1

Tools for *Trans-Splicing* Drug Interference Evaluation in Kinetoplastid

Regina Maria Barretto Cicarelli[1], Lis Velosa Arnosti[1], Caroline Cunha Trevelin[1] and Marco Túlio Alves da Silva[2]

[1]*Universidade Estadual Paulista - Faculdade de Ciências Farmacêuticas - Depto Ciências Biológicas, Rodovia Araraquara-Jaú, São Paulo*

[2]*Universidade De São Paulo – Instituto de Física de São Carlos – Depto Física e Informática, São Carlos*

Brazil

1. Introduction

The scientific progress of the last century has led man to understand every day the intricate mechanisms involved in the transfer of genetic material and how it is interpreted to trigger the most important biochemical processes of the cells for their survival.

It should be noted that the biochemical cell repertoire is conserved in all living organisms on the planet. Since 1990, the scientists observed that eukaryotes have excessively large genomes with hundreds of thousands of introns which were inserted into genes. Most protein-coding genes in human genome are composed of multiple exons interrupted by introns. Advances in the knowledge of genomics and proteomics of mammals confirmed the need for reprogramming of mRNA used to obtain the products of genes and production of proteins and the significance of pre-mRNA splicing, which is an essential step of gene expression by removing noncoding sequences (introns) to ligate together coding sequences (exons). The exons are usually relatively short about 50–250 base pairs, whereas introns are much larger and can be up to several thousands of base pairs. Splicing is a complex nuclear RNA processing event, where different exons from pre-mRNA molecules are joined together. The intron sequences are removed from the pre-mRNA and the exons fused together resulting in the formation of the mature messenger RNA (mRNA), which is subsequently capped at its 5′ end and polyadenylated at its 3′ end, and transported out of the nucleus to be translated into protein in the cytoplasm.

In general, most genes give rise to multiple spliced transcripts by alternative splicing, leading to different mRNA variants and the synthesis of alternative proteins. Utilizing different alternative 5' or 3' splice sites, multiple protein isoforms can be generated from a commom primary transcript (van Santen & Spritz, 1986; Adami & Babiss, 1991; Gattoni et al., 1991; Guo et al., 1991; reviewed by Horowitz & Krainer, 1994; Sharp, 1994, as cited in Eul et al., 1995).

The simple existence of alternatively spliced products greatly increases cellular and organism complexity and may have allowed for evolution by producing additional regulation and diversification of gene function. It is obvious that splicing and alternative splicing must be tightly regulated and executed in time and space not to interfere with the normal cellular and organism physiology. The spliceosome, an intracellular complex of multiple proteins and ribonucleoproteins, is the main cellular machinery guiding splicing. Recently, two natural compounds interfering with the spliceosome were found to display anti-tumour activity *in vitro* and *in vivo*. Therefore, it is conceivable that inhibiting the spliceosome could serve as a novel target for anticancer drug development (Kaida et al., 2007; Kotake et al., 2007, as cited in van Alphen et al., 2009).

Cis-splicing occurs when two exons are initially part of a contiguous RNA, and trans-splicing, where the two exons are initially on two separate RNAs. In the latter case, the partial intron sequences flanking the two exons pair through sequence complementarity to form a catalytic structure joining the associated exons (Will & Lurhmann, 2006).

To direct correct processing of pre-mRNA, the intron sequences contain a number of core splicing signals, notably the conserved splice-site sequences at their extreme 5′ and 3′ ends and a conserved branch point region. The branch point sequence and the branch point itself, usually an adenosine, are located about 20–40 nucleotides upstream of the 3′ splice site. The critical process of recognizing splice sites and the removal of introns and/or exons is the task of the spliceosome (Staley & Guthrie, 1998; Will & Luhrmann, 2001, as cited in van Alphen et al., 2009). The spliceosome consists of five non-coding uridine-rich small nuclear ribonucleoproteins (U snRNPs) and a multitude of associated proteins, creating a network of RNA–RNA, RNA–protein and protein–protein interactions (Zhou et al., 2002; Jurica & Moore, 2003, as cited in van Alphen et al., 2009). See figure 1 for details.

In fact, well over 200 different splicing factors interacting with the spliceosome have been identified, and it is clear that much more research is needed before we fully understand all the intricacies of RNA splicing (Jurica & Moore, 2003; Wang & Burge, 2008, as cited in van Alphen et al., 2009). The various spliceosome components, in particular, the small nuclear RNPs, are sequentially recruited to the splice sites. Next, they are assembled into the spliceosome after which splicing is initiated by a series of two transesterification reactions producing two ligated exons and a liberated intron (Staley & Guthrie, 1998; Wang and Burge, 2008, as cited in van Alphen et al., 2009). See figure 1 for additional details.

Through interactions with various proteins that recognise specific splice site features, the spliceosome components, that is, small nuclear ribonucleoproteins (snRNPs) designated with U1, U2, U4, U5 and U6 are sequentially recruited to the splice site and assembled into the spliceosome. Once completed, splicing is catalysed in two consecutive transesterification reactions. In the initial step, the 2′ OH group of the branch point adenosine upstream of the 3′ end of the intron reacts with the 5′ splice junction, forming a novel 2′, 5′ phosphodiester bond between the branch point and the 5′ terminal nucleotide of the intron, giving rise to a lariat structure. In the second reaction, the 3′ OH of the 5′ exon attacks the 3′ splice junction producing linked 5′ and 3′ exons and liberating the intron. Subsequently, the snRNPs involved are released and recycled in the splicing process. In the top right-hand corner, a detailed view of U2 snRNP with subcomplexes, SF3a and SF3b, is shown. The figure and legend were transcribed from van Alphen et al. (2009).

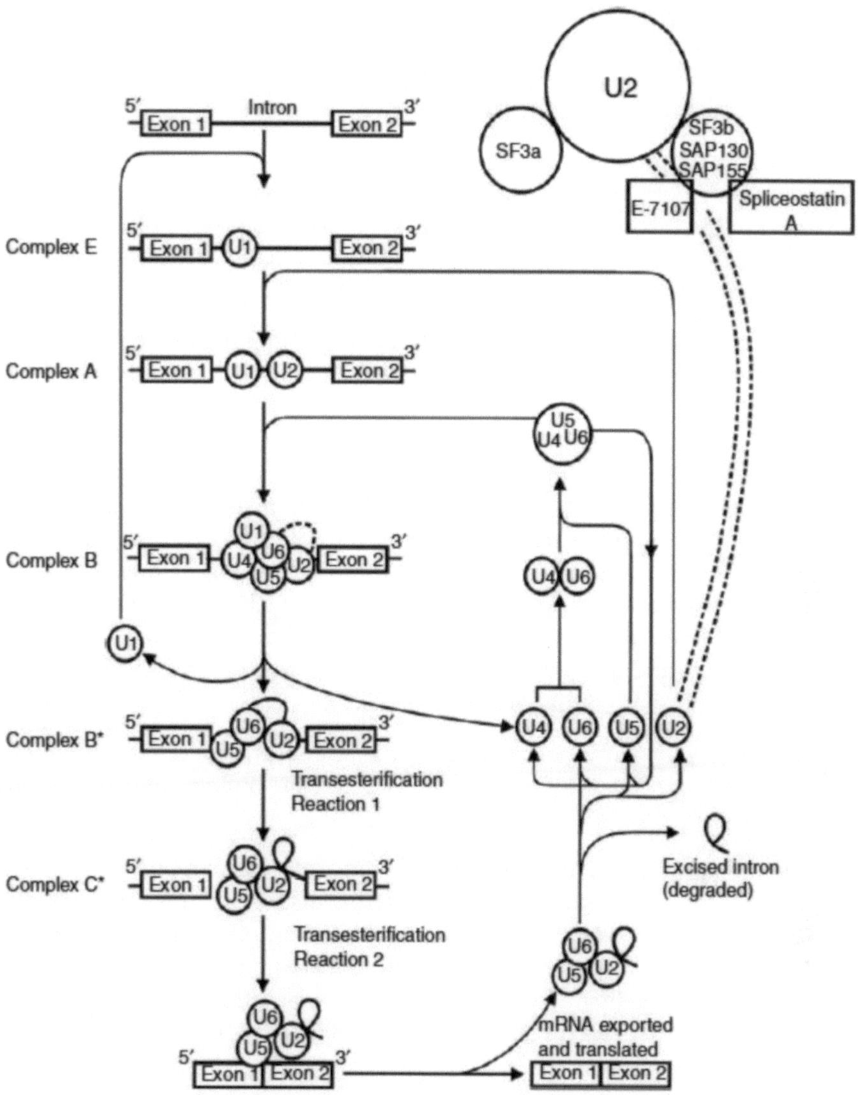

Fig. 1. The spliceosome assembly cycle.

Splicing at different locations in the same pre-mRNA transcript, alternative splicing, enables a gene to produce variant mature mRNAs, and consequently functionally different proteins (House & Lynch, 2008, as cited in van Alphen et al., 2009). The precise mechanisms of and/or triggers for alternative splicing are yet unknown. In higher eukaryotes, like humans, the accuracy of splicing is not solely dictated by base-pairing interactions of the U snRNPs with the pre-mRNA. Owing to degeneracy and poor definition of small splice sites at the end of long introns, splice-site recognition is also influenced by (a) the coupling of splicing with other processes such as transcription, (b) the velocity of the splicing reaction, (c) external stimuli, like the presence of growth factors or oxidative stress and (d) the three-dimensional structure of pre-mRNA itself

(Tazi et al., 2005b; Disher & Skandalis, 2007; House & Kristen, 2008, as cited in van Alphen et al., 2009). In the latter case, the three-dimensional folding of pre-mRNA determines whether a (in pre-mRNA embedded) splice regulator will be located in the vicinity of a splice site (for details see van Alphen et al., 2009).

In trans-splicing, two pre-mRNAs are processed to produce a mature transcript that contains exons from both precursors. This process also involves two trans-esterification steps that result in the linking of the two exons by a normal 3'-5' phosphodiester bond. This process has been described mostly in trypanosomes, nematodes, chloroplasts, and plant mitochondria (Bonen, 1993, as cited in Caudevilla et al., 1998).

Kinetoplastids are a remarkable group of protists. They contain a range of ubiquitous free-living species - pathogens of invertebrates, vertebrates and even some plants. *Trypanosoma* species cause sleeping sickness and Chagas disease, whereas the leishmaniases kill and debilitate hundreds of thousands of people worldwide each year. Furthermore, these morphologically rather simple unicellular organisms are masters at finding unorthodox solutions to the problems of being a eukaryotic cell. Kinetoplastid peculiarities include: (1) complex and energy-consuming mitochondrial RNA editing; (2) a unique mitochondrial DNA architecture; (3) trans-splicing of all mRNA transcripts; (4) the arrangement of genes into giant polycistronic clusters; (5) unprecedented modifications of nucleotides; (vi) the compartmentalization of glycolysis; (vii) evasion of the host immune response using a variable surface coat; and (viii) the ability to escape destruction by migrating out of phagocytic (McConville et al., 2002; Sacks & Sher, 2002).

Trypanosomes are protozoan which intriguing the scientists since a long time for various reasons. Primarily by the pathogenicity followed by the biology and evolution on the phylogenetic tree.

To our studies, *Trypanosoma cruzi* always is a very important model, because it is the etiologic agent of Chagas disease, an endemic parasitic disease in Latin America, discovered by Carlos Chagas in 1909, which still remains without an effective treatment. *T. cruzi* is transmitted by triatomine insects and can also be transmitted by blood transfusion or the placenta, during breastfeeding, through organ transplantation and by processed food contaminated with the insect vector (Lana & Tafuri, 2000; Rey, 2001).

Currently, between 12 and 14 million people are infected and more than 100 million live in endemic areas. Chagas disease is a major neglected diseases considered in the world and affects mainly low-income people. Treatment of infected people in endemic areas has been recommended by the National Health Foundation of Brazil for acute or recent chronic cases as well as for congenital and accidental infections and for children with positive serology (Rey, 2001; WHO, 2005).

The pathogenicity pattern of the disease may be influenced by the characteristics of both human host and the lineage of the *T. cruzi* strain. Thus, the course of infection in susceptible vertebrates is influenced not only by the environmental features or genetic constitution of the human host, but mainly by morphological characteristics of the infecting strains versus host immune response, as well as of therapeutic agents and susceptibility of the *T. cruzi* strain. These are the most challenge limiting the successful treatment and cure of the disease (Teixeira et al., 2006).

In late 1960 and early 70s, two drugs were first used in the treatment of Chagas disease: nifurtimox (NFX - Bayer) and benznidazole (BZ - Roche), sold, respectively, by the trademarks, Lampit® and Rochagan®. Both are more effective to eliminate parasites in the acute phase, reducing the course of infection, since the disease had not affected the cardiovascular system, leading to cure in 78% of patients in acute phase. However, the effectiveness of both drugs in treatment of chronic disease is limited to 8% cure (Coura & de Castro, 2002; Teixeira et al., 2006).

The low efficiency of these drugs with undesirable side-effects imposed limitations on their use. Furthermore, different strains of *T. cruzi* present different levels of susceptibility to benznidazole and nifurtimox, which may explain in part the observed differences in the effectiveness of chemotherapy. In Brazil, nifurtimox was withdrawn of the market due to severe side effects. Thus, the benznidazole became the only alternative for treatment, despite widespread criticism due also to its adverse side effects and low effectiveness in the chronic phase. To date, despite several studies, there is no available vaccine for Chagas disease. Therefore, the identification of new chemotherapeutic and vaccine methods is the biggest challenge for the control of Chagas disease (Issa & Bocchi, 2010).

Several strains of *T. cruzi* were isolated from different countries and geographical areas. Major differences in resistance or susceptibility to the benznidazole in experimental or clinical studies were reported between different strains of the parasite. These findings further complicate the search for new anti-*T. cruzi* drugs. The same approach would be evaluated for vaccine.

Either in Chagas disease as well as other parasitic diseases, cell biology and immunology studies help to understand the mechanisms involved in the ability of certain stages of the parasites (trypomastigotes) invade cells, transforming into replicative forms (amastigotes) which escapes the immune system. Furthermore, the development of new chemotherapeutic attack points takes into account the mechanisms of drug resistance. Thus, the development of work in this field of research may eventually corroborate to minimize or destroy the parasitism, searching for new drugs targeting only the parasites and not cause damage in human cells (Coura & de Castro, 2002). The study of new trypanocidal drugs involves specific objectives related to the structure and RNA processing in *T. cruzi*, which should be first studied on *in vitro* experiments.

Trypanosomatids are early-diverged, protozoan parasites some of them cause severe and lethal diseases in humans, as already described before in *T. cruzi*. To better combat these parasites, their molecular biology has been a research focus for more than 3 decades. Messenger RNA (mRNA) maturation in trypanosomes differs from the process in most eukaryotes mainly because protein-coding genes are transcribed into polycistronic RNAs and processed by trans-splicing in which a common spliced leader sequence (SL) is acquired at the 5'-end to yield mature transcripts. SL trans-splicing has been characterized mainly in trypanosomes and nematodes and requires, in addition to the SL RNP, the small nuclear ribonucleoproteins (U snRNPs) U2, U4/U6, and U5.

Such addition of short, nontranslated leaders to coding transcripts has been observed in representatives from both the protists and animal kingdoms and the phenomenon has been intensively studied particularly in trypanosomes and nematodes, which about 15% of the genes are transcribed by trans-splicing mechanism. To date, the *in vitro* trans-splicing reaction was better study in nematode pre-messenger RNA (Nielsen, 1993).

Until recently, only two snRNP-specific proteins had been studied in trypanosomes, namely, the orthologs of human U2A' (originally termed U2-40K) and the U5-specific PRP8. While the latter was identified by sequence homology, U2A' was copurified with the U2 snRNA in high-stringency U snRNP purifications which typically left only the core structures intact. For a more comprehensive biochemical characterization of U snRNPs and/or of the spliceosome, it was therefore essential to purify the RNA-protein complexes under conditions of lower stringency. A method well-suited for this purpose is tandem affinity purification (TAP), which is based on expressing a known protein factor fused to a composite TAP tag. TAP comprises two consecutive high-affinity chromatography steps which are carried out under nearly physiological conditions. Since the advent of this technology, the TAP tag and the TAP method have been modified in various ways to accommodate different systems, extracts, or protein complexes. For the purification of nuclear protein complexes in trypanosomes, the PTP (protein C epitope-TEV protease cleavage site-protein A domains) modification of TAP has proven to be very useful. One of the first applications of the PTP tag was the purification of the trypanosome U1 snRNP (Günzl 2010). The figure 2 illustrates the different spliceosomal factors of humans and trypanosomes.

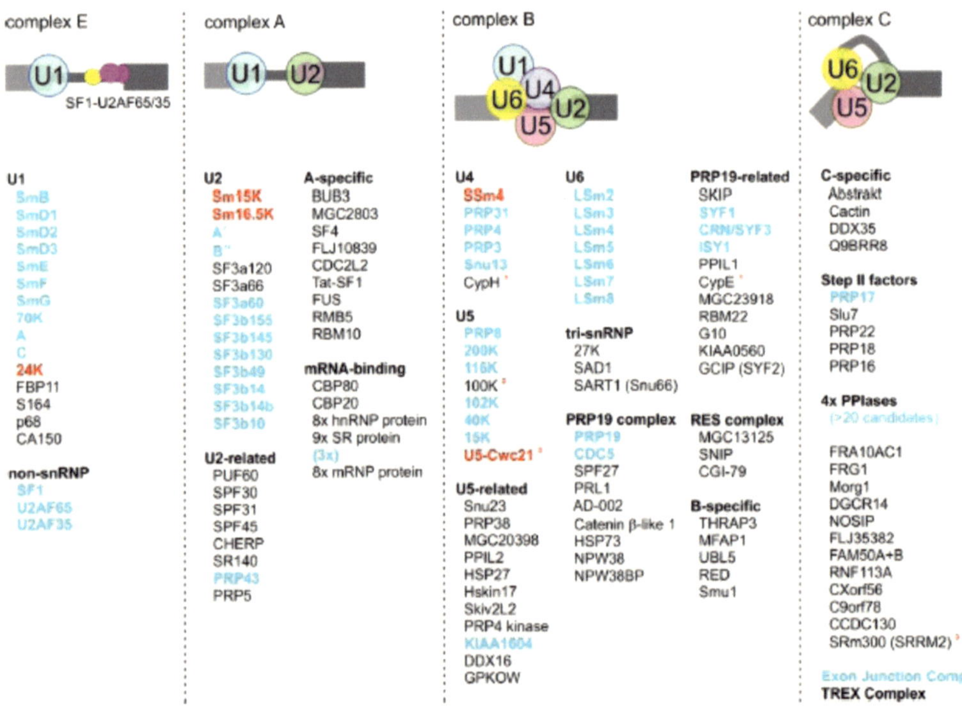

Fig. 2. Comparison of known spliceosomal factors of humans and trypanosomes. For more details the figure was transcribed from Günzl (2010).

2. Trans-splicing and alternative splicing in mammalian cells

Trans-splicing of artificial pre-mRNAs in mammalian cells *in vitro* has been reported but with some limitations. In addition, nematodes or Simian virus 40 spliced leader RNAs can be accurately trans-spliced in transfected COS cells, which revealed functional conservation in the splicing machinery between lower eukaryotes and mammals and demonstrated the potential occurrence of the trans-splicing in mammalian cells (Bruzik & Maniatis, 1992). Studies *in vivo* also have shown that a synthetic pre-mRNA substrate containing an exon and a 5' donor splice site can be efficiently trans-spliced to another synthetic pre-mRNA (3' trans-splicing substrate) if it contains either exonic enhancers or a 5' downstream splice site. Several examples of possible natural trans-splicing in mammalian cells have been reported, but none of these trans-splicing have been demonstrated *in vitro* (Caudevilla et al., 1998).

The hypothesis that trans-splicing is a regular event in mammalian cells was first suggested by Dandekar & Sibbald (1990). Later, the capability of mammalian cells to perform trans-splicing reaction with appropriate foreign RNAs also was demonstrated *in vivo* (Eul et al., 1995). In this work the authors have demonstrated the potential of mammalian cells to generated functional mRNA molecules by trans-splicing. However, there is a competition between cis- and trans-splicing in these cells, which was also demonstrated in nematodes. These worms perform both RNA splice patterns simultaneously (Blumental & Thomas, 1988; Conrad et al., 1993a, b; Nielsen, 1993). In these cells, cis-splicing is dominant when a protein coding precursor RNA contains a valid 5′ and 3′ splice site at its most proximal part. When, however, the 5′ splice site is deleted, cis-splicing is prevented and the remaining 3′ splice site combines with the 5′ splice site of an SL RNA molecule to generate a new mRNA molecule by trans-splicing (Conrad et al., 1991, 1993a). Maybe this is a precursor mechanism of alternative splicing in mammals. Since trypanosomes are protozoan and therefore more primitive eukaryotes, the trans-splicing mechanism occurs more frequently than cis-splicing, although the latter is also present in this cell type as mentioned before.

For trans-splicing in plant mitochondria and plastids, extensive base pairing within the introns of the two pre-mRNAs seems to be essential (Chapdelaine & Bonen, 1991; Knoop et al., 1991; Sharp, 1991, as cited in Eul et al., 1995). These organelles do not contain U snRNAs ans RNPs (Cech, 1986; Saldanha et al., 1993) and the functions of the different snRNAs are replaced by a highly conserved RNA secondary structure specific for all group II introns (Sharp, 1991; Suchy & Schmelzer, 1991; Saldanha et al., 1993).

Caudevilla et al. (1998) have shown that the rat-liver carnitine octanoyltransferase (COT) is a single-copy gene, which is able to be processed in several mature transcripts involving cis- and trans-splicing events. The authors showed the occurrence of three purine rich exonic-splicing enhancers (ESE) in the sequence of exon 2 of the COT gene, which are detected at positions 49 (GAAGAACGAA), 106 (GAAGAA), and 117 (GAAGAAG). This is showed in the figure 3.

The exons are represented by boxes and introns by dotted lines. Sequences 5 '- and 3'-intronic splicing sites are indicated in lowercase. The ESE (exonic-splicing enhancers) is represented in exon 2 in capital letters. Simultaneous cis- and trans-splicing of hepatic mRNA COT are produced. Trans-splicing can be promoted by ESE sequences. Three different transcripts can be produced: one by cis-splicing and two by trans-splicing where exon 2 or exon 2 and exon 3 are repeated. The organization of mature mRNAs is represented at the foot of the figure. The figure was transcribed from Caudevilla et al. (1998).

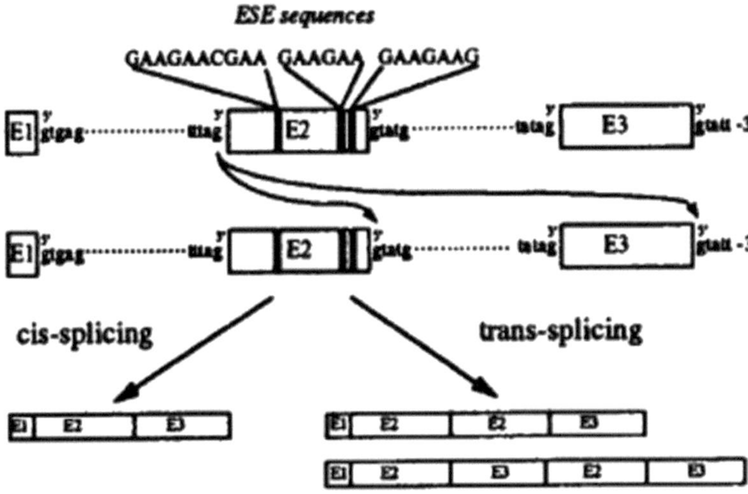

Fig. 3. Model of cis and trans-splicing in mammalian cells (COT pre-mRNA).

Splicing enhancers facilitate the assembly of protein complexes on mRNAs containing a 3′ splice site, and these complexes are sufficiently stable to interact with 5′ splice site located on separate mRNAs.

Conrad et al. (1991, 1993b) demonstrated that a cis-splicing acceptor can act as a trans-splice acceptor if it is moved into a proper context, referred to an outron, which is an intron without a well defined 5' donor splice site. So, in this context, trans-splicing in mammals can be used to reprogram or interfere with specific pre-mRNAs, thus modifying or completely changing the gene expression (Puttaraju et al., 1999; Mansfield et al., 2000, as cited in Codony et al., 2001). In the reprogramming of the target pre-mRNA, it is first necessary to establish which exons of the target pre-mRNA are susceptible to involvement in a trans-splicing reaction. The same principle seems to occur with genes in trypanosomes as well as poly A polymerase, which are cis-spliced, instead of trans-splicing.

Intervening sequences have been described in the Poly A Polymerase (PAP) gene of *Trypanosoma brucei* and *Trypanosoma cruzi,* and a U1 snRNA sequence in *T. brucei,* demonstrating that both cis- and trans-splicing can occur in these organisms, with a prevalence of trans (Mair et al., 2000).

RNA splicing is carried out by the spliceosome, which consists of the five small nuclear ribonucleoprotein particles (snRNPs) U1, U2, U4, U5 and U6, as well as non-snRNP proteins. The ribonucleoproteins are complexes consisting of small uridine-rich RNAs (UsnRNAs), interacting with common Sm proteins and specific proteins for each snRNP. Although well characterized in humans and yeast, little is known about the specific proteins involved in trans-splicing in trypanosomatids (Mayer & Floeter-Winter, 2005). It would be interesting to speculate that the cis-splicing of the poly A polymerase genes can be used as a protozoan mechanism to maintain the viability of their most mRNAs newly trans-spliced.

Many external trans-RNA, like trans-donor or a trans-acceptor that will participate in a trans-splicing reaction, can be synthesized to interfere with other pre-mRNAs (Bruzik & Maniatis, 1995; Chiara & Reed, 1995).

Because of trans-splicing is a post-transcriptional processing event, which was first demonstrated in T*rypanosoma brucei* (Murphy et al., 1986; Sutton & Boothroyd, 1986), in these cells, a 39 nucleotides (nt), "mini-exon", derived from a 140 nt small leader (SL) RNAs is trans-spliced to all pre-mRNA molecules (reviewed by Bonen, 1993; Ullu et al., 1993, as cited in Eul et al., 1995). It was demonstrated that in mammals the cells can utilize a cryptic 5' splice site within the second exon and the conventional 3' splice site, even the cis-splicing is dominant in these cells (Eul et al., 1995). Competition between trans- and cis-splicing has also been demonstrated in nematodes, which perform both RNA splice patterns simultaneously (Blumenthal & Thomas, 1988; Conrad et al., 1993a, b; Nielsen, 1993). In these cells, cis-splicing is dominant when a protein coding precursor RNA contains a valid 5' and 3' splice site at its proximal part. When, however, the 5' splice site is deleted, cis-splicing is prevented and the remaining 3' splice site combines with the 5' splice site of an SL RNA molecule to generate a new RNA molecule by trans-splicing (Conrad et al., 1991, 1993a; Eul et al., 1995).

A diagram comparing the two mechanisms is shown in Figure 4.

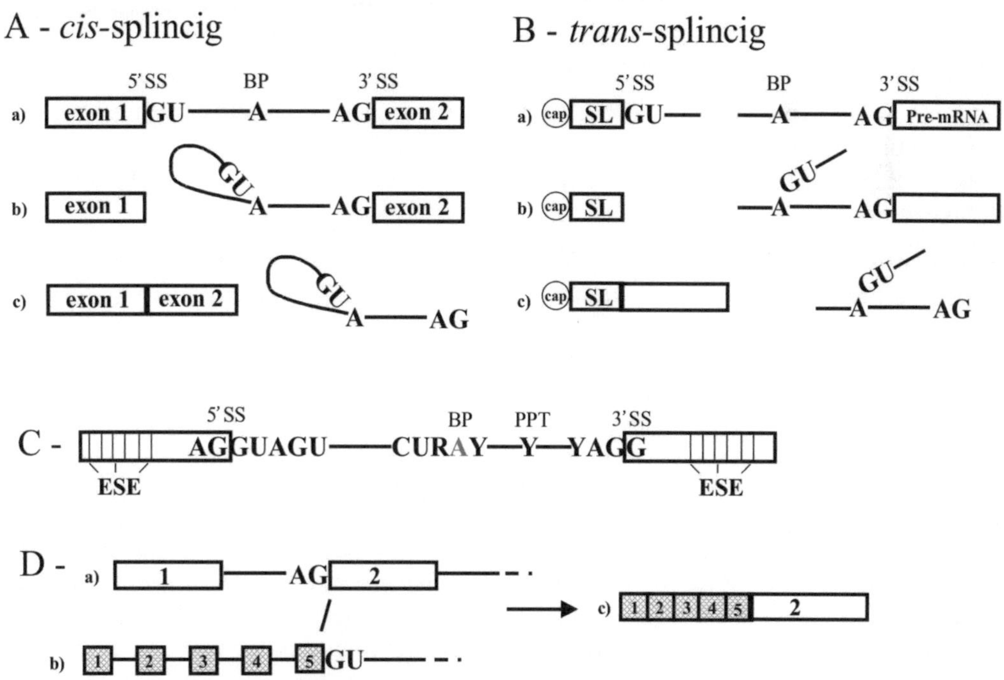

Fig. 4. Schematic representation of cis- and trans-splicing pathways.

A: cis-splicing occurs through a two-step mechanism, each step consisting of a transesterification reaction (Moore et al. 1993, as cited in Mayer & Floeter-Winter, 2005). In the first transesterification (a to b), a nucleophilic attack of a 2'-OH group from an adenosine residue within the intron (branch point, BP) to the phosphorous atom at the 5' splice site (5' SS) generates two intermediates: exon 1 with a free 3'-OH terminus and an intron-exon 2 in a lariat configuration. In the second transesterification (b to c), the 3'-OH group form the exon 1 intermediate acts as a nucleophile and attacks the phosphorous atom at 3' splice site (3' SS), resulting in the displacement of the 3' end of the intron and joining of the 5' and 3' exons. B: SL-addition trans-splicing is very similar to the canonical cis-splicing, except for the use of two substrate molecules, which is the reason for the generation of a Y branched intermediate instead of a lariat. C: cis regulatory elements involved in pre-mRNA splicing. 5' SS, 3' SS, and BP consensus sequences are shown. Polypyrimidine tract (PPT) and exonic splicing enhancers (ESE) are indicated. D: schematic representation of trans-splicing between (a) ABP (androgen-carrier protein produced in the testicular Sertoli cell) and (b) HDC (histidine decarboxylase) pre-mRNAs; (c) represent the mature chimeric mRNA. This figure was transcribed from Mayer & Floeter-Winter, (2005).

Recent research has revealed that alternatively spliced products can be linked to various (genetic) diseases and also may play a role in cancer development (Wang & Burge, 2008, as cited in van Alphen et al., 2009). A systematic approach using large-scale sequencing and splicing-sensitive microarrays gave for the first time a view of the vast spectrum of alternative transcripts (Blencowe, 2006; Ben-Dov et al., 2008, as cited in van Alphen et al., 2009). One or more alternatively spliced exons can be found in transcripts of two-thirds of human genes. In general, the function of the encoded protein remains unchanged. However, some of the alternative protein products may display a malignant phenotype (Blencowe, 2006, as cited in van Alphen et al., 2009). Whether alternative splicing is the cause or result of malignant behavior in cancer cells remains unclear.

However, as alternative splicing affects most genes, it is likely that cell cycle control, signal transduction, angiogenesis, motility and invasion and the metastasis and apoptosis processes that are often impaired in cancer will be affected (Skotheim & Nees, 2007, as cited in van Alphen et al., 2009).

The delineation of splice sites used in alternative splicing or the functional characterization of aberrant proteins expressed as a result of alternative splicing may provide the necessary insight for therapeutic interference. Specific splice-site mutations or proteins might (a) prove to be of predictive value and (b) become potential prognostic markers (Yu et al., 2007, as cited in van Alphen et al., 2009), (c) prove to be targets of future (anticancer) antibody-guided drugs (Orban & Olah, 2003; Heider et al., 2004; Xiang et al., 2007, as cited in van Alphen et al., 2009) or (d) become a target for peptide receptor radionucleotide therapy. An example of the latter is a splice variant of the cholecystokinin receptor found in colorectal and pancreatic cancer that can be targeted by radionuclide therapy (Laverman et al., 2008, as cited in van Alphen et al., 2009). A disease in which an understanding of the alternative splicing process is used for therapeutic purposes is Duchenne's muscular dystrophy (DMD), which is a neuromuscular disease caused by deletions/duplications or point mutations in the 2.4Mb DMD gene, encoding dystrophin, causing disruption of the open reading frame (ORF). The induction of exon skipping, circumventing the mutated exon through intramuscular injection of carefully designed antisense oligonucleotides, corrects the ORF of dystrophin in *in vitro* cell lines, animal models and humans (van Deutekom et al., 2007, as cited in van Alphen et al., 2009). Another example concerns spinal muscular atrophy (SMA) caused by the deletion of SMA1 gene and the inability of the remaining SMA2 gene, which is virtually identical to SMA1, to compensate for the SMA1 loss, as its transcript lacks exon 7 (for review see van Alphen et al., 2009). Maybe a similar approach would help to evaluate the study of drug target in trans-splicing mechanism in parasites.

3. Trans-splicing in mammalian cells versus methodology for detection

Although trans-splicing has been suggested as being a widespread RNA processing system among eukaryotic cells (see references in Eul et al., 1995), no clear experimental evidence has been obtained so far that authentic mRNA molecules and functional proteins are generated in mammalian cells by trans-splicing. However, some results from Eul et al. (1995) supported the hypothesis that trans-splicing is a regular RNA processing mechanism in mammalian cells, since using molecular biology tools in rat cells were able to generate the T1 antigens (for SV-40 virus) by means of trans-splicing. This is not so hard to understanding nowadays, since trypanosomes also use cis-splicing as an alternative mRNA processing.

The best candidates for the trans-splice reaction are those donor pre-mRNA molecules, where 5' splice donor site is not followed by a functional 3' splice site, which would favour a cis-splice reaction. Any candidate for an RNA acceptor molecule must still contain a functional 3' splice acceptor site. In the case of T1 mRNA, donor and acceptor RNA molecules are the same primary transcripts; but it may also be that independent transcripts, derived from different loci, are joined together to generate hybrid protein molecules splice site through trans-splicing (Eul et al., 1995).

The features of an RNA molecule that lead to trans-splicing are still not clear. Caudevilla et al. (2001) in their work assumed that RNA molecules which contain cryptic splice sites that cannot be used for cis-splicing, are good candidates for heterologous trans-splicing. Cryptic splice sites can be a genuine feature of a gene (e. g. HIV-nef) or they can be generated and activated by point mutation. It is noteworthy that splice site mutations are frequently associated with human genetic diseases. One interesting question in heterologous trans-splicing is how RNA molecules that are transcribed from different genes find each other, differently on the trypanosomes trans-splicing mRNAs which have always the 39 nucleotides in 5′ end. The model in mammals proposes that the splice sites from stable complexes with ribonucleoproteins and with splice factors such as SR proteins (Fu & Maniatis, 1992; Staknis & Reed, 1994, as cited in Caudevilla et al., 2001) that mediate the association of the two RNA molecules by protein-protein interaction (Eul et al., 1995). SR proteins have both exon-dependent and independent functions in pre-mRNA splicing (Hertel & Maniatis, 1999, as cited in Caudevilla et al., 2001). These proteins bind to purine-rich sequences called exon splicing enhancer (ESE), promoting both the assembly of the pre-spliceosomal complex (Staknis & Reed, 1994, as cited in Caudevilla et al., 2001) and the subsequent splicing steps (Chew et al., 1999, as cited in Caudevilla et al., 2001). The importance of these purine-rich sequences for trans-splicing *in vivo* was further confirmed by analyzing COT mRNA processing in Cos7 monkey cells. In contrast to the rat COT gene, the second exon of the monkey COT gene lacks an ESE and the cells do not perform homologous COT trans-splicing. Moreover, direct RNA-RNA association via complementary sequences may additionally facilitate heterologous trans-splice efficiency as it was shown for ribozyme trans-splicing (Koehler et al., 1999; Puttaraju et al., 1999, as cited in Caudevilla et al., 2001) and for homologous SV40 T-antigen trans-splicing (Eul et al., 1995).

The mechanism of the trans-splicing process presumably is more similar to cis-splicing than the trans-splicing process in trypanosomes, nematodes and plant cell organelles, requiring the formation of an equivalent pre-spliceosomal complex. Formation of the pre-spliceosomal complex may be facilitated by a direct base pairing between the two precursor mRNA molecules (Eul et al., 1995). In analogy to cis-splicing, the U1 snRNP could bind via its snRNA to the 5′ cryptic splice site on the first pre-mRNA (molecule A) and the U2 snRNP to the branch site of the second pre-mRNA (molecule B) The donor 5′ splice site and the branch site of the two RNA molecules are brought together by a U1/U2 snRNP interaction/association (Mattaj et al., 1986; Chabot & Steitz, 1987; Lutz & Alwine, 1994, as cited in Eul et al., 1995).

Although trans-splicing has been suggested as being widespread RNA processing system among eukaryotic cells (Konarska et al., 1985; Solnick, 1985; Sharp, 1987; Dandekar & Sibbald, 1990; Joseph et al., 1991; Nigro et al., 1991; Shimizu et al., 1991; Sullivan et al., 1991, as cited in Eul et al., 1995), no clear experimental evidence has been obtained that authentic mRNA molecules and functional proteins are generated in mammals cells by trans-splicing. But the results obtained by Eul et al. (1995) supported the hypothesis that trans-splicing is a regular RNA processing mechanism in mammalian cells, since they showed that the best candidates for the trans-splice reaction are those donor pre-mRNA molecules, where the 5′ splice donor site is not followed by a functional 3′ splice site, which would favour a cis-splice reaction. Any candidate for an RNA acceptor molecule must still contain a functional 3′ splice acceptor site (Eul et al., 1995).

Excision of intronic sequences from pre-mRNAs (pre-mRNA splicing) is an obligatory step for the expression of the majority of higher eukaryotic genes and requires the function of a complex molecular machinery, the spliceosome, which is composed of five small nuclear ribonucleoprotein (snRNP) complexes and more than 200 proteins (for review, see Wahl et al., 2009, as cited in Corrionero et al., 2011). The function of the spliceosome relies on an intricate network of protein–protein, protein–RNA, and RNA–RNA interactions that undergo significant conformational and compositional rearrangements to facilitate intron excision (for review, see Smith et al., 2008; Wahl et al., 2009, as cited in Corrionero et al., 2011). These interactions can be modulated to allow the generation of alternative patterns of splicing, a phenomenon reported to occur in the majority of human genes (for review, see Chen & Manley, 2009; Nilsen & Graveley, 2010, as cited in Corrionero et al., 2011). Alternative splicing plays important roles in the development of multicellular organisms and in numerous pathologies, including cancer (for review, see Cooper et al., 2009; David & Manley, 2010, as cited in Corrionero et al., 2011).

The efficiency and precision required for intron removal is in contrast to the limited sequence consensus at intron/exon boundaries, a feature likely connected to the establishment of mechanisms of splice site regulation mediated by a diverse array of auxiliary sequences and cognate factors (for review, see Wang & Burge, 2008; Barash et al., 2010, as cited in Corrionero et al., 2011).

In higher eukaryotes, the 39 end of the intron is characterized by a polypyrimidine-rich sequence (the pY-tract) followed by a conserved AG as the intron 39-most dinucleotide. Upstream of the pY-tract is the branch point, which functions optimally when it coincides with the invariant yeast sequence UACUAAC (Zhuang et al., 1989, as cited in Corrionero et al., 2011), but which corresponds to the loose consensus YUNAY in higher eukaryotes (Y representing pyrimidines, R purines, N any nucleotide, and the A represents the invariant adenosine that engages in a 29–59 phosphodiester bond with the 59 end of the intron after the first catalytic step of the splicing reaction) (Gao et al., 2008; for review, see Wahl et al., 2009, as cited in Corrionero et al., 2011). Initial recognition of the 39 splice site sequences involves cooperative binding of the branch point-binding protein (BBP/SF1) to the branch point, and of the U2 snRNP auxiliary factor (U2AF) 65-kDa and 35-kDa subunits to the pY-tract and the AG dinucleotide, respectively (Ruskin et al., 1988; Zamore et al., 1992; Berglund et al., 1997; Merendino et al., 1999; Wu et al., 1999; Zorio & Blumenthal, 1999; Liu et al., 2001; Selenko et al., 2003, as cited in Corrionero et al., 2011). RNA–protein and protein–protein contacts involving these factors are believed to enforce a unique RNA structure that triggers subsequent events in 39 splice site recognition (Kent et al., 2003, as cited in Corrionero et al., 2011). These interactions, together with recognition of the 59 splice site by U1 snRNP and possibly other contacts across the intron, establish the earliest ATP-independent (E) complex that commits the pre-mRNA to the splicing pathway (Michaud & Reed, 1991, 1993, as cited in Corrionero et al., 2011).

The next step in 39 splice site recognition is the recruitment of U2 snRNP, which is composed of U2 snRNA and several polypeptides, including two protein subcomplexes (SF3a and SF3b), which are part of the 17S U2 snRNP complex (for review, see Wahl et al., 2009, as cited in Corrionero et al., 2011). SF3a is composed of three subunits of 60, 66, and 120 kDa, while SF3b is composed of at least eight subunits of 10, 14a, 14b, 49, 125, 130, 140, and 155 kDa (for review, see Wahl et al., 2009, as cited in Corrionero et al., 2011). U2 snRNP recruitment involves at least two separable steps. U2 snRNP has been detected in E complexes, but U2 binding in this complex is not stable and does not require the presence of a branch point (Hong et al., 1997; Das et al., 2000; Donmez et al., 2004, 2007, as cited in Corrionero et al., 2011). Stable binding of U2 snRNP to form pre-spliceosomal complex A requires ATP and depends on base-pairing interactions between the branch point and a region of U2 snRNA known as the branch point recognition sequence (bprs) (Parker et al., 1987; Nelson & Green, 1989; Wu & Manley, 1989; Zhuang & Weiner, 1989, as cited in Corrionero et al., 2011). Base-pairing between the branch point and the bprs bulges out the branch point adenosine, which facilitates the first catalytic step (Query et al., 1994; Smith et al., 2009, as cited in Corrionero et al., 2011). It has been proposed recently that initial interaction of the bprs with the branch point requires a stem–loop structure in U2 snRNA, which is subsequently disrupted to facilitate stable base-pairing between the branch point and the bprs (Perriman & Ares, 2010, as cited in Corrionero et al., 2011). This rearrangement of RNA–RNA interactions could be mediated by Prp5, a member of the RNA-dependent DExH/D-box family of ATPases/helicases involved in fidelity of splice site recognition and other key spliceosomal transitions (for review, see Konarska et al., 2006, as cited in Corrionero et al., 2011), because the ATPase activity of Prp5 has been linked to kinetic proofreading of branch point/bprs base-pairing interactions (Xu & Query, 2007, as cited in Corrionero et al., 2011).

U2 snRNP binding serves as a platform for additional RNA–RNA and protein interactions, leading to the recruitment of the tri-snRNP U4/U5/U6 and formation of mature spliceosome complexes, within which numerous RNA rearrangements and changes in protein composition facilitate splicing catalysis (for review, see Smith et al., 2008; Wahl et al., 2009, as cited in Corrionero et al., 2011). A recent report by Roybal and Jurica (2010) concluded that spliceostatin A (SSA) inhibits spliceosome assembly subsequent to pre-spliceosome formation, impeding the transition between complex A and B, implying a role for SF3b in maturation steps of the spliceosome after its established function in early U2 snRNP recruitment.

4. Drug targeting aspects for parasite infection and trans-splicing in human cells could be target by similar therapies

Since all trypanosomatid mRNAs are trans spliced and trypanosomatid genes typically do not harbor introns, it was long thought that these organisms use RNA splicing exclusively for SL transfer, and accordingly, trypanosome-specific deviations of splicing factors were hypothesized to be trans splicing specific. It therefore came as a surprise when the *T. brucei* PAP gene (TriTryp database [TriTrypDB] accession no. Tb927.3.3160), encoding poly (A) polymerase, was shown to harbor a single intron that was removed by conventional cis-splicing. The search for further introns revealed only one more gene in *T. brucei* (Tb927.8.1510), encoding a putative RNA helicase, whose pre-mRNA was shown to be cis spliced. Interestingly, a recent characterization of the *T. brucei* transcriptome by high-throughput RNA sequencing strongly indicates that there are no other introns disrupting protein-coding genes (Mair et al., 2000).

Since differences were observed in the machinery of cis- and trans-splicing, the latter mechanism would represent an alternative to development of new drugs more potent and with fewer side effects. Because of this, several techniques have been developed to detect possible interference in the process of trans-splicing. The first studies involving the union of distinct sequences in transcripts were done in 1985, where by using the machinery of HeLa cells was possible to combine two independent exons transcribed into molecules (Konarska et al., 1985, Solnick, 1985).

Only a few years later, Ullu and Tschudi (1990) established the reaction using permeable cells, aiming to study transcription and trans-splicing in *Trypanosoma brucei* cells. These cells can be treated with lysolecithin that makes the parasites permeable to triphosphate and radioactive nucleotides, as well as other molecules, and were able to synthesize the mature mRNAs. The detergent treatment is relatively mild and the overall cellular morphology and integrity of the plasma membrane are retained. Nevertheless, after exposure to lysolecithin, trypanosome cells become permeable not only to nucleotide triphosphates but also to other macromolecules like DNAse I, which readily penetrates the nuclei and digests the nuclear DNA and DNA to oligomers up to 23 nt long. These observations suggest that the intercalation of lysolecithin in the lipid bilayer can cause profound effects on the permeability characteristics of the cellular membranes.

Using permeable parasites was possible to incorporate other elements on the reaction as well as the radioactive nucleotide, usually [α-^{32}P] UTP and ATP, GTP, CTP, creatine kinase and creatine phosphate. After this step, followed by electrophoresis in 6% acrylamide gel with urea, it can be revealed the abundance of newly synthesized mRNA during the incubation time. This is an important parameter because it indicates RNA is degraded (Figure 4). It was demonstrated by permeable cell system that the efficiency synthesis and accumulation of various cellular RNAs is severely affected by the concentrations of monovalent ion and, to a lesser extent, of divalent ions. Potassium concentrations greater than 20 mM were strongly inhibitory for the synthesis of SL, U4, and 7SL RNAs and magnesium ions have less dramatic effects than potassium ions on the overall synthesis of SL, 7SL, U4 and tubulin mRNAs. However, above 3 mM [Mg++] occured accumulation of a 3' end shortened form of the SL RNA (SL RNA 130) (Ullu & Tschudi, 1990).

To determine if trans-splicing is taking place in permeable cell system, was necessary to determine the structure of newly synthesized SL RNA sequences by RNAse protection experiments, using a transcript containing antisense sequence to SL RNA as a probe, followed by enzymatic treatment with RNases A and T1, which degraded non-hybrid mRNAs and allowed the localization of SL exon and intron, respectively. The probe used in this kind of experiment was an unlabelled antisense SL RNA, which is complementary to nucleotides 7 to 128 of the SL RNA. It was possible detected four fragments with approximate motilities of 129, 123, 90, and 39 nt. The 123 nt RNA species had the correct size expected for protection of SL RNA which had not been cleaved at the 5' splice site. The 129 nt RNA was longer than the fragment expected for full protection of the probe (123 nt) and may be derived from incomplete cleavage of intact SL RNA by ribonuclease A and TI. This would be the case if the 129 nt SL RNA fragment has a fully methylated cap structure (in which the first four nucleotides adjacent to the cap are methylated), and therefore the ribonucleases would not be able to cleave the 5' end sequence. Therefore, both the 123 and 129 SL RNA fragments represented SL RNA which had not been cleaved at the 5' splice site (Ullu & Tchudi, 1990). On the other hand, the 90 nt and 39 nt long SL RNA fragments had the sizes consistent with their identity as the SL intron and the SL exon, respectively (Figure 5).

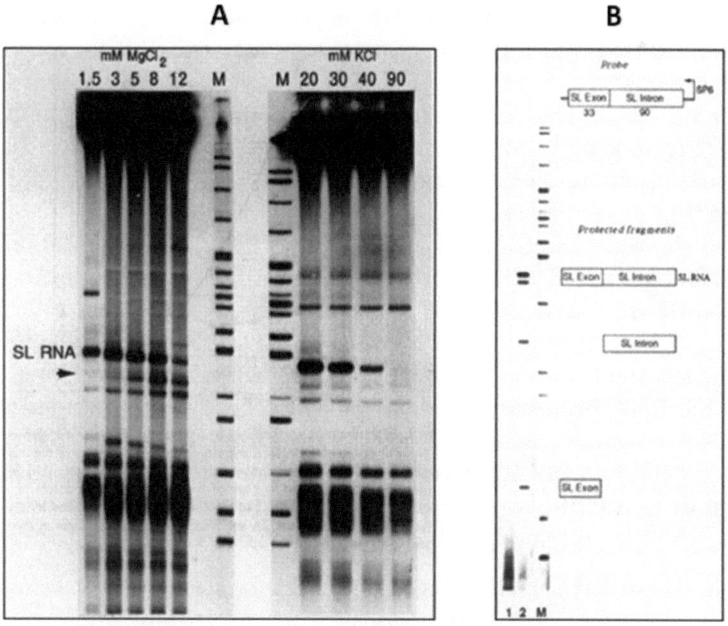

Fig. 5. Trans-splicing in *T. brucei* permeable cells and RNase protection.

A: RNA synthesis. Radiolabelled RNA was synthesized for 8 min. in permeable cells using variable amounts of $MgCl_2$ and KCl, as indicated above each lane (mM). Aliquots from each reaction were fractionated by electrophoresis on a 6% polyacrylamide-7 M urea gel and ^{32}P-RNA was detected by authoradiography. The position of the SL RNA is indicated and a solid arrowhead indicates the position of the SL RNA 130 (see text for details). M, end labelled MspI fragments of pBR322 as molecular weight markers. B, Fractionation of radiolabelled RNA fragments protected from RNAse digestion by the antisense SL RNA probe. Radiolabelled RNA from 6x 10^6 cells was analyzed by RNAse mapping in the absence (lane 1) or presence (lane 2) of 200 ng of unlabelled SL antisense RNA essentially as described (3) except that 40% formamide was included in the hybridization solution and hybridization was carried out at 37°C. The products of digestion were analyzed by electrophoresis as described in Figure 1. M, molecular weight marker. The structures of the antisense SL RNA probe and of the expected products of RNAse digestion are shown on the right. This figure was transcribed from Ullu & Tschudi, (1990).

Experiments using S-adenosyl-L-homocysteine (Ado-Hcy) were pioneers in demonstrating the use of permeable cells as a model to study substances capable of interfering with the reaction of trans-splicing (Ullu & Tschudi, 1990). The use of Ado-Hcy inhibited trans-splicing reaction by competitive inhibition of S-adenosyl-L-methionine (Ado-Met) mediated by 5'end methylation reactions and it allowed the analysis of the methylation as a rule for trans-splicing reaction. Its addition in the transcription/trans-splicing reaction mix, following by RNase protection as described before, allowed the localization of methylated-SL exon + SL intron (figure not showed).

Ambrósio and co-workers (2004) demonstrated that standardization of trans-splicing reaction with *T. cruzi* epimastigote forms (Y strain) permeable cells facilitates the study of RNA processing in these trypanosomatids and can be used as a model of study drug activity on trans splicing mechanism. The authors also demonstrated that pro-drug NFOH-121, derived from nitrofurans (Chung et al., 2003), was able to interfere with RNA processing this parasite, although the reaction of trans-splicing has not been affected (Ambrósio et al., 2004). The nitrofurans are compounds with the capacity to inhibit trypanotiona reductase, an important enzyme involved in the antioxidant metabolism of *T. cruzi*. To develop more selective drugs with low toxicity and more specific targets, a reciprocal prodrug of nitrofurazone, the hydroxymethylnitrofurazone (NFOH-121), was developed and showed higher trypanocidal activity than nitrofurazone and benznidazol in all stages (Chung et al., 2003). In order to analyze the drug activity in *T. cruzi* RNA processing, NFOH-121 was added to the mixture of reagents in different final concentrations. The bands which were revealed in electrophoresis acrylamide gel (Figure 6) decreased when higher concentrations of the drug were used suggesting that the drug would affect the RNA processing in these parasites. However, the presence of double band (SL RNA methylation) shows that even if the drug interferes in mRNA processing, the trans-splicing reaction still occurred, even the protein would not be active. This would mean that the drug activity was prominent at level of the mRNA processing in these parasites and maybe by interfering in the transcription rate (Figure 6, panel A).

Recent data also show that the technique of permeable cells/RNAse protection can be used in assessing the activity of natural compounds on the mRNA processing machinery/trans-splicing (Figure 6, panels B and C). (−)-Cubebin, a compound extracted from the dry seeds of the Asian pepper (*Piper cubeba* L.) and leaves of *Zanthoxylum naranjillo*, seems to provide treatments with little collateral effect as compared to benznidazole, evaluated by *in vitro* (cells) and *in vivo* (mice) tests (Bastos et al., 1999). Partial synthesis of (−)-cubebin resulted in (−)-6,6′- Dinitrohinokinin (DNH) and (−)-hinokinin (HQ) which were also tested in *T. cruzi* parasites and HQ showed to be a potential candidate for the development of a new drug to treat Chagas' disease (Saraiva et al., 2007, 2010). It showed higher trypanocidal activity than benznidazole against epimastigote forms and similar activity against amastigote forms (De Souza et al., 2005; Saraiva et al., 2007). Furthermore, *in vivo* assays showed significant parasitemic reduction after administration of HQ in mice infected, and it was observed that the groups treated with HQ displayed better survival rates than that treated with benznidazole. However, DNH presented less activity than benznidazole (Saraiva et al., 2007, 2010). It was also demonstrated that HQ and DNH were not capable to cause strong interference in the RNA processing by trans-splicing in *T. cruzi*, as observed by the RNase protection reaction. HQ, mainly, leads to an increase dose-dependent of mRNA synthesis which demonstrates the parasites attempt to remaining viable. This result was also observed in Bolivia strain but at lower concentration, which seems to reinforce the higher Bolivia resistance than Y strain and would indicate a strain-dependent activity of the substances. In both, Y and BOL strains, after the addition of the substances, there was no blocked of the trans-splicing processing, therefore it was continued observing the methylated SL RNA bands in gel, which were related to the capping reaction, as well as the exon and intron bands, referring to trans-splicing reaction. These results showed that the substances might have interfered in any step of the RNA transcription, promoting alterations in the RNA synthesis, even though the RNA processing mechanism still occurs (Andrade e Silva et al., 2011).

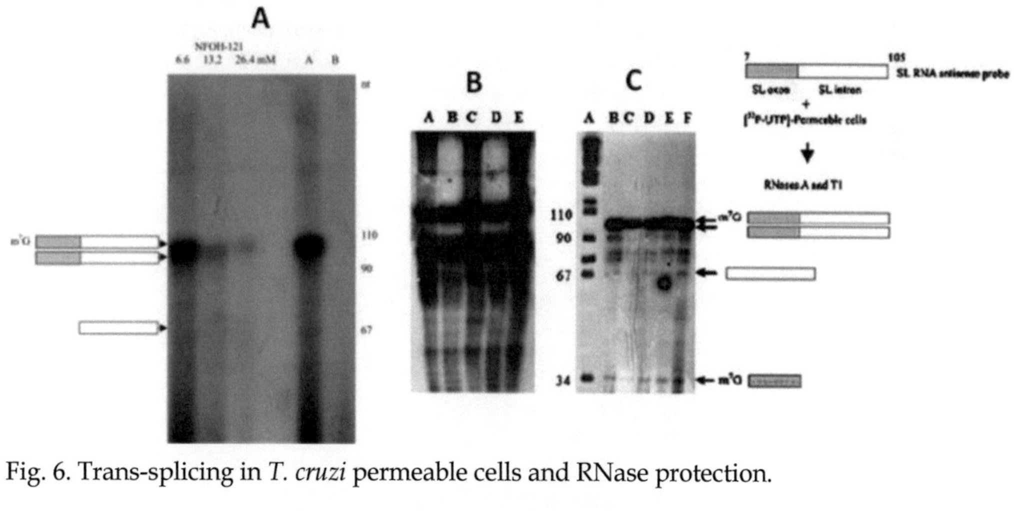

Fig. 6. Trans-splicing in *T. cruzi* permeable cells and RNase protection.

Panel A: RNase protection reaction with Trypanosoma cruzi Y strain using NFOH-121 and electrophoresed on a 10% polyacrylamide - 7M urea gel and detected by autoradiography. The concentrations of NFOH-121 are indicated in the figure. The bands correspondent to SL exon + SL intron methylated, non-methylated and SL intron are indicated in the figure by the symbols and arrows; control with no NFOH-121 (A) and RNase control in the absence of SL antisense probe (B) are indicated. The molecular weight in nucleotides (nt) is indicated in the figure; m7G: 7-methylguanosine. Transcribed from Ambrosio et al. (2004). Panel B: Permeable cells experiments with *T. cruzi* Y strain, electrophoresed on a 10% polyacrylamide–7 M urea gel and detected by autoradiography. A, control (without substances); B, 1 mM DNH; C, 2 mM DNH; D, 1 mM HQ; E, 2 mM HQ. Panel C: RNase protection experiments with *T. cruzi* Y strain permeable celss, electrophoresed on a 10%polyacrylamide–7 M urea gel and detected by autoradiography. A, pBR322 digested with MspI labeled with [32P]-dCTP; B, control (without substances); C, 1 mM DNH; D, 2 mM DNH; E, 1 mM HQ; F, 2 mM HQ. The bands correspondent to SL exon+SL intron methylated, non-methylated, SL intron, and SL exon are indicated in the figure by the symbols and arrows, and the bands non-indicated are different sizes of intron structures. m7G 7-methylguanosine. Transcribed from Andrade e Silva et al. (2011).

Experiments using permeable cells have to use radioactive material, making more difficult to use the technique, because besides the high cost of material, it requires specific license to obtain the material and trained personnel to establish the method in the laboratory. Based on this view, Barbosa et al. (2007) developed a rapid test to detect interference from molecules in the reaction of trans-splicing using the permeable cell model and traditional silver staining. They replaced the isotope by a nonradioactive nucleotide. It was possible to observe reduction of specific bands on polyacrylamide gels stained with silver staining method. Figure 7 shows the gel and snRNAs bands. Reducing costs and simplifying the method, it was possible to observe the interference of trypanocida molecules in the processing of messenger RNA in different strains of *T. cruzi,* taking into account the phenotypic and genotypic diversity of this species. Tests made using the prodrug NFOH-121 (Figure 6, panel A) demonstrated a reduction of the band U2, U1, U4, U5, U6 snRNAs in different strains of *T. cruzi* (Y, NCS and Bolivia strains). All six bands analyzed in the gel showed decreased when higher concentrations of NFOH-121 were used, suggesting that the drug did affect RNA processing, mainly in the Y and NCS parasite strains. However, the drug showed no effect on the Bolivia strain. The activity of NFOH-121 compared with the parental drug NF (nitrofurazone, Andrade & Brener, 1969) was evaluated either by direct biological activity on the parasites or reducing RNA processing, showing that NFOH-121 drug's activity is dose-dependent (Barbosa et al., 2007).

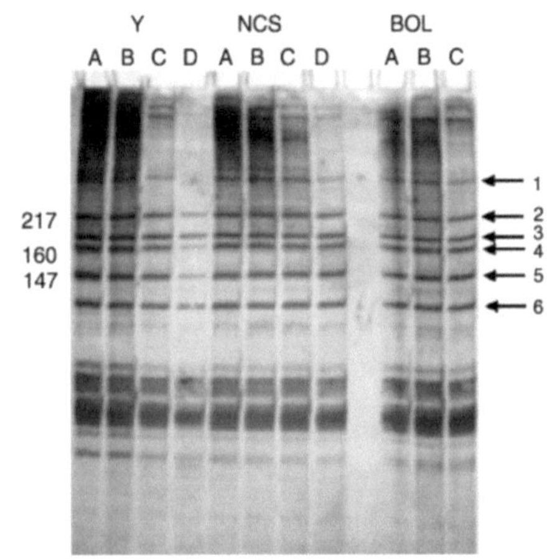

Fig. 7. RNAs (1 trough 6) from *T. cruzi* permeable epimastigote cells from Y, NCS, and BOL strains.

Cells were treated with the hydroxymethylnitrofuran (NFOH-121) and electrophoresed on 10% polyacrylamide-7 M urea gel. A, Control without NFOH-121; B, 2 μM NFOH-121; C, 5 μM NFOH-121; D, 12.5 μM NFOH-121. 1, Unrelated small nuclear RNA; 2, U2; 3, U1; 4, U4; 5, U5; 6, U6 small nuclear RNAs. Molecular weights in base pairs are given on the left. Silver-stained gel. This figure was transcribed from Barbosa et al. (2007).

More recent data, using the combination of RNA interference (RNAi) of some proteins involved in splicing reactions and reverse transcriptase-polymerase chain reaction (RT-PCR) demonstrate the possibility of a relatively simple tests being used in evaluation of the splicing reaction in trypanosomatids. The discovery of RNAi in *T. brucei* occurred unexpectedly and simultaneously with the some findings made in *Caernorhabditis elegans*, in which the parasites transfected with expression vectors for proteins showed multiple morphological phenotypes, including multiple nucleous and kinetoplasts. These observations showed that a hairpin similar to RNA 5'-UTR of alpha-tubulin (α-tubulin) was the element responsible for the new phenotypes. Transfections with double-stranded RNA (dsRNA) constructed with T7 RNA polymerase generated parasites with the same characteristics mentioned earlier (Ketting et al., 2003).

Currently, the mechanism of RNAi is a powerful tool to studying the molecular biology of parasitic trypanosomatids, allowing the specific interference of endogenous genes. Due to the nature of this type of silencing (post-transcriptional and dominant), this mechanism of interference constitutes a particularly useful technique for silencing gene expression in diploid organisms, where the traditional knockout of target genes would be highly costly and, in the case of essential genes, virtually impossible (Ullu & Tschudi, 2003). By the other hand, studies using this mechanism in *T. brucei*, allowed to extrapolate the results obtained for other species of trypanosomatids in which the machinery of RNAi silencing is not competent, for example, in *T. cruzi*.

Having in account that the RNAi approaches described above were transient, vectors were constructed to achieve long-lasting RNAi response expressing dsRNAs under control of tetracycline-inducible promoters. At present, two types of vectors are available that afford regulated expression of either hairpin RNA or dsRNA transcribed from opposing T7 RNA polymerase promoters. Both vectors types are stably integrated in the genome by homologous recombination at the nontranscribed spacer of the ribosomal DNA (rDNA) locus and require a recipient trypanosome cells expressing T7 RNA polymerase ant *tet* repressor. In the hairpin-type vector, dsRNA is produced from a sense and antisense fragment of the gene of interest cloned upstream and downstream from a stuffer fragment, respectively. The purpose of the stuffer fragment is to stabilize the plasmid for replication in bacteria. The double T7 vector contains two opposing T7 polymerase promoters, each of them followed by two T7 terminators arranged in tandem. A portion of the gene of interest is cloned between the two promoters (Ullu & Tschudi, 2003).

After the discovery of RNAi in trypanosomes, different authors have used this tool to check whether different genes and their protein products are potentially involved in splicing reaction. The first information was obtained about the essentiality of the gene for the parasite viability (Shi et al. 2000). In most cases, gene silencing proved to be essential for survival, as demonstrated by growth curves of induced RNAi cells compared to the non-induced controls.

To check the interference of the splicing reaction of a set of RT-PCR can be designed, using primers directed to the processed and unprocessed gene as Poly-A polymerase (cis-splicing) and alpha-tubulin (trans-splicing). The primers synthesized for specific regions of PAP (Figure 8) are capable of binding to the exons flanking the single intron found in this gene. During the induction time with appropriate antibiotic it was observed accumulation of unprocessed transcripts of PAP (band around 780 bp), and reduced level of mature transcripts (band of approximately 130 bp), demonstrating the interference in cis-splicing in these trypanosomatids (Figure 8). Similarly, a semi-quantitative reaction of RT-PCR, using oligos targeted to specific regions of alpha-tubulin was able to detect reduction of non-processed transcript (band of approximately 750 bp) and accumulation of non-throughput (band of about 150 bp), as shown in Figure 8.

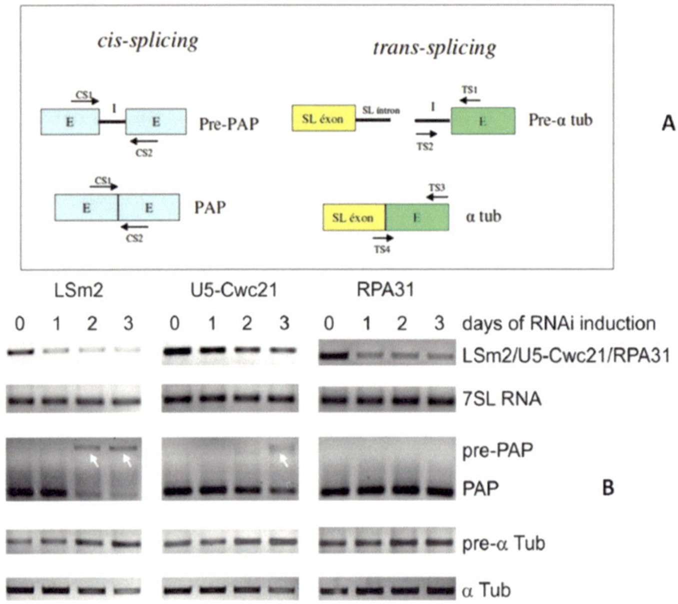

Fig. 8. *In vitro* evaluation of cis- and trans-splicing reaction in *T. brucei.*

A. Schematic diagram of the annealing regions of primers used in functional analysis of cis- and trans-splicing reactions. CS1 and CS2 anneal to the exon transcribed from the poly A polymerase unprocessed (pre-PAP) and processed (PAP); TS1 and TS2 anneal to the exon and intron of the transcript not processed for α-tubulin (Pre-α-tub). To evaluate the processing of α-tubulin, TS3 binds to another region of the exon of α-tubulin, while TS4 anneals to both the SL exon and α-tubulin exon (α-tub). E, exon ; I, intron. (B) Semi-quantitative RT-PCR analysis of RNA abundance in total RNA preparations from cells in which dsRNA synthesis was induced for 0, 1, 2, or 3 days. As a control, the knockdown of the RNA polymerase I subunit RPA31 was co-analyzed. The first panels show the knockdown of the respective mRNAs and the second panels the analysis of 7SL RNA which is not sensitive to splicing defects. The third panels show a competitive PCR of the PAP pre-mRNA/mRNA. The white arrows point to the pre-mRNA amplification products. Pre-mRNA (pre-α Tub) and mature mRNA of α-tubulin (α-Tub) were amplified in the fourth and fifth panels, respectively. The figure 8 B was transcribed from Ambrósio et al. (2009).

Newly discovered genes have been characterized for their participation in the splicing using the tests described above. Cwc21 protein, which was described being exclusive of trypanosomatids, proved to be essential for survival of the parasite and its silencing caused inference in both cis- and trans-splicing (Ambrósio et al, 2009). Several other examples are presented in the literature as highly conserved protein of U5 snRNP, U5-15K (da Silva et al., 2011) and recently described SMN (Palfi et al., 2009) from *T. brucei*, whose participation in splicing was detected using semi-quantitative RT-PCR.

Although different molecules are still to be tested for interference on the reaction of trans-splicing, in theory, it can be possible to employ semi-quantitative RT-PCR for this purpose. In this case, it would require molecules with features for passage through cell membranes to reach the splicing machinery.

After two decades of unsuccessful attempts in establishing an *in vitro* trans-splicing system, such a system was recently established by Shaked et al. (2010). The failure to date to establish an *in vitro* system in trypanosomes lies in the use of radiolabeled pre-mRNA substrates that were extensively degraded, and the deficiency in essential factor(s) in the extract. The degradation could not be eliminated even if the mRNA was capped at the 50-end or at the 30-end with pCp. The success in detecting the trans-spliced product in lied in three parameters: (i) the extract used was crude but contain all the factors necessary for the reaction. It is prepared very rapidly to eliminate the potential inactivation of essential factors. However, because the extract is not purified, it contains enzymes that may inactivate essential factors, thus reducing the reaction efficiency. (ii) A large amount of pre-mRNA is added to the reaction, leaving sufficient amounts of substrate (after its immediate degradation) to assemble into an active complex. The amount of pre-mRNA (4 pmol) is 50-fold higher than the amount of SL RNA in the extract (~80 fmol). Indeed, it was demonstrated that increasing the amount of pre-mRNA increases the reaction efficiency. (iii) The assays were the most critical parameter that made it possible to detect the trans-spliced product. Three different assays were used. In all the assays, only the end-product but none of the intermediates are monitored. The reaction efficiency, roughly calculated by the RNase protection assay, is ~1–2% of the input pre-mRNA utilizing almost 50% of the SL RNA present in the extract. Thus, the limiting factor in this system is the SL RNA (Shaked et al., (2010).

Although the traditional assays to monitor splicing so far are based on the use of radiolabeled substrate, the real-time PCR assay represents a much desired substitute. It avoids the use of radiolabeled materials; it is quantitative, and is able to quantitatively detect the amount of trans-spliced product even at levels less than a few fentomoles. In addition, the assay is convenient relative to the RNase protection assay.

An additional parameter that was essential for establishing the *in vitro* system was the choice of pre-mRNA substrate. The results indicated that the TIR pre-mRNA (pNS21-TIR carrying the beta-tubulin intergenic region) was a better substrate than the PIR pre-mRNA (EP-2-3, (Tb927.6.520), positions 226182-227114 on chromosome 6, in fusion with the luciferase gene). The poor performance of the PIR substrate *in vitro* might stem from its size. The larger substrate appeared more vulnerable to degradation. In other splicing systems, it was demonstrated that shortening both the exons and the introns resulted in a substrate that is spliced more efficiently (Shaked et al., 2010; for review and more details also see Michaeli, 2011).

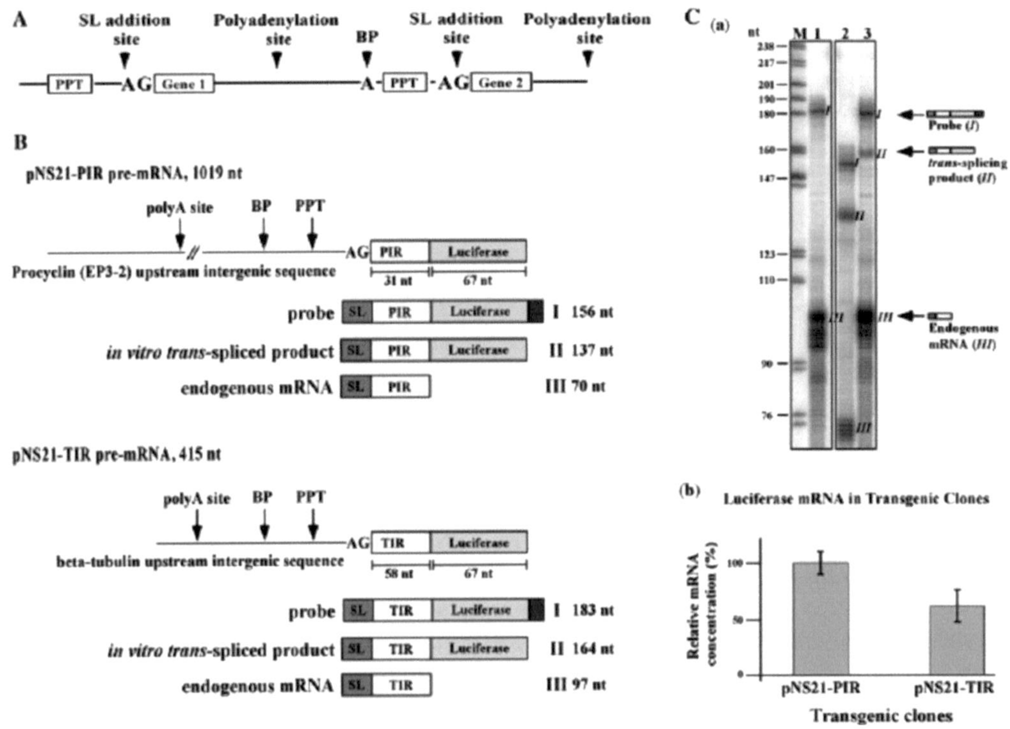

Fig. 9. *In vitro* trans-splicing reaction using RNase protection assay.

(A) Schematic representation of a trypanosome polycistronic pre-mRNA. The significant sequence elements essential for trans-splicing are indicated. (B) Pre-mRNA substrates used in trans-splicing establishment. Schematic representation of the pre-mRNA substrates highlighting the significant sequence elements: polyadenylation site (polyA site), polypyrimidine tract (PPT) and AG splice site. The lengths of the PIR and TIR UTRs as well as the Luciferase ORF are indicated. Underneath each pre-mRNA, the respective probe, in vitro trans-spliced product and endogenous mRNA are shown, along with the expected size of the protected fragments after RNase protection. (C) RNase protection assay to monitor the expression of the TIR and PIR constructs. (a) Thirty micrograms of total RNA was hybridized with labeled antisense probe, complementary to the trans-spliced product. Protected RNA products were separated on a 6% sequencing gel. M- DNA marker, labeled pBR322 DNA MspI digest. The size of the marker is indicated on the left. Lane contents are as follows: 1, RNA from parental strain; 2, RNA from transgenic parasites expressing the pNS21-PIR construct; 3, RNA from transgenic parasites expressing the pNS21-TIR construct. The scheme on the right hand side of the gel indicates the structure of the probe and the protected fragments. (b) Relative expression of the tubulin-luciferase or the EP-luciferase to the endogenous tubulin and EP transcripts. The figure was transcribed from Shaked et al. (2010).

5. Conclusions

From the data presented above, it appears that there are still many difficulties to overcome in the sense that scientists can adequately and favorably control the trans-splicing reaction either in mammals or parasites.

Curiously, although the trypanosomes process virtually all their mRNAs by trans-splicing, the establishment of this reaction *in vitro* using cell-free extracts still presents some methodological obstacles, unlike the reaction in mammalian cells, which was relatively rapidly set up *in vitro* a few years ago.

Thus, efforts should be made to obtain a very similar *in vitro* methodology in parasite trypanosomatids as in mammalian cells to better understand the reaction itself and study all the requirements similarly to evaluation already done in mammals, which would help in the study of interesting and more specific therapeutic targets for parasites. One of the advantages of specific targets to block the trans-splicing reaction in these parasites would be that the drug action it is independent on the parasite strain and also its life stage.

However, based on current studies, some of them reported in this chapter, there are some interesting points in the trans-splicing reaction that could be targets for drug action and could be different from mammalian cells and parasites. For the latter, drugs that interfere or prevent the binding of the SL RNA/SL RNP in the pre-mRNA, ie, which act in the first transesterification reaction, it would become very attractive because they probably block all mRNA processing in the parasite. This type of drug would be highly selective for the parasites and possibly will not affect the host cell.

Regarding to potential drugs that interfere with the trans-splicing reaction in mammals, in this chapter we mentioned that spliceostatin A, an anti-tumor drug, interfered in the fidelity of the recognition of U2 snRNP to the pre-mRNA, leading to interference in the formation of the cis-spliceosome. Although these results referred to the alternative splicing studies and, we may question the extent to which alternative splicing occurring in mammalian cells would not be compared to the trans-splicing in the same cells? In this particular case, as described before, the SR proteins appear to play an important role in this reaction *in vivo* as well as ESE (exonic-splicing enhancers), which bind to SR proteins and probably helps the cryptic 5′ splice site becomes the donor site. A drug which interfering in SR-ESE binding probably would destabilize the complex and the trans-splicing reaction in mammals.

6. Acknowledgment

We thank Dr. Montse Bach-Elias, from CSIC, Barcelona, Spain, who has transmitted all your knowledge about cis- and trans-splicing and showed up how interesting would be this issue.

7. References

Ambrósio, D. L., Barbosa, C. F., Vianna V. F., Cicarelli, R. M. B. (2004). *Trypanosoma cruzi*: establishment of permeable cells for RNA processing analysis with drugs. *Memórias do Instituto Oswaldo Cruz*, Vol. 99, No. 6, pp (617-620), ISSN 6074-0276.

Ambrósio, D. L., Lee, J. H., Panigrahi, A. K., Nguyen, T. N., Cicarelli, R. M. B., Günzl, A. (2009). Spliceosomal proteomics in *Trypanosoma brucei* reveal new RNA splicing factors. *Eukaryotic Cell*. Vol. 8, No. 7, pp (990-1000), ISSN 1535-9778.

Andrade e Silva, M. L., Cicarelli, R. M. B., Pauletti, P. M., Luz, P. P., Rezende, K. C., Januário, A. H., Da Silva, R., Pereira, A. C., Bastos, J. K., De Albuquerque, S., Magalhães, L. G., Cunha, W. R. (2011). *Trypanosoma cruzi*: evaluation of (-)-cubebin derivatives activity in the messenger RNAs processing. *Parasitol Res*, published online, ISSN 0932-0113.

Andrade, Z. A., Brener Z. (1969). Action of nitrofurazone (5-nitro-2-furaldehyde-semicarbazone) on the intracellular forms of *Trypanosoma cruzi* in experimental Chagas disease. *Rev Inst Med Trop São Paulo*, Vol. 11, pp (222-228), ISSN 0036-4665.

Barbosa, C. F., Okuda, E. S., Chung, M. C., Ferreira, E. I., Cicarelli, R. M. B. (2007). Rapid test for the evaluation of the activity of the prodrug hydroxymethylnitrofurazone in the processing of *Trypanosoma cruzi* messenger RNAs. *Brazilian Journal of Medical and Biological Research*, Vol. 40, pp (33-39), ISSN 0100-879X .

Bastos, J. K., Albuquerque, S., Silva, M. L. A. (1999). Evaluation of the Trypanocidal Activity of Lignans Isolated from the Leaves of *Zanthoxylum naranjillo*. *Planta Med*, Vol. 65, No. 6, pp (541-544), ISSN 0032-0943.

Blumenthal, T. & Thomas, J. (1988). *Cis* and *trans* mRNA splicing in *C. elegans*. *Trends Genetics*, Vol. 4, No.11, pp (305-308), ISSN 0168-9525.

Bruzik, J.P. & Maniatis, T. (1995). Enhancer-dependent interaction between 5' and 3' splice sites in *trans*. *Proc. Natl. Acad. Sci*, Vol. 92, pp (7056-7059), ISSN 1091-6490.

Bruzik, J. & Maniatis, T. (1992). Spliced leader RNAs from lower eukaryotes are trans-spliced in mammalian cells. *Nature*, Vol. 360, pp (692-695), ISSN 0028-0836.

Caudevilla, C., Da Silva-Azevedo, L., Berg, B., Guhl, E., Graessmann, M. & Graessmann, A. (2001). Heterologous HIV-nef mRNA trans-splicing: a new principle how mammalian cells generate hybrid mRNA and protein molecules. *FEBS Letters*, Vol. 507, No. 3, pp (269-279), ISSN 0014-5793.

Caudevilla, C., Serra D., Miliar, A., Codony, C., Asins, G., Bach M. & Hegardt, F. G. (1998). Natural trans-splicing in carnitine octanoyltransferase pre-mRNAs in rat liver. *Proc. Natl. Acad. Sci.*, Vol. 95, pp (12185-12190), ISSN 0027-8424.

Cech, T. R. & Bass, B. L. (1986). Biological catalysis by RNA. *Annual Reviews of Biochemistry*, Vol. 55, pp (599-629), ISSN 0066-4154.

Chiara, M. D., Reed R. (1995). A two-step mechanism for 5′ and 3′ splice-site pairing. *Nature*, Vol.375, pp (510 - 513), ISSN 0028-0836.

Chung, M. C., Guido, R. V. C., Martinelli, T. F., Gonçalves, M. F., Polli, M. C., Botelho, K. C. A., Varanda, E. A., Colli, W., Miranda, M. T. M., Ferreira, E. I. (2003). Synthesis and in vitro evaluation of potential antichagasic hydroxymethylnitrofurazone (NFOH-121): a new nitrofurazone prodrug. *Bioorg Med Chem* Vol. 11, No. 22 pp (4779-4783), ISSN 0968-0896.

Codony, C., Uil S., Caudevilla, C., Serra, D., Asins, G., Graessmann, A., Hegardt, F. G., Bach-Elias, M. (2001). Modulation in vitro of H-ras oncogene expression by trans-splicing. *Oncogene*, Vol. 20, pp (3683-3694), ISSN 0950-9232.

Conrad, R., Liou R. F. & Blumenthal, T. (1993a). Conversion of a trans-spliced C.elegans gene into a conventional gene by introduction of a splice donor site. *The EMBO Journal*, Vol. 12, No. 3, pp (1249-1255), ISSN 0261-4189.

Conrad, R., Liou R. F. & Blumenthal, T. (1993b). Functional analysis of a C.elegans trans-splice acceptor. *Nucleic Acids Research*, Vol. 21, No.4, pp (913-919), ISSN 0305-1048.

Conrad, R., Thomas, J., Spieth J. & Blumenthal, T. (1991). Insertion of part of an intron into the 5' untranslated region of a Caenorhabditis elegans gene converts it into a trans-spliced gene. *Molecular and Cellular Biology*, Vol. 11, No.4, pp (1921-1926), ISSN 027-7306.

Corrionero, A., Minana, B. & Valcarcel, J. (2011). Reduced fidelity of branch point recognition and alternative splicing induced by the anti-tumor drug spliceostatin A. *Genes and Development*, Vol. 25, No. 13, pp (445-459), ISSN 0890-9369.

Coura, R. J., Castro, S. L. (2002). A critical review on Chagas disease chemotherapy. *Memórias do Instituto Oswaldo Cruz*, Vol. 97, No. 1, pp (3-24), ISSN 6074-0276.

Dandekar, T. & Sibbald, P. (1990). *Trans*-splicing of pre-MRNA is predicted to occur in a wide range of organisms including vertebrates. *Nucleic Acids Research*, Vol. 18, pp (4719-4725), ISSN 0305-1048.

Da Silva, M. T., Ambrósio, D. L., Trevelin, C. C., Watanabe, T. F., Laure, H. J., Greene, L. J., Rosa J. C., Valentini, S. R., Cicarelli, R. M. B. (2011). New insights into trypanosomatid U5 small nuclear ribonucleoproteins. *Mem Inst Oswaldo Cruz*, Vol. 106, No. 2, pp (130-138), INSS 6074-0276.

De Souza, V. A., Da Silva, R., Pereira, A. C., Royo, V. A., Saraiva, J., Montanheiro, M., De Souza, G. H. B., Da Silva Filho ,A. A., Grando, M. D., Donate, P. M., Bastos, J. K., Albuquerque, S., Silva, M. L. A. (2005). Trypanocidal activity of (−)-cubebin derivatives against free amastigote forms of *Trypanosoma cruzi*. *Bioorg Med Chem Lett*, Vol.15, pp (303–307), ISSN 0960-894X.

Eul, J., Graessmann, M. & Graessmann, A. (1995). Experimental evidence for RNA trans-splicing in mammalian cells. *The EMBO Journal*, Vol. 14, No. 13, pp (3226-3235), ISSN 0261-4189.

Gunzl, A. (2010) The Pre-mRNA Splicing Machinery of Trypanosomes: Complex or Simplified? *Eukariotic Cell*, Vol. 9, No. 8, pp (1159–1170), ISSN 1535-9778.

Issa & Bocchi. (2010). Antitrypanosomal agents: treatment or threat? *The Lancet*, Vol. 376, No. 9743, pp (768), ISSN 0099-5355.

Ketting, R. F., Tijsterman, M. & Plasterk, R. H. A. (2003). RNAi in Caenorhabditis elegans, In: RNAi a Guide to Gene Silencing, editing by Gregory, J. Hannon, pp (65-85), *Cold Spring Harbor Laboratory Press*, ISBN 0-87969-641-9, USA.

Konarska, M. M., Padgett, R. A., Sharp, P. A. (1985). *Trans*-splicing of mRNA precursors in vitro. *Cell*, Vol. 42, pp (165-171), ISSN 0092-8674.

Lana, M. & Tafuri, W. L. (2000). *Trypanosoma cruzi e Doença de Chagas*, in: Parasitologia Humana, Neves D. P., pp (73-96), Atheneu, ISBN 85-7379-787-1, BR.

Mair, G., Shi, H., Li H., Djikeng, A., Aviles, H. O., Bishop, J. R., Falcone, F. H., Gavrilescu, C., Montgomery, J. L., Santori, M. I., Stern, L. S., Wang, Z., Ullu, E., Tschudi, C. (2000). A new twist in trypanosome RNA metabolism: cis-splicing of pre-mRNA. *RNA*, Vol. 6, pp (163-169), ISSN 1355-8382.

Mayer, M. G., Floeter-Winter, L. M. (2005). Pre-mRNA trans-splicing: from kinetoplastids to mammals, an easy language for life diversity. *Mem Inst Oswaldo Cruz*, Vol. 100, No. 5, pp (501-513), ISSN 6074-0276.

McConville, M. J., Mullin, K. A., Ilgoutz, S. C., Teasdale, R. D. (2002). Secretory pathway of trypanosomatid parasites. *Microbiology and Molecular Biology Reviews*, Vol. 66, No. 1, pp (122-54), ISSN 10985557.

Michaeli, S. (2011). Trans-splicing in trypanosomes: machinery and its impact on the parasite transcriptome. *Future Microbiol*, Vol. 6, No.4, pp (459–474), ISSN 1746-0913.

Murphy, W. J., Watkins, K. P., Agabian, N. (1986). Identification of a novel Y branch structure as an intermediate in trypanosome mRNA processing: evidence for trans-splicing. *Cell*, Vol. 47, pp (517-525), ISSN 0092-8674.

Nielsen, T. W. (1993). Trans-Splicing of Nematode Premessenger RNA. *Annual Review of Microbiology*, Vol. 47, pp (413-440), ISSN 0066-4227.

Palfi, Z., Jaé, N., Preusser, C., Kaminska, K. H., Bujnicki, J. M., Lee J. H., Günzl, A., Kambach, C., Urlaub, H., Bindereif, A. (2009). SMN-assisted assembly of snRNP-specific Sm cores in trypanosomes. *Genes Dev*, Vol. 23, pp (1650-1664), ISSN 0890-9369.

Rey, L. (2001). *Tripanossomíase por Trypanosoma cruzi: A doença*, in: Parasitologia, 3.ed, pp (161-178), Guanabara Koogan, ISBN 978-85-277-1406-8, BR.

Roybal, G. A. & Jurica, M. S. (2010). Spliceostatin A inhibits spliceosome assembly subsequent to prespliceosome formation. *Nucleic Acids Research*, Vol. 38, No. 19, pp (6664-6672), ISSN 0305-1048.

Sacks, D., Sher, A. (2002). Evasion of innate immunity by parasitic protozoa. *Nature Immunology*, Vol. 11, No. 3, pp (1041-1047), ISSN 15292908.

Saldanha, R., Moh,r G., Belfort M. & Lambowitz A. M. (1993). Group I and group II introns. *FASEB Journal*, Vol. 7, No.1, pp (15-24), ISSN 0892-6638.

Saraiva, J., Lira, A. A., Esperandim, V. R., Da Silva, F. D., Ferraudo, A. S., Bastos, J. K., Silva, M. L. E., De Gaitani, C. M., De Albuquerque, S., Marchetti, J. M. (2010). (−)-Hinokinin-loaded poly(D,-lactideco-glycolide) microparticles for Chagas disease. *Parasitol Res* Vol. 106, No. 3, pp (703–708), ISSN 0932-0113.

Saraiva, J., Vega, C., Rolon, M., Silva, R., Silva, M. L. A., Donate, P. M., Bastos, J. K., Gomez-Barrio, A., Albuquerque, S. (2007) .In vitro and in vivo activity of lignan lactones derivatives against *Trypanosoma cruzi. Parasitol Res,* Vol. 100, pp (791–795), ISSN 0932-0113.

Shaked, H., Wachtel, C., Tulinski, P., Yahia, N. H., Barda, O., Darzynkiewicz, E., Nilsen, T. W. & Michaeli, S. (2010). Establishment of an in vitro trans-splicing system in *Trypanosoma brucei* that requires endogenous spliced leader RNA. *Nucleic Acids Research,* Vol. 38, No. 10, pp (1-17), ISSN 0305-1048.

Sharp, P. A. (1991). "Five easy pieces". *Science,* Vol. 254, No. 5032, pp (663), ISSN 0036-8075.

Shi, H., Djikeng, A., Mark, T., Wirtz, E., Tschudi, C. & Ullu, E. (2000). Genetic interference in *Trypanosoma brucei* by heritable and inducible double-strandec RNA. *RNA,* Vol. 6, pp (1069-1076), INSS 1355-8382.

Solnick, D. (1985). *Trans*-splicing of mRNA precursors. *Cell,* Vol. 42, pp (157-164), ISSN 0092-8674.

Suchy, M. & Schmelzer, C. (1991). Restoration of the self-splicing activity of a defective group II intron by a small *trans*-acting RNA. *Journal of Molecular Biology,* Vol. 222, No. 2, pp (179-187), ISSN 0022-2836.

Sutton, R. E. & Boothroyd, J. C. (1986). Evidence for Trans-splicing in Trypanosomes. *Cell,* Vol. 47, No. 4, pp (527-535), ISSN 0092-8674.

Teixeira, A. R. L., Nitz, N., Guimaro, M. C., Gomes, C., Santos-Buch, C. A. (2006). Chagas disease. *Postgrad. Med. J.,* Vol. 82, pp (788-798), ISSN 0022-3859.

Ullu, E. & Tschudi, C. (2003). An siRNA ribonucleoprotein is found associated with polyribosomes in *Trypanosoma brucei. RNA,* Vol. 9, pp (802-808), ISSN 1355-8382.

Ullu, E. & Tschudi, C. (1990). Permeable trypanosome cells as a model system for transcription and trans-splicing. *Nucleic Acids Research,* Vol. 18, No. 11, pp (3319–3326), ISSN 0305-1048.

Van Alphen, R. J., Wiemer, E. A. C., Burger, H. & Eskens, F. A. L. M. (2009). The spliceosome as target for anticancer treatment. *British Journal of Cancer,* Vol. 100, No. 2, pp (228–232), ISSN 0007-0920.

Wahl, M. C., Will, C.L., Luhrmann, R. (2009). The spliceosome: design principles of a dynamic RNP machine. *Cell,* Vol. 136, No. 4, pp (701–718), ISSN 1535-9778 .

WHO 2005, WHO - World Health Organization on behalf of the Special Programme for Research and Training in Tropical Diseases, Seventeenth Programme Report, ISSN 1010-9609.

Will, C. L. & Luhrmann, R. (2006). *Spliceosome Structure and Function,* In: The RNA World: the nature of modern RNA suggests a prebiotic RNA, Raymond, F. Gesteland, Thomas, R. Cech, John, F. Atkins, pp (369-400), Cold Spring Harbor Laboratory Press, ISBN 0-87969-739-3, USA.

2

Innovation of the Parasitic Cycle of *Coccidioides* spp.

Bertha Muñoz-Hernández[1], Ma. De los Angeles Martínez- Rivera[2], Gabriel Palma-Cortés[1] and Ma. Eugenia Manjarrez[1]
[1]*Instituto Nacional de Enfermedades Respiratorias Ismael Cosío Villegas*
[2]*Escuela Nacional de Ciencias Biológicas, Instituto Politécnico Nacional*
Mexico

1. Introduction

Coccidioides immitis and *C. posadasii* are etiologic agents of coccidioidomycosis. Major endemic zones are arid and semi-arid climates in North America, such as the northern Mexican states and the southwestern United States. *Coccidioides* spp. is a dimorphic fungus that forms arthroconidia during its mycelial phase while growing in soil. *Coccidioides* spp. enters the lungs through airways and causes an infection and the inhalation of arthroconidia by a susceptible host, initiates the parasitic phase. The infection is usually benign, however, the infection is sometimes severe and lethal, particularly in immunocompromised patients. Elderly persons are at greater risk of developing severe pulmonary disease, while disseminated infection is more frequent in black patients and pregnant women. Transplant patients on immunosuppressive therapy or with human immunodeficiency virus infection have a higher risk of developing severe and progressive coccidioidomycosis. In the host the arthroconidia is transformed into endospore-containing spherules, which are classically found in *Coccidioides* spp. infected tissue. Although parasitic mycelial structures have been identified in some cases, these non classic mycelial structures of *Coccidioides* spp. have not been observed in human tissue or fluid, but when fungal structures are examined, hyphae can be found in up to 50% of specimens. Parasitic mycelial forms have been observed mainly in specimens from lung tissue, sputum, cerebrospinal fluid, and nervous tissue. Parasitic mycelial forms of *Coccidioides* spp. are less frequently observed in pleural fluid, and gastric lavage product. Pulmonary coccidioidomycosis shares clinical manifestations with other pulmonary pathologies, including other mycoses, neoplasia, and tuberculosis. Diagnosis of pulmonary coccidioidomycosis is a multidisciplinary effort.

2. Epidemiology and geotyping

Coccidioidomycosis was described for the first time in 1892 by Alejandro Posadas, a medical student, who reported the case of Domingo Escurra, a soldier whose death is attributed to this disease. The etiological agent was considered to be a protozoan of the genus *Coccidia*. Gilchrist and Rixford studied the first case in the U.S. Later, Stiles denominated the etiological agent: *Coccidioides immitis* (coccidia-like). It was in 1896 that Opülus and Moffitt discovered the fungal origin of the pathogen. In Mexico in 1932, Cicero and Perrín presented the first case and they later described diverse cases in patients residing in northern Mexico and the southern U.S., the main endemic zones of coccidioidomycosis. Also, in Argentina (1967), 27 cases of the disease had been described. *Coccidioides immitis*, the etiological agent of this mycosis represented the unique species recognized of this genus. Baptista et al., utilizing U.S. environmental variables and geospatial reference points of the U.S. and Mexico, reported that the main ecological niche for *Coccidoides* is found in the arid deserts of North America (Hirschmann 2007; Baptista-Rosas et al., 2007).

2.1 Epidemiology

Coccidioidomycosis is the most frequent and serious respiratory mycosis in endemic areas inhabited by the fungus. The infection is acquired via the respiratory pathway by exposure to the infectious propagules (arthroconidia) of the fungus. Person-to-person transmission has not been described; however, intrauterine transmission has been (Charlton et al., 1999). *Cocciddioides* spp. is the causal agent of coccidioidomycosis or "Valley fever,". The fungus infects at least 150,000 people annually, whom develop a pulmonary infection. Sixty to seventy percent of individuals who have been in contact with the fungus present the infection asymptomatically, while only 1% develops the disseminated infection. The male/female ratio is 4:1; the disease affects persons of any age, from children (newborns) to elderly individuals aged ≥80 years. It is an occupational disease: archeologists, agricultural workers, soldiers, and construction workers, as well as specialists in microbiological diagnosis, can acquire the infection. Animal species inhabiting endemic areas, such as horses, field mice, armadillos, donkeys, foxes, dogs, and cats acquire the infection and disseminate it to surrounding zones (Negroni 2008; Sharpton et al., 2009).

Discovery of the teleomorphic state of *Coccidioides* complicated the classification of this ascomycete until the similarity was discovered between the asexual spores of *C. immitis* and aleuroconidia of the mitosporic genus *Malbranchea.* Philogenetic studies suggest a close relationship of this pathogen with *Uncinocarpus reesii*; in its anamorphous state, both produce barrel-shaped arthroconidia, generally placing them in *Coccidioides* genus, Onygenaceae order. Sharpton and coworkers considere *Coccidioides* species are not soil saprophytes, but that they have evolved to remain associated with their dead animal hosts in soil, and that *Coccidioides* metabolism genes, membrane-related proteins, and putatively antigenic compounds have evolved in response to interaction with an animal host (Sharpton et al., 2009).

2.2 Geotyping

Coccidioides spp. is found in the Western Hemisphere at latitudes between 40ºN and 40ºS from California to Argentina. Distribution of these organisms is patchy. It is endemic in Southwestern U.S., including Arizona (where the incidence in humans is particularly high), parts of New Mexico, Texas (west of El Paso), and in Central and Southern portions of California, especially the San Joaquin Valley. The endemic area extends into Mexico, and foci of infection have been detected in Central and South American countries including Argentina, Colombia, Guatemala, Honduras, Venezuela, Paraguay, and Brazil (Sharpton et al., 2009).

On investigating the intraspecific relations of this fungus, the authors compared the Restriction fragment length polymorphism (RFLP) of the total genomic DNA of the different isolates of patients, of the environment, and of a sea lion, observing different profiles (Zimmermann et al., 1994). The separation of *C. immitis* into two main groups, Group I and Group II, was reported for the first time by Zimmerman and colleagues in 1994. The two groups are referred by Koufopanou and cols and other investigators: *C. immitis* CA (Concentrated in California) clade, and *C. posadasii* non-CA (represented by clinical isolates from Arizona, Texas, Mexico, and Argentina) clade. Biogeographic distribution of *Coccidioides* has been reported by Fisher and Taylor in populations from endemic zones in the U.S., (Central and Southern California, Arizona, and Texas), North, Central, and Southern Mexico, and South America (Venezuela, Brazil, and Argentina). *C. immitis* seems to be restricted to California, but it might exist in some adjacent areas of Baja California (Mexico) and Arizona. *C. posadasii* is found in the remaining regions (Koufopanou et al., 1997; Fisher et al., 2002; Taylor & Fisher 2003; Sharpton et al., 2009).

3. Parasitic polymorphism of *Coccidioides* spp.

Taylor and Fisher in 2002, using molecular biology technologies, separated two *Coccidioides* species. Data on biological cycle or pathology prior to this date are referred as the *Coccidiodes immitis* species; after this date, information appears as *Coccidioides immitis* or *Coccidioides posadasii*. However, no knowledge is available on whether both species are similar or whether they share the same characteristics. All information refers to *C. immitis* or *C. posadasii*, but not to both species; thus, from this point on, we will refer both species as *Coccidioides* spp. for events described for either of the two species (Taylor & Fisher, 2002).

Coccidioides spp. is a dimorphic fungus. The saprobic phase grows as mycelia in desert and semi-arid soils, and disturbances in the soil facilitate the dispersal of arthroconidia, which are the infectious propagules. These become airborne as the result of the action of the wind or some other disturbance of the soil. Susceptible humans acquire the infection by inhalation of arthroconidia, which differentiate into large, endosporulating spherules that are found in the typical parasitic-phase form. Observation of these structures in pathological specimens is considered as diagnosis of the disease. In addition, we describe different mycelial forms and chronic pulmonary coccidioidomycosis in patients with diabetes (Figure 1a). Also, these mycelial forms were described in chronic and cavitary pulmonary, ventriculoperitoneal shunt, and different cases of Central nervous system (CNS) infections by other researchers (Dolan et al.,1992; Hagman et al., 2000; Heidi et al., 2000; Klenschmidt-DeMasters et al., 2000; Meyer et al., 1982; Muñoz et al., 2004; Muñoz-Hernández et al. 2008; Nosanchuk et al., 1998; Wages et al., 1995; Zepeda et al., 1998).

In addition, mycelial parasitic forms have been described in coccidioidoma, and fungal ball as a spheroid mass of hyphae. *Coccidioides* is established in pulmonary cavities and the fungus is in direct contact with the air, modifying O_2/CO_2 relation, favoring mycelial grow. This fungal mass is similar to a macrocolony of highly branched hyphal elements with no host cells inside the fungal ball (Figure 1b).

4. Host risk factors for arthroconidia and parasitic mycelial forms development

Coccidioides spp. can infect immunologically competent individuals. The disease exhibits protean manifestations, ranging from an inapparent or benign pulmonary infection to a progressive and often lethal disseminated form that most commonly involves the CNS, skin, and bones. This spectrum includes the following: i) an inapparent infection; ii) primary respiratory disease (usually with uncomplicated resolution), but one half of these patients develop an atypical pneumonia, iii) cutaneous infection; iv) valley fever; v) stabilized or progressive chronic pulmonary disease, and vi) extrapulmonary dissemination that is acute, chronic, or progressive. The degree of severity varies considerably within each syndrome and depends on the dose of inhaled arthroconidia, fungus virulence factors, the genetic predisposition of the host, and the host's immune response. In this chapter, we analyze the relationship between clinical spectrum, fungus virulence factors, mycelial parasitic forms, and host immune response in chronic pulmonary coccidioidomycosis, due to that we found these arthroconidia and parasitic mycelial structures in specimens from patients with diabetes with chronic and cavitary pulmonary coccidioidomycosis (Muñoz-Hernández et al., 2008).

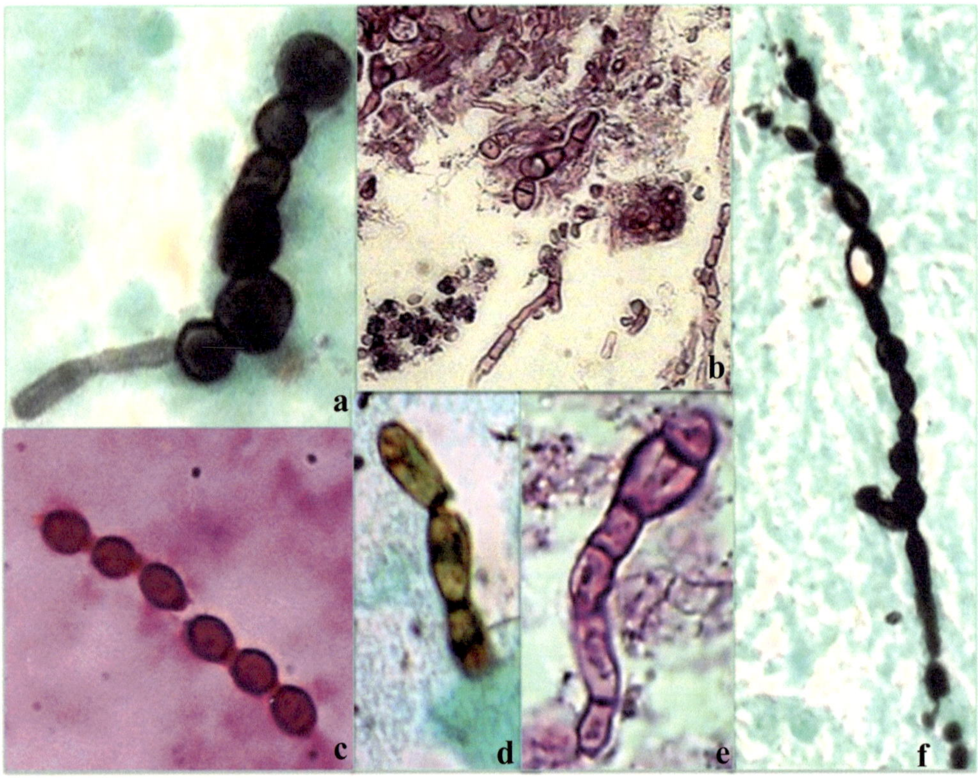

Fig. 1a. *Coccidioides* spp. parasitic hyphal phenotypic diversity. a) and f) Hyphae forming ovoid and spherical cells. b) Pleomorphic cells producing septate hyphae. c) Chain of ovoid cells. d) Separation of arthroconidia. e) Septate hyphae forming a barrel-shaped cells. a), d) and f) Grocott stain of sputum. b), c) and e) Lung tissue stained with periodic acid-Schiff.

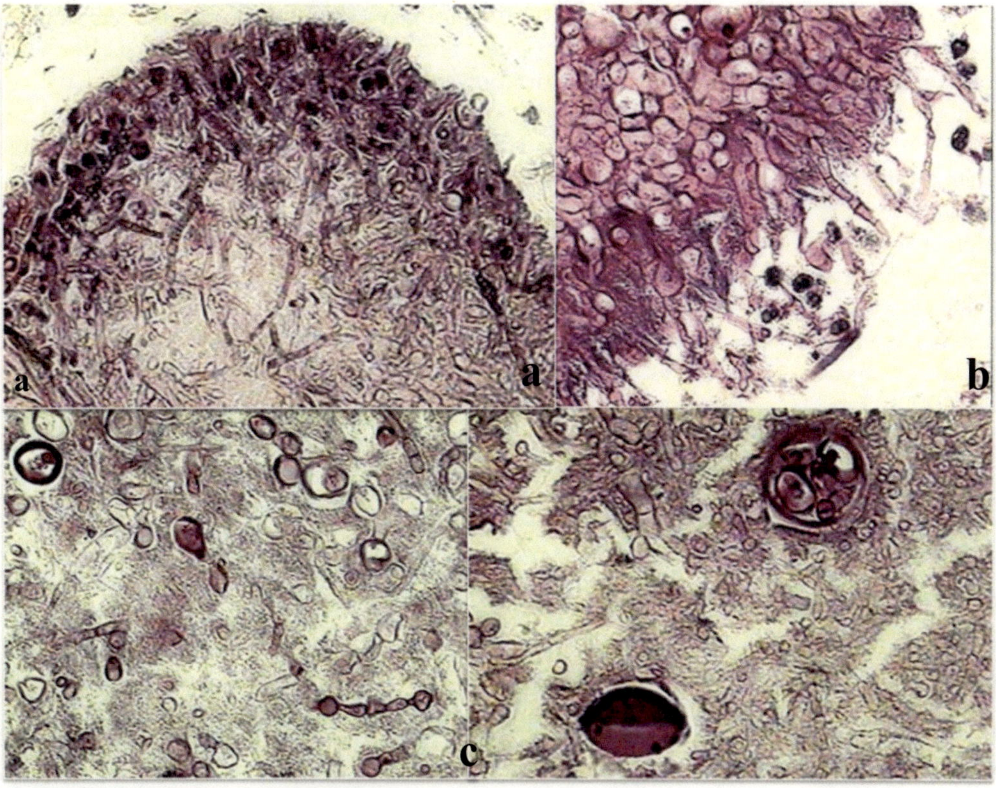

Fig. 1b. *Coccidioides spp*. a) Mycelium fungal ball with septate hyphae and spherules b) Arthroconidia fungal ball forming barrel-shaped and globose cells, both predecessors of spherules. c) presence of septate hyphae in the fungus ball forming arthroconidia, endospore filament, immature spherules, and endospores. Lung tissue stained with periodic acid schiff.

4.1 Pulmonary coccidioidomycosis

Individuals with primary coccidioidomycosis develop persistent pulmonary coccidioidomycosis in 5% of cases, manifested by chronic progressive pneumonia, miliary disease, pulmonary nodules, or pulmonary cavitation. Pulmonary nodules are usually benign but can become cavitary. A classic radiologic finding is the presence of a thin-walled cavity, which typically fails to exhibit a surrounding-tissue reaction; it is strongly suggestive of coccidioidomycosis. The majority of patients have cavities, multiple or multilocular; one half of cavities eventually close spontaneously. Possible complications of cavitation include hemorrhage, secondary infection, progressive increase in size, and, if located peripherally, bronchopleural fistulae. Cavities are formed during acute pneumonia and tend to grow intensively. Infection with this fungus may be asymptomatic, but approximately 50% of immunologically competent persons develop an atypical pneumonia characterized by a cough, fever, and pleuritic chest pain that is often accompanied by rashes, sore throat, cephalea, arthralgia, myalgia, or anorexia (Cole et al., 2006; Cox & Magee 2004).

A few patients develop chronic progressive pulmonary involvement, with symptoms of cough, weight loss, fever, hemoptysis, dyspnea, and chest pain that may persist for years. Radiographic results include inflammatory infiltrates, biapical fibronodular lesions, and multiple cavities. Chronicity is an essential factor in the development of mycelial forms in lung coccidioidomycoses. In our study, all patients with mycelial parasitic forms presented cavitary lesions (Figure 2). Another risk factor is the concomitant diseases that alter the patient's immune response; these forms have also been observed in patients with CNS and chronic pulmonary coccidioidomycosis. We do not know whether Mexican population possesses the Human leukocyte antigen system (HLA), which is related with the control of or which favors the development of arthroconia and parasitic mycelial forms of Coccidoides. In our studies, all patients were born in Mexico. We found a close association between evolution time of coccidioidomycosis and presence of parasitic mycelial forms, suggesting that chronicity is an essential factor in the development of arthroconidia and mycelial forms. We formulated a comprehensive definition based on the results as follows: patients with pulmonary coccidioidomycosis with an evolution >8 months, cough, hemoptysis, radiological evidence of cavitary lesion, and type 2 diabetes mellitus develop arthroconidia and mycelial forms of *Coccidioides* spp. Based on microscopic images of patient's specimens and descriptions of chronic pulmonary or CNS coccidioidomycosis, we propose incorporating mycelial forms into the parasitic phase of *Coccidioides* spp. (Figure 3) (Muñoz-Hernández et al., 2008).

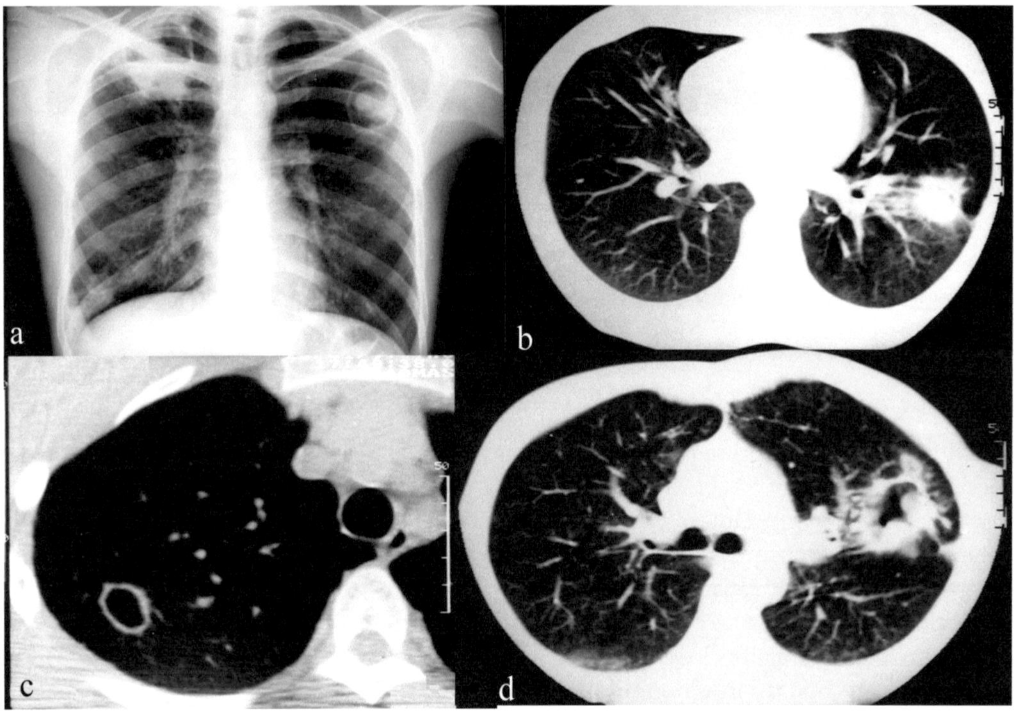

Fig. 2. Radiological evidence of pulmonary coccidioidomycosis. a) Right apical pulmonary cavity with abscess and fluid levels. Left apical cavity occupied. b) Left lobe region coccidioidoma peripheral calcifications and fibrosis, bilateral micronodules. c) Coin shaped lesion with fibrous reaction and scattered micronodules. d) Left lobe cavitary lesion occupied with fibrous reaction.

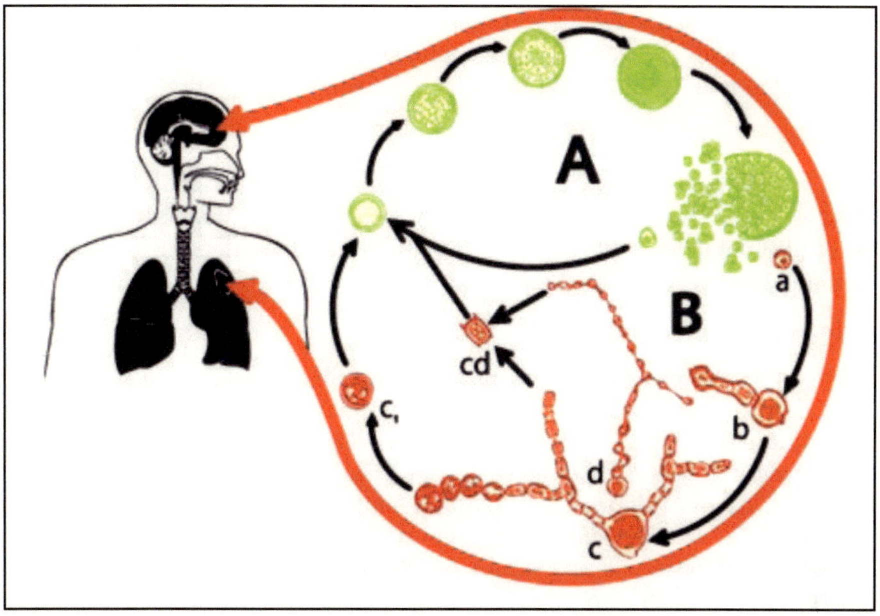

Fig. 3. Mycelial forms and spherules during the parasitic phase of *Coccidioides* spp. in diabetic patients with chronic cavitary pulmonary coccidioiddomicosis. Also observed in patients with CNS infection. With permission.

4.2 Virulence factors, immune response, and microenvironment

We think that interactions between virulence factor traits associated with *Coccidioides* spp. and the host immune response determine the clinical form of infection, which in our studies comprises chronic pulmonary coccidioidomycosis and integrates the microenviroment that will permit the development of diverse parasitic fungal forms, including spherules, endospores, arthroconidia, and different mycelial forms. Indeed, the microenviroment will favor the predominance of some of these parasitic forms, or their co-existence.

4.2.1 *Coccidioides* spp. virulence factors

Adhesins

Coccidioides spp. is a dimorphic fungus that has a saprobic phase characterized by mycelia that produce enterothallic arthroconidia; the latter are typically barrel-shaped, measuring 2.5 a 4 µm in width and 3 a 6 µm in length. Thus, they are sufficiently small to reach the alveoli of the lungs when inhaled. Adhesion to laminin and collagen type IV, which act as interlinking molecules. Adhesins are present on spherules and endospores. During isotropic growth, there is intense synthesis of a Spherule outer wall glycoprotein (SOWgp), a specific component of the parasitic phase, which has shown to be important in *Coccidioides* pathogenicity. SOWgp is located in the wall of the endospores and is transported by exocytic vacuole to the spherule's extracellular outer wall. Expression of SOWgp during pathogen growth appears to be restricted to spherule-endospore formation stages, but it is present only in the spherule. SOWgp in the *Coccidioides* spp. spherule form binds to host ECM proteins. In addition, this glycoprotein is an immunodominant antigen that is capable of eliciting both humoral and cellular responses in infected patients. Thus, SOWgp acts as an adhesin and modulates the host immune response (Hung et al., 2002; 2005; 2007; Klein & Tebbets 2007; Mendes-Giannini et al., 2005).

Dimorphism

Within the mammalian host, *Coccidioides* spp. effects arthroconidia differentiation into spherule-phase cells. This process is unique to *Coccidioides* spp. Dimorphism is an adaptive response of the fungus to a hostile host, modifying its parasitic structures as well as its microenvironment.

Protein kinases

Dimorphism is triggered by exposure to host conditions, particularly temperature, and the fungus leads to the programs required for adaptation to the host environment, including expression of genes for survival and associated virulence factors. Potential signals for histidine kinase sensing in dimorphic fungi include temperature, osmotic or oxidative stress, nutrient deprivation, redox potential, and host-derived factors such as hormones like 17-β-estradiol, which induces germ tubes in *Candida albicans* and blocks the mold-to-yeast transition of *Paracoccidioides brasiliensis*. The histidine kinase system senses host signals and triggers the mold-to-yeast transition and also regulates cell-wall integrity, sporulation, drug resistance, and the expression of virulence genes *in vivo*. Histidine kinase regulates sensing of environmental changes required for morphogenesis in *C. albicans*, *Blastomyces dermatitidis*, *Histoplasma capsulatum*, *Coccidioides* spp., and *Aspergillus fumigatus*. System signaling pathway components are often similar in fungi, but system structures and mechanisms of activation may differ from species to species. These pathways have recently been implicated in environmental sensing and cell development in eukaryotes; phosphorylation/dephosphorylation cycles represent a major mechanism for switching cellular pathways in response to changing microenviromental factors, both internal developmental cues and external environmental stimuli. Histidine kinase functions as a global regulator of dimorphism and virulence in pathogenic fungi. Protein phosphorylation is generally accepted as playing a key role in transducing the signals involved in several processes such as cell adhesion, internalization, and killing of pathogens (Johannesson et al., 2006; Mendes-Giannini et al., 2005; Nemecek et al., 2006, 2007). We suggest that histidine kinases sense environmental signals such as temperature, CO_2 concentration, and pH and that they play key roles regulating *Coccidioides* spp. phase transition and dimorphism, allowing for the following in parasitic polymorphism: arthroconidia; mycelial forms, and spherules or spherules/endospores in lung tissue as a result of the balance generated by histidine kinases.

CO_2, trehalose, and nitrate redactase

Dimorphism is an adaptive response of the fungus to a hostile host. Temperature (between 34 and 41°C), CO_2 (20%), and a partial pressure of 20 a 80 mm of Hg are essential for development of the parasitic phase of *Coccidioides* spp. The aforementioned conditions are present in pulmonary tissue. Dimorphism initiates with isotropic growth characterized by spherical-cell enlargement and the rounding and swelling of the cells followed by synchronous nuclear divisions and segmentation (Lones & Peacock 1960).

The central portion of the young spherule is occupied by a vacuole. Progressive compartmentalization of the cytoplasm surrounding the vacuole gives rise to uninucleate compartments reproducing by mitosis and differentiating into endospores. The mature spherule measures 30-100 μm in diameter and can contain 200-400 endospores. At maturity, the spherule ruptures, releasing the endospores (Figure 4), which measure 2-4 μm in diameter. The high fecundity of *C. immitis* is a feature that contributes to the aggressive nature of this primary human fungal pathogen (Mendes-Giannini et al., 2005). Thus, at any given point, the infected host is exposed to immature, mature, and rupturing spherules, newly released endospores, arthroconidia, and mycelial forms (Figure 5). These parasitic forms can disseminate from the lungs to multiple other body organs. We think that, in pulmonary cavities, O_2/CO_2 exchange is inefficient; CO_2 partial pressure will be near 0 mm Hg and there additionally, there is tissue damage. Both CO_2 concentration and tissue damage could permit the co-existence of these polymorphic parasitic forms. When Coccidioidoma is developed, fungus can colonize the pulmonary cavity; in these microhabitats, alterations are increased, favoring the growth of hyphae; thus, there is plentiful mycelial growth.

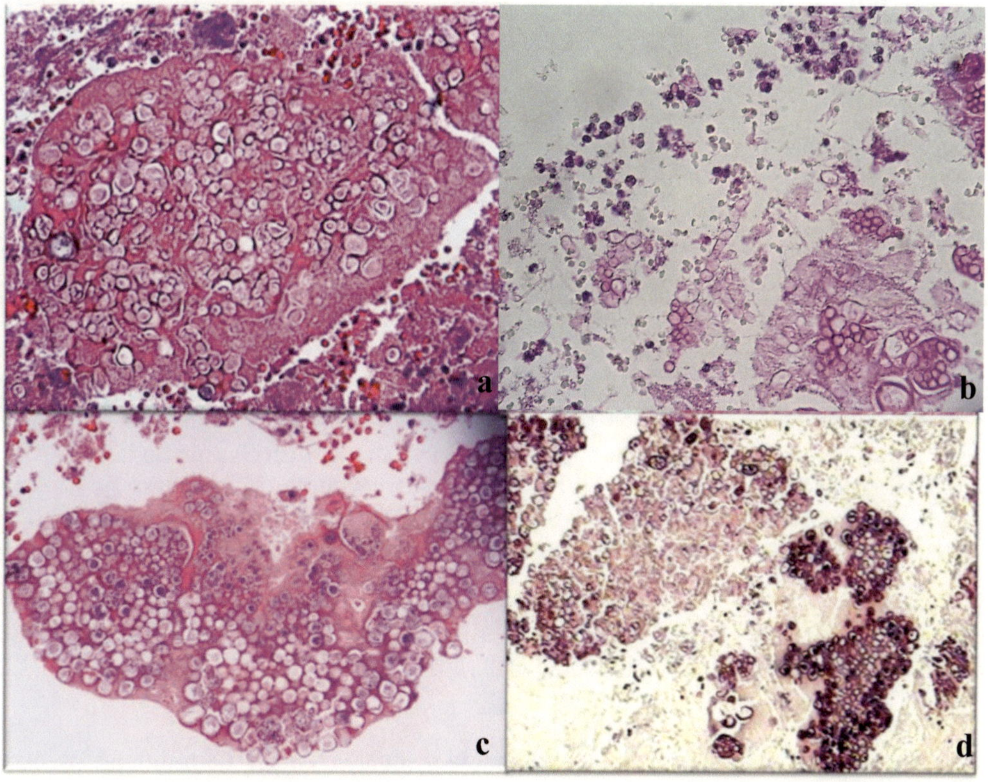

Fig. 4. *Coccidioides* spp. lung tissue: a) Young spherules differentiated, b) Hyphae, spherules with endospores and presence of inflammatory infiltrate; c) Immature spherules and spherules rupture expelling endospores, d) Dissemination of spherules in lung tissue. a, b, c) Staining with hematoxylin-eosin, d) Stained with periodic acid-Schiff.

In addition, the nitrate reductase (*nir*) gene is expressed during the parasitic phase growth in *Coccidioides* infection. This gene is likely to be an important virulence factor in *Coccidioides* because it allows fungi to grow under anoxic conditions. Several fungi that are considered as obligate aerobes could be facultative anaerobes, due to their presence in the host's microhabitat, inside of an abscess or in a granuloma, if they possess and express the *nir* gene (Moran et al., 2011).

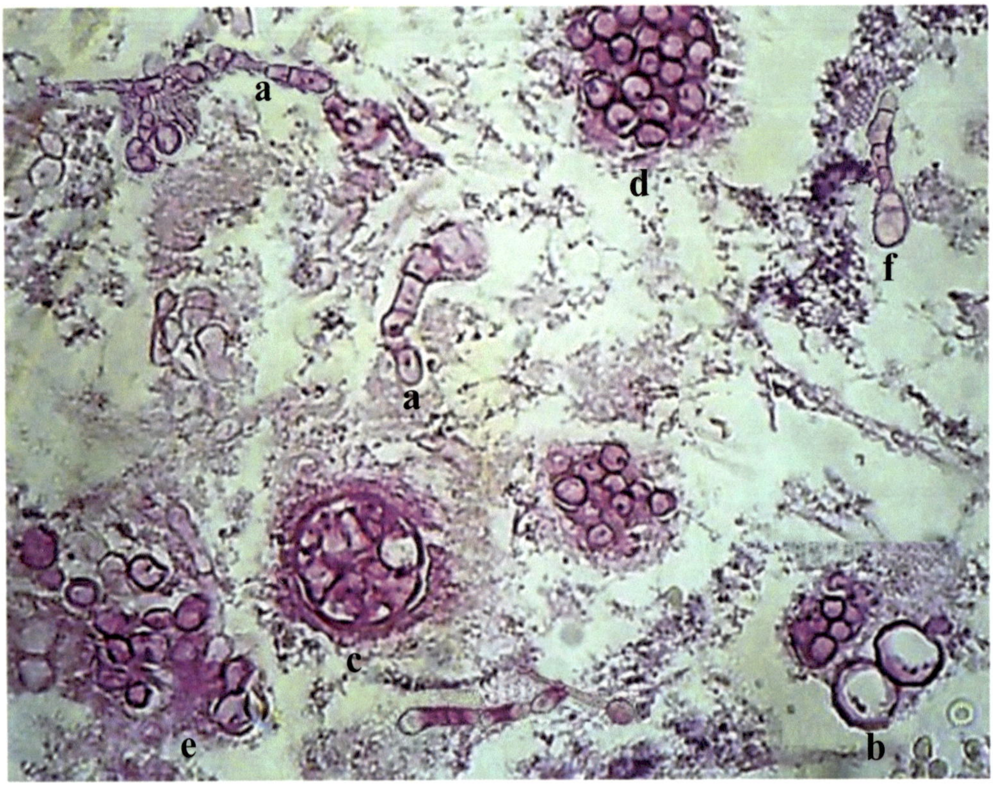

Fig. 5. Parasitic forms of *Coccidioides* spp. observed in patients with chronic cavitary pulmonary coccidioidomycosis. a) Hyphae forming arthroconidia, b) Immature spherules, c) spherules with endospores, d) Morulares forms, e) Alone endospores. f) Endospores filament. Lung tissue stained with periodic acid-Schiff.

Also, in the *Coccidioides* spp. parasitic phase, genes involved in trehalose synthesis are increased. Trehalose can protect fungi against thermal stress (heat, cold), desiccation, and oxidation (Johannesson et al., 2006; Moran et al., 2011).

Melanin

Melanins are multifunctional polymers that are negatively charged, hydrophobic pigments with a high molecular weight. Melanin is considered a virulence factor for human pathogenic fungi such as *Cryptococcus neoformans*, Aspergillus species, *Exophiala dermatitidis*, *Sporothrix schenckii*, *P. brasiliensis*, *H. capsulatum*, *B. dermatitidis*, *C. albicans* and *Coccidioides* spp. Melanin or melanin-like compounds are present in *Coccidioides* arthroconidia, spherules, and endospores *in vitro* and *in vivo*, but not in hyphae. Melanin is deposited in the cell wall and cytoplasm. Melanin protects fungi against diverse insults, including extremes temperatures, Ultraviolet (UV) light, solar or gamma radiation, oxidants, hydrolytic enzymes, antifungal drugs, microbicidal peptides, enzymatic degradation, and killing by macrophages (preventing the respiratory burst). Melanins are immunologically active; they affect macrophages, reduce proinflammatory cytokines, and can downregulate the afferent immune response. Melanin production may promote fungal survival in different environments, increasing their resistance to immune effector responses in the infected host and reducing their susceptibility to antifungal drugs (Nosanchuk et al., 2007; Taborda et al., 2008).

Enzymatic activities

Enzymatic activities from host and fungus, together with the host immune response, play the following key roles in the fate of the infection: death of the pathogenic infection; establishment of chronic infection, or dissemination of the fungus. It is not possible to separate fungal virulence factors from the host immune response, due to that there is a close interaction between these.

Metalloproteinase

Metalloproteinase (*MEP1* gene) activity has been found from the crude Spherule outer wall (SOW) fraction isolated from first-generation, parasitic-phase cultures during the endospore-differentiation phase. SOWgp disappears from the endospore surface under the control of a specific metalloproteinase. SOWgp is present only in the spherule wall's outer membranous and amorphous layers. Endospores (diameter size, 2 a 4 µm) that emerge from ruptured spherules do not possess glycoprotein; thus, they are not recognized by SOWgp antibodies and evade immune response when they are most vulnerable to killing by host phagocytes, whereas the surfaces of mature spherules are coated with the immunodominant antigen and demonstrate high affinity for the anti-SOWgp antibody. However, Polymorphonuclear neutrophils (PMN), macrophages, or Dendritic cells (DC) cannot kill spherules due to that they are too large (40 a 100 µm in diameter) to be rendered phagocytic by these cells. It is possible, therefore, that the SOW complex provides protection to the pathogen against the host innate immune system's phagocytic and fungicidal activities. This evasive mechanism contributes significantly to the survival of the pathogen within lung tissue and potentially to the establishment of a persistent coccidioidal infection in the host (Hung et al., 2005, 2007).

Arginase

L-arginine is generated by both host and fungus. Macrophages express two arginase isoforms: arginase I, and arginase II. Arginase I is located in the cytosol of macrophages, while arginase II is a mitochondrial enzyme. Arginase activity from pathogens interferes with and competes in host L-arginine pathways. In *Coccidioides* infection, arginase can play multiple roles related to fungus metabolism and evasion of the immune response. Some of these are described as follows.

Urease

Urease activity has been reported in *Coccidioides;* it hydrolyzes the urea molecule to release [NH_4/NH_3], pH 8. The urease protein has been localized to the spherule cytoplasm and vesicles and to the large central vacuole. L-arginine is the arginase substrate and catalyzes the break of arginine in ornithine + urea. Urease hydrolyzes the urea molecule to release [NH_4/NH_3]; therefore, *Coccidioides* generates its own alkaline environment due to the release of ammonia (Figure 6). Enzymatically active urease is released from the contents of mature spherules during the parasitic cycle's endosporulation stage. The enzyme subsequently associates with the surface of intact endospores (Klein & Tebbets 2007). Urease activity of *Coccidioides in vivo* may contribute to the generation of an alkaline microenvironment near the fungal pathogen's surface, as well as stimulation of the host inflammatory response to the extracellular protein and exacerbation of the severity of coccidioidal infection by contributing to a compromised immune response and damage at infection foci of the host tissue. In *Helicobacter pylori* infection, the persistent inflammatory response causes damage to mucosal tissue and exacerbates the ulcerated condition. Some studies have suggested that engulfment of urease-producing bacteria by macrophages in the presence of exogenous urea results in intraphagocytosis of ammonia, which has an inhibitory effect on the macrophage surface expression of major histocompatibility complex class II molecules. In *Coccidioides* infection, there could be similar consequences: both an alkaline microenviroment, and an intense inflammatory response with the production of proinflammatory cytokines; if these are generated at high levels and in a persistent manner, they cause an intense inflammatory

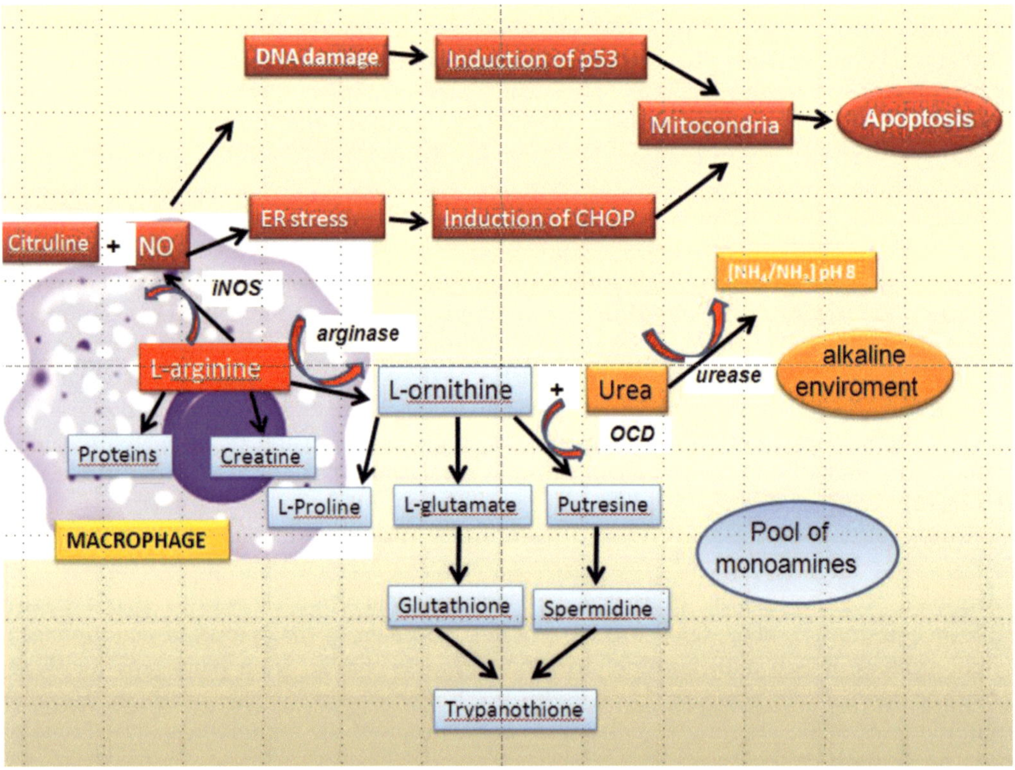

Fig. 6. Enzimatic activity in *Coccidioides* spp. Induction of elevated production of host arginase I and coccidioidal urease, which contribute to tissue damage at focus infection. Arginase I compete with iNOS in macrophages for the common substrate, L-arginine, and thereby reduces nitric oxide (NO) production and increases the synthesis of host orinithine and urea. Excess of NO induce apoptosis mediated by ER involving CHOP. Abbreviations: NO, nitric oxide; ODC, ornithine decarboxylase; CHOP, C/EBP homologous protein; inducible nitric oxide synthase, iNOS); ER endoplasmic reticulum. Modified from Vincendeau, et al., 2003.

response localized at the infection site. Urease released from spherules during the *Coccidioides* spp. parasitic cycle contributes to host-tissue damage, which further exacerbates the severity of coccidioidal infection. This damage may be mediated both by the pathogen and the host. PMN are the dominant cells in this response, although macrophages are also present. However, these cells only partially disable *Coccidioides* growth and are unable to kill it (Vincendeau et al., 2003; Mirbod-Donovan 2006; Hung et al., 2007).

Polyamines

L-ornithine is generated by arginase activity and is the substrate for Ornithine decarboxylase (ODC), which is a key enzyme in polyamine biosynthesis (Figure 6). Host-derived L-ornithine may promote pathogen growth and proliferation by providing a monoamine pool, which could be taken up and used for polyamine synthesis via the parasitic cells' metabolic pathways. Polyamines possess the following multiple roles: stabilizing nucleic acid and membranes; regulating cell growth and the cell differentiation pathway, and regulating *Coccidioides* parasitic-cell differentiation. Polyamines can also regulate the cellular death process, known as apoptosis. In extreme cases, high exogenous polyamine concentrations can lead to cell death. Effects of the polyamines comprise both induction and inhibition of biosynthetic and catabolic enzyme activities, which are associated with the increase and decrease of apoptosis (Figures 6 and 7) (Vincendeau et al., 2003; Wallace et al., 2003).

Nitric oxide (NO) synthesis

Arginase I competes with inducible Nitric oxide synthase (iNOS) in macrophages in order for the common substrate, L-arginine, to produce NO following macrophage activation by microbial products and antigen-specific, T-cell-derived cytokines. Therefore, the Th1/Th2 balance could also be considered as a mechanism whereby the immune system regulates and limits NO production (Figure 6) Dendritic cells (DC) have also been shown to upregulate arginase I expression and arginase activity on Th2 stimulation. This leads to the depletion of L-arginine, a substrate of NOS, resulting in lower levels of cytotoxic NO and increased production of polyamines. Expression of NOS creates a cytotoxic environment, promoting microbiostasis and favoring vasodilatation, which might be important in the early wound-healing phase, and arginase activity produces an environment favorable to fibroblast replication and collagen production and is therefore required for tissue repair (Vincendeau et al., 2003; Wallace et al., 2003). The concentration of L-arginine is crucial in determining the effect of NO-dependent parasite killing by macrophages. NO is a messenger molecule functioning in vascular regulation, host immunity, defense, neurotransmission, and other systems. ODC and polyamine uptake are negatively regulated by NO, given that host-arginase activation may result in decreased levels of NO production in macrophages and may permit intracellular survival of the fungal pathogen. In macrophages, a Th1 response, mainly Interferon (IFN)-γ, induces NO synthesis and parasite killing, whereas Th2 cytokines, Interleukin (IL)-4 and IL-10 inhibit NO synthesis and favor parasite growth. Th1 and Th2 cytokines regulate iNOS/arginase equilibrium in macrophages. Parasite survival appears to be related with the host's ability to mount an effective granulomatous response to the pathogen, which leads to clearance of fungal cells from infected lung tissue (Figure 6) (Wallace et al., 2003).

Apoptosis

High production of arginase I results in increased polyamine synthesis, decreased NO production, and alkalinization of the microenvironment as a consequence of the increased urea concentration and microbial urease activity at infection sites. These metabolic events contribute to the survival of *Coccidioides* in the hostile environment of the host. Low concentrations of NO protect cells from apoptosis. NO-induced apoptosis is mediated by the Endoplasmic reticulum (ER) stress pathway involving C/EBP homologous protein (CHOP) induction. ER stress has been implicated in a variety of common diseases such as diabetes, ischemia, and neurodegenerative disorders (Figure 7). Excess NO induces programmed cell death (apoptosis) in several cell types. ER stress and induction of the p53 pathway-mediated apoptosis have been described in *Coccidioides* spp. (Figures 6 and 7) (Hung et al., 2007; Vincendeau et al., 2003).

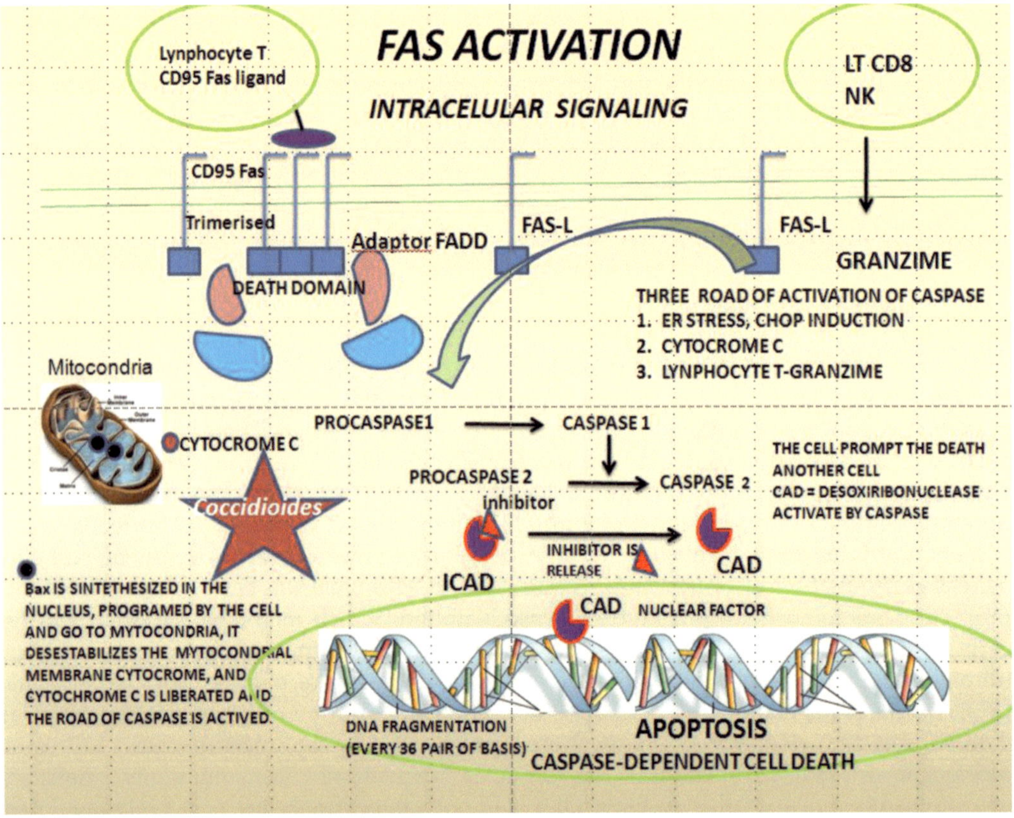

Fig. 7. Apoptosis via Fas activación. *Coccidioides* spp. induce apoptosis by ER stress or mitocondria (cytocrome C) pathway activate by caspase. Abreviations: APO-1/CD95, encodes a transmembrane type I receptor.

5. Immune response

The immune system comprises the innate immune response (constitutive) and the adaptative immune response (induced and specific). Both immune-response types share cells and cytokines (inductors and effectors), but they also possess specific components of every type of immune response. In chronic progressive pulmonary coccidioidomycosis, the integral result of the immune response (innate and adaptative) can be observed in tissue imaging. In coccidioidal infection, there are microabscesses with abundant

Polymorphonuclear neutrophils (PMN) and mononuclear cells. In addition, there is an increase in the size of endothelian cells, with intense perivascular infiltrators. Spherules and spherules/endospores are significant increased in patients with poor prognosis for recovery (Figure 4). Granulomas are also present, with abundant Langhans cells, lymphocytes, and monocytes, and scant eosinophils, plasmocytes, and epitheliod cells surrounding the spherules and spherules/endospores. When *Coccidioides* infection has progressed, there are plentiful fungal structures. Granuloma a fibrous wall with a necrotic center, in which are found spherules (Figure 8) (Winn et al., 1994).

5.1 Innate immunity

Innate immunity in *Coccidioides* spp. protects healthy individuals from coccidioidal infection in 70% of cases; thus, it is highly efficient in healthy subjects. However, this response is not sufficiently efficient to kill arthroconida-infectant propagules. The major members responsible for the innate immune response in *Coccidioides* infection are PMNL, monocytes/ macrophages, Natural killer (NK) cells, DC, and Surfactant protein A (SP-A).

PMNL

These comprise the first cellular influx into the arthroconidia. This response may be attributable to chemotactic components released by the arthroconidia. Arthroconidium phagocytosis is enhanced in the presence of immune serum. Ingestion of arthroconidia is followed by a respiratory burst, but <20% of arthroconidia are killed by the encounter. Transformation of arthroconidia into spherules prevents phagocytosis and the killing of these by PMNL, owing in part to the increased spherule size (60-80 μm) relative to that of the PMNL (12 μm). Rupture of spherules and release of endospores newly trigger a PMNL influx. The host mounts an intense inflammatory response to the released products. Neutrophils are the dominant innate cells found associated with endosporulating spherules, although macrophages are also present (Figure 8).

Monocytes/macrophages

Both *Coccidioides* spp. arthroconidia and endospores are phagocytized by monocytes/ macrophages, but <1% of phagocytized cells are killed. *Coccidioides* appears to inhibit the fusion of arthroconidia- or endospore-containing phagosomes with lysosomes. However, a significant increase in phagosome-lysosome fusion was observed in macrophages when adaptative immunity was specifically activated with fungus antigens. This increase in fusion correlated with the ability of the macrophages to kill *Coccidioides* spp.

Natural killer cells

NK cells comprise a major component of innate immunity. They can migrate to inflammation sites in response to chemokines. NK cells secrete cytokines, IFN-γ, and chemokines, which induce inflammatory responses and control monocyte and granulocyte growth.

Dendritic cells

These are potent Antigen-presenting cells (APC) and play a pivotal role in innate and adaptive immunity. On initial infection, precursor DC are recruited from the blood to inflammatory sites, where they transform into immature DC. In the initial interaction, the pathogen binds to pattern-recognition receptors, notably Toll-like receptors (TLR), which recognize structurally conserved pathogen-associated microbial products. This initial recognition leads to induction of proinflammatory cytokines, which include Tumor necrosis factor alpha (TNF-α) and Interleukin (IL) -1, IL-6, and IL-8. The spherule-phase antigen induces maturation of peripheral blood-derived DC from healthy, nonimmune subjects. When immature DC are exposed to the coccidioidal antigen, this encounter can generate anergy in patients with systemic infection.

Surfactant protein A

The pulmonary surfactant is a complex mixture of lipids and proteins that reduces surface tension at the air-liquid interface within alveoli. The most abundant protein component of alveolar surfactant is Surfactant protein A (SP-A). This protein binds to macrophages, generating diverses phenotypical and functional alterations into macrophage biology-increased phagocytosis through complement receptors (FcR); there is altered production of proinflammatory cytokines such as TNF-α and IL-1 and decreased production of NO in response to stimuli. Thus, in the lung, macrophages produces Reactive oxygen intermediates (ROI) promote host defense and avoid host damage. Therefore, SP-A inhibits ROI production through NADPH oxidase by human macrophages in response to stimuli by reducing NADPH oxidase activity. In addition, SP-A contributes to the alternate activation phenotype of alveolar macrophages and to the maintenance of an anti-inflammatory environment in the healthy lung (Crowther et al., 2004).

5.2 Adaptive immunity

Adaptative Cell-mediated immune response directly correlates with specific resistance to *Coccidioides* spp. infection, whereas susceptibility correlates with expression of Th2-associated cytokines, which potentiate the production of IgE and IgG1 antibodies and suppress macrophages and T-cell responses. Disseminated coccidioidomycosis is associated with T-cell anergy and the production of exaggerated levels of anti-*Coccidioides* immunoglobulin (Ig)G and IgE antibodies. The mechanisms that induce CMI responses in coccidioidomycosis are probably under genetic control. Persons with Asian, Afro-american, or Hispanic ancestry are at higher risk for developing disseminated coccidioidomycosis than those with Caucasian ancestry.

5.2.1 Cell-Mediated Immunity (CMI)

Cell-mediated immunity has been related with induction of Th1-associated immune responses (IL-2, IL-12, TNF-α, and IFN-γ). The cumulative response includes processing and presentation of critical antigens by macrophages and/or DC, leading to the induction of T-cells to produce IFN-α and other Th1-associated cytokines. These cytokines provide the signals for recruiting and activating immune effector cells. One example is that activation of immature DC leads to their secretion of chemokines and maturation of DC into highly efficient APC, which function in T- and B-cell response regulation. APC interact with T- and B-cells. Mature DC induces and triggers multiple events to develop the cellular and humoral adaptive immune response. The Cell-mediated immunity response comprises the following: i) cutaneous delayed-type hypersensitivity; ii) cytokine production, and (iii) cytokine activation of monocytes (Cox & Magee, 2004; Xue et al., 2005)

Cutaneous delayed-type hypersensitivity

The classic antigen preparation, a soluble broth-culture filtrate of mycelial cells (coccidioidin) or the culture of the spherule-endospore phase *in vitro* (spherulin), both are employed as a coccidioidin skin-sensitivity test. Persons with primary, asymptomatic, or benign disease characteristically have strong skin-test reactivity to coccidioidin and low or nondemonstrable levels of anti-*Coccidioides* complement fixation (CF) antibody. Skin-test reactivity persists in the majority of persons who recover from primary infection, and these persons are endowed with immunity to exogenous reinfection. Patients who develop progressive or chronic pulmonary coccidioidomycosis manifest a reaction to the coccidioidin skin-sensitivity test. Low or nonresponse to the latter test denotes poor prognosis for recovery. Anergy occur in patients who have severely disseminated disease involving multiple infection foci.

Cytokine production

Cytokines and chemokines are host factors that guide Th1- and Th2-cell differentiation. Th1/Th2 cytokine profiles correlate with resistance and susceptibility to *Coccidioides* infection, respectively.

TNF-α

This is a cytokine produced by a large variety of cells, including macrophages, DC, and T- and B- lynphocytes. In patients with active coccidioidomycosis, TNF-α is responsible for many of the biological and physiological consequences of acute infection, immunological reactions, and tissue injury. Additionally, TNF-α is required for control of acute infection and formation and maintenance of granulomas, but, on the other hand, it has been implicated as a major component in host-mediated destruction of lung tissue (Figure 8).

IFN-γ

Is another cytokine that is produced in coccidioidal infection. Lymphocytes from patients with pulmonary disease secreted IFN-γ levels comparable to those of healthy persons. In contrast, in patients with disseminated disease, IFN-γ was significantly lower than in healthy persons with the coccidioidin skin-sensitivity test. The mechanism by which IFN-γ and TNF-α can activate macrophages is generating NO and related reactive nitrogen intermediates via nitric oxide synthase, using L-arginine as substrate (loVelle 1987; Hung et al., 2002; Magee & Cox 1995).

Production of these cytokines was at the infection site and generally revealed quantitative rather than qualitative differences. Although IFN-γ production is assigned to Th1 T-cells, natural killer cells also produce abundant levels of this cytokine. One mechanism by which IFN-γ might mediate resistance to *C. immitis* is by activating macrophages to inhibit or kill the fungus (Magee & Cox 1995).

SOW (without glycoprotein)

Is rich in lipid complexes with high amounts of phospholipids; this fraction is highly immunogenic and induces high amounts of IFN-γ. The principal functions of IFN-γ *in vivo* are activation of macrophages and increased expression of the Major histocompatibility complex (MHC), which can result in stimulation of a host immune-response Th1 pathway.

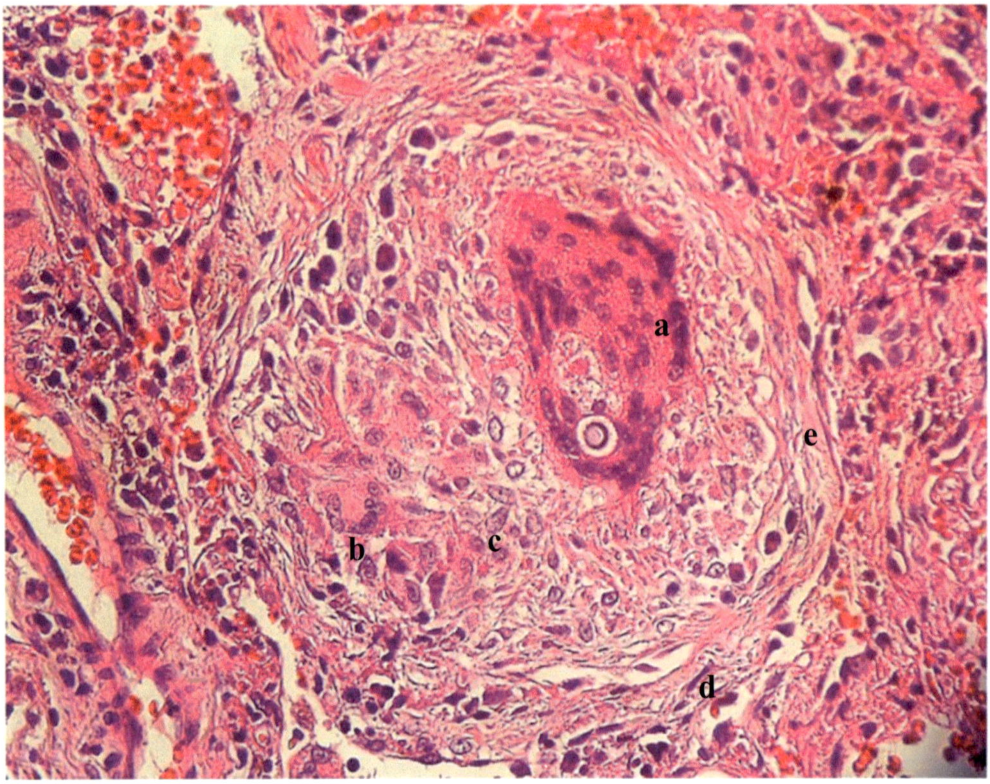

Fig. 8. *Coccidioides* granuloma in inflammatory infiltrate. a) Spherule embedded in a cell of Langhans; b) Langhans cell with nuclei arranged in a horseshoe shape; c) epithelioid cells; d) fibroblasts; e) fibrin. Hematoxylin-eosin staining in lung tissue.

IL-2

This has been shown to modulate early development of Th1 vs. Th2 responses. IL-12 plays a role as an important control mechanism for developing protective host defenses against coccidioidal infection. IL-12 possesses multiple functions, such as stimulation of T-lymphocyte and NK cell proliferation, promotion of cytolytic activity of macrophages, and induction of the secretion of other cytokines, including IL-2, TNF-γ, and IFN-α. It has also been correlated with the induction of a protective TH1 immune-response pathway against systemic fungal infections (Magee & Cox 1995).

Cytokine activation of monocytes

Phagocytized, non-activated (innate immunity) monocytes do not kill *Coccidioides* arthroconidia or endospores. Fungi might survive intracellularly by employing inhibition of phagosome-lysosome fusion. In contrast, monocytes specifically activated by IFN-γ or TNF-α (adaptative immunity) augmented the fungicidal capabilities for killing *Coccidioides* spp. structures.

5.2.2 Humoral immunity

The Th2 immune response compromises host protection against coccidioidomycosis and exacerbates the disease course, while Th2-type immune response produces high levels of IL-4, IL-5, IL-6, and IL-10, which in turn stimulate the B-cells to produce antibodies; this type of response exacerbates the disease course. In addition, there is no evidence that this response protects the host from coccidioidal infection. High amounts of IL-6 correlate with intense inflammatory response to *Coccidioides* infection, which may contribute to host-tissue damage and exacerbation of disease too (Hung et al., 2005, 2007).

Antibodies

High antibody titers to *Coccidioides* in patients with this respiratory disease typically correlate with poor clinical outcome. Chronic or progressive coccidioidomycosis is associated with polyclonal B-lymphocyte activation, and Th2 response, as evidenced by elevated levels of IgG, IgA, and IgE in serum. Serum IgG levels directly correlate with disease progression; highest titers are present in patients with multifocal involvement. The serum IgA level is elevated in patients with chronic pulmonary disease. In addition, there is IgE hyperproduction, with highest incidence occurring in patients with disseminated disease. SOWgp is the major cell-surface antigen of *Coccidioides* that elicits both antibody-mediated and cellular immune responses in patients with coccidioidal infections. SOWgp may contribute to a bias in Th1 vs. Th2 pathways during the course of *C. immitis* infection. The SOWgp antigen exerts an influence on the host to react to *Coccidioides*-associated respiratory diseases by activation of a T-helper 2 (Th2) pathway (Hung et al., 2002, 2007).

Immune complexes

Circulating C1q-binding immune complexes have been detected in sera from patients with coccidioidomycosis and were shown to correlate with disease severity 7). Whereas 33% of sera from patients with the disease involving a single-organ system had elevated immune complex levels, 67% of sera from patients with disseminated multifocal disease demonstrated circulating immune complexes. Analyses of immune complexes in serum from a patient with severe disseminated disease revealed *Coccidioides* antigen, C1q, and anti-*Coccidioides* IgG antibody (Hung et al., 2002, 2007).

6. Diagnosis

Coccidioidomycosis can be clinically and radiologically confused with other respiratory apparatus pathologies such as neoplasms, fungal and bacterial infections, and mainly with tuberculosis; in tissue slices, histophatological images are found that are similar to those of other mycotic or bacterial infections. Laboratory diagnosis is complicated if no typical spherules/endospores are observed in the pathological specimens. Therefore, in order to arrive at the correct analysis of this disease, the collaboration is necessary of a multidisciplinary group of health professionals in which Clinicians, Epidemiologists, Radiologists, Mycologists, and currently Molecular Biologists, who have contributed considerably to the identification of the etiological agent and in the diagnosis of this mycosis.

Coccidioides is a dimorphic fungus; it grows in its saprobic or vegetative phase as a mycelium, forming a large amount of arthroconidia, and in its parasitic phase, it is differentiated in structures denominated spherules, which generate in its interior hundreds of endospores. They are considered diagnosis for active infection. However, a parasitic phenotypic diversity has been observed in the transition of arthrocondia to spherules/endospores; in this variation are included the parasitic mycelial forms of *Coccidioides,* which have been observed in >50% of patients with chronic pulmonary coccidioidomycos (Figures 1, 2, 4, and 5) (Muñoz-Hernández et al., 2004, 2008). Notwithstanding microscopic observation of hyphae and arthroconidia of *Coccidioides,* these are not diagnosed; it is necessary to have knowledge of their presence in this mycosis and to recognize them in biological samples. This morphological diversity can generate errors in fungal identification due to the morphological similarity that these can possess with other fungi, or parasites, and even with artifices present in pathological specimens. All of these characteristics of the pathogen considerably complicate the final diagnosis of this disease. In addition, it is considered the most infectious and virulent of the mycoses, and difficult to treat. Therefore, the laboratory diagnosis is relevant.

In order to perform a specific diagnosis, it is important to work with an adequate sample, which should derive from the lesion site, to have a sufficient amount, and to transport it immediately to the laboratory for its processing. It is suggested to analyze a minimum of three pathological specimens. Muñoz-Hernández and colleagues report that the most frequently analyzed biological product was sputum, achieving a good result without the need of using invasive methods during specimen-taking, followed by bronchial lavage and brushing (Muñoz-Hernández et al., 2004, 2008).

The most customary methods for laboratory diagnosis comprise microscopic analysis, whether by observing the product in its fresh state with KOH or in histopathological preparations with different stains, in which diverse parasite forms can be observed: from arthroconidia and septate hyphae with multiple morphologies, to conidia transition, spores to mature spherules and endospore-releasing spherules (Figures 1, 2, 4, and 5). This technique is the most rapid and the result can be given on the same day that the sample is received in the laboratory. Isolation of the etiological agent is the best test for identification of this infectious agent. Identification of the fungus is performed by recognizing the macro- and microscopic phenotypic characteristics of the fungus. For management of cultures and all material containing *Coccidioides* spp. arthroconidia, the use of level 3 biosafety hoods is recommended (Ampel, 2010; Soubolle, 2007). Genus confirmation from the culture is detected by means of exoantigens and through the use of a genetic probe (Accuprobe, GenProbe, San Diego, CA, USA). Characterization of C. immitis and C. *posadasii species* is carried out employing molecular methods. Serology is a useful auxiliary method for diagnosis and prognosis of the disease; however, the sensitivity of this test is not ideal. Determination of coccidioidal galactomannan is commercially available for detecting the antigen in urine, this tool is highly sensitive and it is recommended in patients with more severe forms of coccidiodomycosis (Durkin, et al., 2008). Molecular methods had been proved useful to Coccidioides identification. Darko Vucicevic considered PCR successful when culture is negative. However, few laboratories can provide these techniques (Darko, 2010; De Aguilar et al., 2007; Galgiani et al., 2011).

7. Conclusions

Coccidioides is a fungal pathogen that causes diseases ranging from mild to severe infection, the knowledge of their parasitic cycle, virulence factors and host immune response are important for understanding its pathogenesis and effect the accurate diagnosis. The subregistry of this mycosis is closely linked to clinical and laboratory diagnosis. Laboratory diagnosis is very important, since coccidioidomicosis may be confused with pulmonary tuberculosis or other lung diseases.

Typical parasitic forms of *coccodioides ssp* are spherules and spherules/endospores, however, other parasitic structures have been reported. It is important identify the diverse parasitic morphological forms of *Coccidioides* spp., they are spherules, spherules/endospores and mycelial forms. Mycelial forms are pleomorfic cells and can present as: hyphae forming ovoid and spherical cells, pleomorphic cells producing septate hyphae, chain of ovoid cells, arthroconidia, and septate hyphae forming a barrel-shaped cells. We thing different parasitic forms of *Coccidioides* spp. are present in function of:

- Virulence factors
  - Quorung- sensing.- protein kinases sensing host conditions and dimorphism is triggered by exposure to temperature, pH, and CO_2 concentration, so the fungus leads diferenciation and dimorphism: Parasitic forms, Spherules and spherules/endospores
  - Tissue damage with inflammatory infiltrate.- urease activity of *Coccidioides in vivo* can contribute to the generation of an alkaline microenvironment near the fungal pathogen's surface, as well as stimulation of the host inflammatory and exacerbation of the severity of coccidioidal infection, lead to generate apoptosis, cavity lesion with relation O_2/CO_2 exchange inefficient: Parsitic forms, spherules/endospores and mycelial forms
- Clinical form
  - Chronic pulmonary coccidioidomycosis, central nervous system coccidioidomycosis, chronic and cavitary pulmonary coccidioidomycosis (>8 months), ventriculoperitoneal shunt and fungal ball: Parasitic forms, spherules, spherules/endospores and mycelial forms.
- Comorbidity
  - Diabetes mellitus type 2 and chronic pulmonary infection: Parsitic forms spherules, spherules/endospores and mycelial forms
- Cellular immune response
  - CMI responses in coccidioidomycosis are probably under genetic control. Persons with Asian, Afro-american, or Hispanic (possibly HLA) ancestry are at higher risk for developing disseminated coccidioidomycosis than those with Caucasian ancestry: Parsitic forms, spherules and spherules/endospores and mycelial forms.
  - Granulomas are present, with abundant Langhans cells, lymphocytes, and monocytes, and scant eosinophils, plasmocytes, and epitheliod cells surrounding the parasitic fungal: Parsitic forms, spherules and spherules/endospores.

Based on microscopic images of patient specimens and on observations of mycelial structures in our studies, as well as those reported by various authors in coccidioidal infection in the lung and central nervous system, we propose that mycelial forms should be incorporated into the parasitic phase of the *Coccidioides* spp.

8. Acknowledgements

The authors acknowledge the financial support from CONACYT (SALUD-2011-1-161897). We are grateful to Miguel Angel Escamilla González for the illustration of the parasitic life cycle; to EDD/IPN and COFAA/IPN and SNI/ CONACYT programs; and the ethics and scientific committees revise and approve the chapter.

9. References

Baptista-Rosas RC, Hinojosa A, Riquelme M. 2007. Ecological Niche Modeling of *Coccidioides spp.* in Western North American Deserts. *Ann. N.Y. Acad. Sci.* 1111: 35–46.

Charlton V, Ramsdell K, Sehring S. 1999. Intrauterine transmission of coccidioidomycosis . Pedriat Infect Dis. J. 18: 561-563.

Cole GT, Xue J, Seshan K, Borra P, Borra R, Tarcha E, Schaller R, Yu JJ, Hung CY. 2006. Virulence mechanisms of *Coccidioides*. In: *Molecular Principles of Fungal Pathogenesis*. Joseph Heiman, Filler Scott, John Edwards, Aaron Mitchell. ASM Press. ISBN-13: 987-1-55581-368-D; ISBN-10: 155555813682, Washington, D.C. USA.

Cox R & Magee D. 2004. Coccidioidomycosis: Host Response and Vaccine Development. *Clin Microbiol. Rev.* 17(4): 804–839.

Crowther JE, Kutala V, Kuppusamy P, Ferguson JS. et l. 2004. Production in Response to Stimuli by Reducing Macrophage Reactive Oxygen Intermediate Pulmonary Surfactant Protein A Inhibits NADPH Oxidase Activity. *J Immunol.* 172: 6866-6874.

Darko V. 2010Chain Reaction Testing in the Clinical Setting, Mycopathologia. 170(5): 345-351.

De Aguiar Cordeiro R, Nogueira Brilhante RS, Gadelha Rocha MF, Araújo Moura FE, Pires de Camargo Z, Costa Sidrim JJ. 2007. Rapid diagnosis of coccidioidomycosis by nested PCR assay of sputum. Clin Microbiol Infect. 13(4):449-51.

Dolan MJ, Lattuada CP, Melcher R, Zellmer R, Allendoerfer R, Rinaldi MG. 1992. *Coccidioides immitis* presenting as a mycelial pathogen with empyema and hydropneumothorax. *J Med Vet Mycol* 30: 249–255.

Durkin M , Connolly P, Kuberskia T, Myers R , Kubak BM , Bruckner D, Pegues DL. 2008. Diagnosis of Coccidioidomycosis with Use of the *Coccidioides* Antigen Enzyme Immunoassay *Clin Infect Dis. 47 (8): e69-e73. doi: 10.1086/592073.*

Fisher MC, Koenig GL, White TJ, Taylor JW. 202. Molecular and phenotypic description of *Coccidioides posadasii* sp. previously recognized as the non-California population of *Coccidioides immitis. Mycologia.* 94(1): 73–84.

Hagman HM, Madnick EG, D'Agostino AN et al. 2000. Hyphal forms in the central nervous system of patients with coccidioidomycosis. *Clin Infect Dis* 30:349–353.

Heidi MH, Madnick EG, D'Agostino AN et al. 2000. Hyphal forms in the central nervous system of patients with coccidioidomycosis. *Clin Infect Dis* 30:349–355.

Hirschmann JV. 2007. The Early History of Coccidioidomycosis: 1892–1945. *Clin Infect Dis.* 44(9): 1202-1207.

Hung CY, Yu JJ, Kalpathi R, Utz R, Cole GT. 2002. A Parasitic Phase-Specific Adhesin of *Coccidioides immitis* Contributes to the Virulence of This Respiratory Fungal Pathogen. *Infect and Immun.* 70 (7): 3443–3456.

Hung CY, Seshan K, Yu JJ, Schaller R, Xue J, Basrur V, Gardner MJ, Cole GT. 2005. A Metalloproteinase of *Coccidioides posadasii* Contributes to Evasion of Host Detection. *Infect and Immun*. 73 (10): 6689–6703.

Hung CY, Xue J, Cole GT. 2007. Virulence Mechanisms of *Coccidioides. Ann. N.Y. Acad. Sci.* 1111: 225–235.

Galgiani JN, Kauffman CA, Thorner AR. 2011. Laboratory diagnosis of coccidioidomycosis. Last literature review version 19.2: This topic last updated: abril 21, 2011.

Johannesson H, Kasuga T, Schaller RA, Good B, Gardner MJ. et al. 2006. Phase-speciphic gene expression underlying morphological adaptations of the dimorphic human pathogenic fungus, *Coccidioides posadasii. Fungal Genet Biol.* 43:545-559.

Klein BS & Tebbets B. 2007. Dimorphism and virulence in fungi. *Curr Opin Microbiol.* 10:314–319.

Klenschmidt-DeMasters BK, Mazowiecki M, Bonds LA, Cohn DL, Wilson ML. 2000. Coccidioidomycosis meningitis with massive dural and cerebral venous thrombosis and tissue arthroconidia. *Arch Pathol Lab Med.* 124:310–314.

Koufopanou V, Burt A, Taylor JW. 1997. Concordance of gene genealogies reveals reproductive isolation in the pathogenic fungus Coccidioides immitis. *Proc Natl Acad Sci USA.* 94(10):5478-82.

Lones GW. & Peacock CL. 1960. Role of carbón dioxide in the dimorphism of *Coccidioides immitis. J Bacteriol.* 79(2): 308–309.

loVelle B. 1987. Fungicidal Activation of Murine Macrophages by Recombinant Gamma Interferon *Infec Immun.* 55(12): 2951-2955.

Magee D & Cox R. 1995. Roles of Gamma Interferon and Interleukin-4 in Genetically Determined Resistance to *Coccidioides immitis. Infect Immun.* 63(9): 3514–3519.

Mendes-Giannini MJ, Pienna SCh, Leal J, Ferrari P. 2005. MiniReview Interaction of pathogenic fungi with host cells: Molecular and cellular approaches. *FEMS Immunol Med Microbiol.* 45: 383–394.

Meyer PR, Hui AN, Biddle M. 1982. *Coccidioides immitis* meningitis with arthroconidia in cerebrospinal fluid: report of the first case and review of the arthroconidia literature. *Hum Pathol.* 13:1136–1138.

Mirbod-Donovan F, Schaller R, Hung CY, , Utz RJ, Cole GT. 2006. Urease Produced by *Coccidioides posadasii* Contributes to the Virulence of This Respiratory Pathogen. *Infect Immun.* 74: (1): 504-515.

Moran GP, Coleman D, Sullivan D. 2011. Comparative Genomics and the Evolution of Pathogenicity in Human Pathogenic Fungi. *Eukaryotic Cell.* 10(1): 34–42.

Muñoz-Hernández B, Castañón LR, Calderón I, Vázquez ME, Manjarrez ME. 2004. Parasitic mycelial forms of *Coccidioides* species in Mexican patients. *J Clin Microbiol* 42:1247–1249.

Muñoz-Hernández B, Martínez-Rivera MA, Palma Cortés G, Tapia-Díaz A, Manjarrez ME. 2008. Mycelial Forms of *Coccidioides* spp. in the Parasitic Phase Associated to Pulmonary Coccidioidomycosis with Type 2 Diabetes Mellitus. *Eur J Clin Mcrobiol Infect Dis.* 27(9):813-20.

Negroni R. 2008. Evolución de los conocimientos sobre aspectos clínico-epidemiológicos de la Coccidioidomycosis en las Américas. *Rev Arg Microbiol.* 40: 246-256.

Neil AM. 2010. The diagnosis of coccidioidomycosis, F1000 Medicine Reports. 2: (2) 1-4.

Nemecek JC, Wurthrich M, Klein BS. 2006. Klein. Global Control of Dimorphism and Virulence in Fungi. *Sci.* 312 (5773):583-8

Nemecek JC, Wurthrich M, Klein BS. 2007. Detection and measurement of two-component systems that control dimorphism and virulence in fungi. *Methods Enzymol.* 422:465-487.

Nosanchuk JD, Snedeker J, Nosanchuk JS. 1998. Arthroconidia in coccidioidoma: case report and literature review. *Int J Infect Dis* 3:32–35.

Nosanchuk JD, Yu JJ, Chiung-Yu H, Casadevall A, Cole GT. 2007. *Coccidioides* posadasii produces melanin in vitro and during infection. *Fungal Genet Biol.* 44: 517–520.

Ramsdell V, & Sehring S. 1999 intrauterine transmission of coccidioidomycosis . *Pedriat Iinfect Dis J.* 18:561-563.

Saubolle MA. 2007. Laboratory aspects in the diagnosis of coccidioidomycosis. Ann N Y Acad Sci. 1111: 301-14.

Sharpton TJ, Jason ES, Steven DR, Malcolm JG, Vinita JS, et al., 2009. Comparative genomic analyses of the human fungal pathogens *Coccidioides* and their relatives. *Genomic Res.* 19: 1722-1731.

Taborda C, da Silva M, Nosanchuk JD, Travassos LR. 2008. Melanin as a virulence factor of *Paracoccidioides brasiliensis* and other dimorphic pathogenic fungi: a minireview. *Mycopathol.* 165(4-5): 331–339.

Taylor JW & Fishery MC. 2003. Fungal multilocus sequence typing — it's not just for bacteria. *Curr Opin Microbiol.* 6:351–356.

Taylor JW & Fisher MC. 2003. Fungal multilocus sequence typing — it's not just for bacteria. *Curr Opi Microbiol.* 6:351–356.

Vincendeau P, Gobert AP, Dauloue ´de S, Moynet D, Mossalayi MD. 2002. Arginases in parasitic diseases. *Trends in Parasitol.* 19 (1): 9-11.

Vucicevic D, Blair JE, Binnicker MJ, McCullough AE, Kusne S, Vikram HR, Parish JM, Wengenack NL. 2010. The utility of Coccidioides polymerase chain reaction testing in the clinical setting. Mycopathologia. 170(5):345-51.

Xue J, Hung CY, Yu JJ, Cole GT. 2005. Immune response of vaccinated and non-vaccinated mice to *Coccidioides posadasii* infection. *Vaccine.* 23: 3535-3544.

Wages DS, Helfend L, Finkle H. 1995. *Coccidioides immitis* presenting as a hyphal form in a ventriculoperitoneal shunt. *Arch Pathol Lab Med.* 119:91–93.

Wallace HM, Fraser AV, Hughes A. 2003. A perspective of polyamine metabolism Review article. *Biochem J.* 376: 1–14.

Winn RE, Jhoson R, Galgiani JN, Butler C, Pluss J. 1994. Cavitary coccidioidomycosis with fungus ball formation. Diagnosis by fiberoptic bronchoscopy with coexistence of hyphae and spherules. *Chest.* 105:412–416.

Zepeda MR, Kobayashi GK, Applerma MD, Navarro A. 1998. *Coccidioides immitis* presenting as a hyphal form in cerebrospinal fluid. *J Nat Med Assoc.* 90:435–436.

Zimmermann CR, Snedker CJ, Pappagianis D. 1994. Characterization of Coccidioides immitis Isolates by Restriction Fragment Length Polymorphisms. *J Clin Microbiol.* 32(12): 3040-3042.

3

Biological Control of Parasites

Khodadad Pirali-Kheirabadi
Department of Pathobiology, Faculty of Veterinary Medicine
and Research Institute of Zoonotic Diseases,
Shahrekord University, Shahrekord
Iran

1. Introduction

As a rule, all species of animals are regulated by other living organisms (antagonists) which are not under manipulation by man but they are naturally occurring in our surrounding environment. The process called natural biological control when man attempts to use naturally occurring antagonists to lower a pest population which would cause losses to plant or animals. Biological control is an ecological method designed by man for lower a pest or parasite population to keep these populations at a non harmful level. In practice, applied biological control has no direct application to internal animal parasites especially in their parasitic stages which may be indirectly regulated by intermediate, paratenic or transport vectors even free living larval stages. Many organisms such as viruses, bacteria, turbellarians, earthworms, tardigrades, fungi, spiders, ants, insects, rodents, birds, and other living things are found to contribute significantly toward limiting parasite populations such as arthropods, protozoans and helminthes of domesticated animals. Numerous pathogens and predator of parasites (arthropods) have been known for decades, but few biocontrol programs have been developed. Parasites are controlled almost exclusively by chemical acaricides. The development of resistance to acaricides and their harmful to the environment necessitate alternative control strategies such as habitat modification, use of pheromones and hormones, improvement of host resistance and biological control. Research on the potential use of pathogens, parasitoids, or predators for the biological control of animal parasites lags for behind for plant pests. Among the discouraging remarks are statements that natural enemies are not efficient for biological control, because the population of parasites is so large and that there is little potential for biological control (Cole., 1965). Because the fecundities of predators appear to be below the level required to respond to the explosive increase in example tick numbers which follow certain types of weather such statements may explain partly the longtime neglect of this field and similar arguments were also expressed during the first steps of plant pest biocontrol.

2. Pathogens and their potential in biological control

Most pathogens enter arthropods via contaminated food. This means of entry is however not efficient for introducing pathogens into sucking arthropods such as ticks. Even so, some entomopathogenic fungi, as well as nematodes can penetrate the host via the integument.

Most pathogens are effective against arthropods only at relatively high humidity. The efficiency of pathogens to invade an arthropod depends to a large extent on the arthropod density. However when an area is artificially over flooded with a pathogen, it may reduce a pest population nearly to zero.

2.1 Fungi

2.1.1 Entomopathogenic fungi

The kingdom fungi is a monophyletic assemblage which at present comprises four major phyla: A; Chytridiomycota, B; Zygomycota C; Basidiomycota and D; Ascomycota. (Berbee & Taylor., 1999). The chytridiomycota contains few entomopathogenic species, but includes two genera (Coelomomyces and coelomycidium that kill the larvae of haematophagous diptera and have been studied fot the biocontrol of mosquitoes and black flies (Tanada and Kaya., 1993). The entomophthorales (zygomycota) include some important obligate entomopathogens that cause natural epizootics in a range of agricultural pests , and contain some key species that can not be grown readily *in vitro*. (MacCoy et al., 1988). The most widely studiesd genera of entomophthoraleans fungi, associated with pest control , include Conidiobolus, Entomophthora, Erynia and neozygites. Also Basidiomycota include a limited number of entomopathogens (MacCoy et al ., 1988). The Ascomycota contains many of the major plant pathogens and, together with the mitosporic fungi they also constitute the majority of the entomopathogens. The laboulbeniales (Ascomycota) comprise a larg number of commensal species that are confined to the exoskeleton of insects. The mitosporic fungi include many species of most important entomopathogens and members of the mitosporic entomopathogens are the most widely used for biological pest control.

Important genera of fungi are reported to be major pathogens of some parasites (insects) (Hall and Papierok 1982) because of their wide dispersal, their wide spectrum of hosts and their ability to efficiently enter into the cuticle. Entomopathogenic fungi require high humidity for propagule germination and hyphal penetration. At low temperature and low humidity they may parasitize the ticks via the anus and the fungus hyphae invade the ticks via the genital pore. The most commonly investigated entomopathogenic fungi belonged to the genera *Metarhizium* and *Beauveria*, and to the less extend to *Verticillium* and *Paecilomyces*. We reported for the first time the pathogenic effects of *Lecanicillium psalliotae* against *Boophilus annulatus* (Pirali-Kheirabadi et al., 2007 a,b). Entomopathogenic fungi are used against terrestrial insects, because of their wide geographic spread and host range as well as their unique ability to germinate even at a relatively low humidity. Fungi can remain active on cattle ears for 1-3 weeks in field trial. (Kaaya et al., 1996). The effect of a lot numbers of entomopathogenic fungal species has not yet been tested on different acari or insects. Entomopathogenic fungi attack insects by fungal propagules and affect their host via mycelia as well as by mycotoxins. In a study, application of extracts from 158 fungal strains in 29 genera on engorged females of *Booophilus microplus* tick (Acari ixodidae) revealed that only *Aspergillus niger* was able to prevent egg laying (Connole., 1969). Fungi from the genera *Metarhizium* and *Beauveria* are used increasingly in commercial formulations against insects. Their value as commercial biocontrol agents has yet to be proven but their high genetic variability and possible alternative ways to improve their formulations can made them promising candidates for future use as commercial biocontrol agents. In a comprehensive study, the pathogenicity of 11 strains of fungi including *Metarhizium anisopliae* (3 strains),

Beauveria bassiana (6 strains) and *Lecanicillium psalliotae* (2 strains) against various developmental stages of *Boophilus annulatus* was evaluated for the first time in Iran (Pirali-Kheirabadi et al., 2007.a). The authors introduced the fungus *L. psalliotae* as a novel biocontrol agent of *Boophilus annulatus, in vitro.* Fig. 1 shows detailed information about destructive effects of tested fungi on different developmental stages of *B. annulatus.* In another report, the susceptibility of different developmental stages of *R. (B.) annulatus* to the Iranian strains of Entomopathogenic fungi *B. bassiana* and *M. anisopliae* and *L. psalliotae* were studied (Pirali-Kheirabadi et al., 2007.b). These fungi have global distributions and can be mass produced readily. Over 15 mycopesticides formulated from these genera are now available commercially for the management of a reng of pests in the homoptera, Coleoptera, Lepidoptera , Diptera, and orthoptera (Shah & Goettel., 1999).

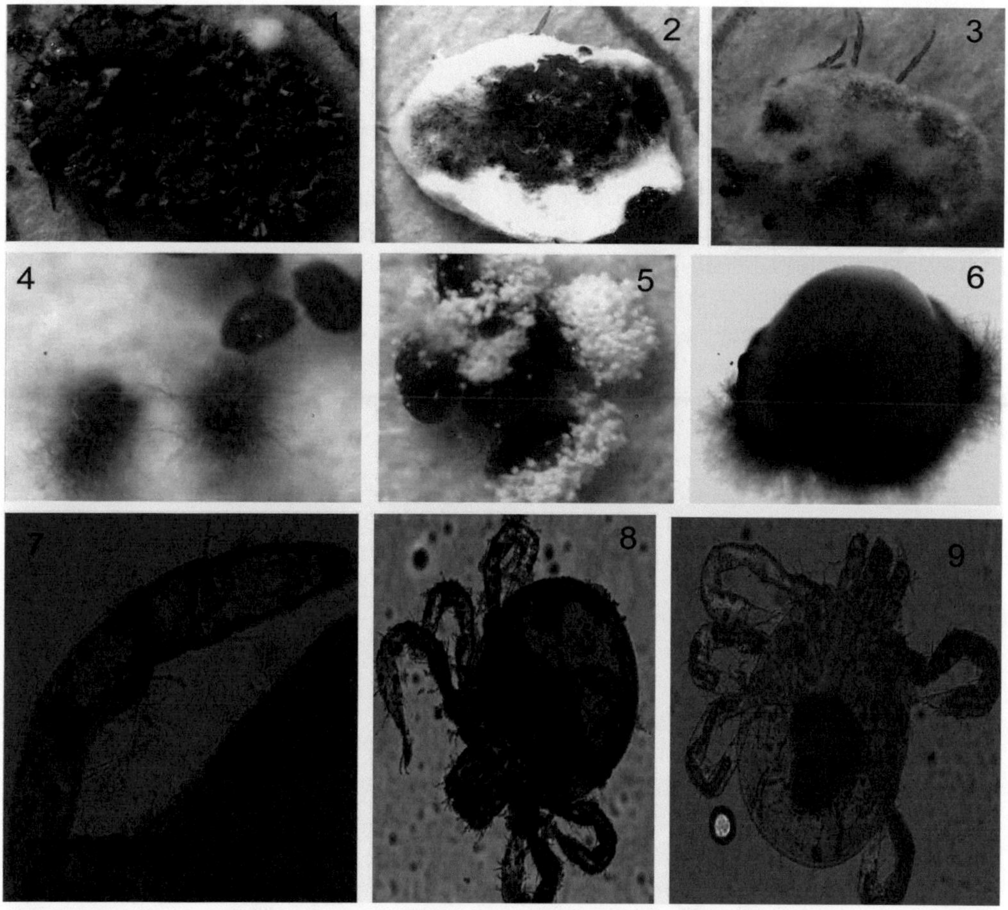

Fig. 1. Effect of fungal strains on engorged females (Figs. 1-1, 1-2 and 1-3), eggs (1-4, 1-5 and 1-6) and larvae (1-7, 1-8 and 1-9) of *Rhipicephalus annulatus. M. anisoplae* in Figs. 1-1, 1-4 and 1-7, *B. bassiana* in Figs. 1-2,1-5 and 1-8 and *L. psalliotae* in Figs. 1-3, 1-6 and 1-9.

A few entomopathogenic fungi have been tested against mosquitoes led to obtaining different results. However, only small-scale experiments have been carried out. The protective effect of two isolates of an entomopathogenic fungus, *Metarhizium anisopliae*

(DEMI 002 and Iran 437 C) on bee (*Apis mellifera*) colonies from the adult stage of *Varroa destructor* was evaluated in comparison with fluvalinate strips in the field by Pirali-Kheirabadi et al. (Unpublished data) and demonstrated that Isolate DEMI 002 can be considered as a possible non-chemical biocontrol agent for controlling bee infestation with *V. destructor* in the field.

2.1.2 Nematopathogenic fungi

Nematopathogenic fungi commonly called nematode-destroying fungi are a widespread ecological group of more than 150 species of microfungi which are able to invade nematodes. They maybe divided in to three groups. Most species are found within the group of nematode trapping fungi. Species of this group produce nematode-trapping organs such as constricting (active) or non constricting (passive) rings, sticky hyphae, sticky knobs (as shown in Fig. 2 for *Arthrobotrys candida*), sticky branches or sticky networks (as shown in Fig. 3 for *A. oligospora*), at intervals along the length of a widely distributed vegetative hyphal system. The anchoring of the nematode to the traps is followed by hyphal penetration of the nematode cuticle. Inside the nematode host, trophic hyphae grow out and fill the body of the nematode and digest it. Another group, the endoparasitic fungi, infects nematodes by spores. Inside the host, they develop an infectious thallus which absorbs the body contents. Endoparasitic fungi have no extensive hyphal development outside the body of the host except fertile hyphae such as evacuation tubes or conidiophores that release the spores. A third group may be defined as fungal parasites of cyst and root-knot nematodes. They invade eggs or females by in growth of vegetative hyphae the last two groups should be called endopathogenic fungi and fungal pathogens of cyst and roar-knot nematodes, respectively.

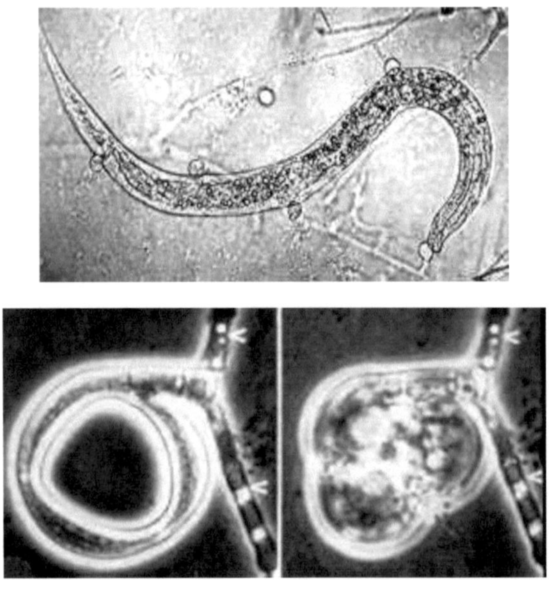

Fig. 2. Sticky knobs of *Arthrobotrys candida* and trapping fungi before and after constriction (Baron 1977).

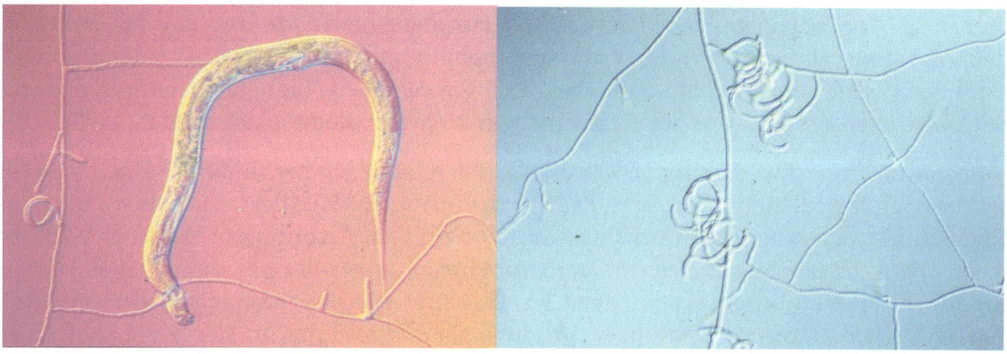

Fig. 3. Sticky ring and branches of *Arthrobotrys oligospora* (Jaffee 1990).

In a survey, the effect of temperature, incubation time and in vivo gut passage on survival and nematophagous activity *Arthrobotrys oligospora* var. *oligospora* and *A. cladodes* var. *macroides* was studied in order to show the potential of these fungi in management of parasitic nematodes infections of ruminants in field condition (Ranjbar Bahadori et al., 2010).

2.2 Nematodes and earthworms

Numerous nematodes are either obligate or facultative parasites of insects. To date, hundreds of antagonistic organisms of nematodes have been described which are found within the group of viruses, bacteria, fungi, amoeba, earthworms, tardigrades, copepods, dang beetles and mites. Infection may take place by penetration of the cuticle, invasion through spiracles or anus or after ingestion by the host insect. Promising entomoparasitic nematodes are members of the genera Steinernema (Neoaplectana) and Heterorhabditis. Apparently, it is not the nematodes themselves, but the symbiotic bacteria they carry which are released in to the insect body that cause septicaemia and death. Mermitid nematodes can infected some ticks. For example among *Ixodes ricinus* ticks collected in denemark, 6% were infected. The length of juvenile nematodes was up to 20 mm and their exact taxonomic status is not known (Lipa, et al., 1997). Their fetal effect on their hosts is primarily due to a large hole left in the cuticle when they exist the host. With the success of mass cultivation, entomopathognic nematodes like Heterorhabditidae and Steinernematidae have been used commercially against various insects during the last decades. (Martin., 1997). Because their infective juveniles live in the upper layer of the soil, they are used mostly against insects living in this layes, e.g. ground-inhabiting stages of fleas. (Henderson et al., 1995). Engorged females of numerous other ticks species were killed by these nematodes. (El-Sadawy., 1994; Kocan., et al., 1998; Mauleon et al., 1993., Samish et al., 1996; Zhioua et al., 1995). The 50% lethal concentration values obtained with engorged *Boophilus annulatus* are similar to those achieved with nematode preparations against insect. *Steinernema* strain is active at 20-30 °C, but less infective at 15 °C, whereas a sub population of the some strain was efficient between 15-30 °C (Samish and Glazer., 1992, Zhioua et al., 1995). Soil-filled buckets with more silt, more manure or less moisture reduced the virulence of the nematodes (Samish et al., 1998). Nematodes may become a successful tool against ticks because many ticks drop off the host are highly susceptible to nematodes and most engorged ticks hide for days in dark and humid upper layers of the soil. Finally, nematodes could be readily applied either by irrigation or by spraying from the ground or air at low cost and they remain infective in humid soil for long periods. (Martin., 1997) However nematode use may be limited to defined ecological niches because of the susceptibility of nematodes to low humidity, high manure or high silt concentration, the need for relatively high temperatures and the difference in susceptibility of tick stages and species to nematodes (Samish et al., 1998).

Nematodes from the families Heterorhabditidae and Steinernamatidae are used in commercial formulations but non field experiments to kill ticks and their value as commercial biocontrol against ticks has yet to be proven. According to Williams 1985, the entomoparasitic nematode, *Steinernema (Neoaplectana) carpocapsae* has shown some success against mosquitoes on an experimental level. A host specific entomoparasitic nematode, *Heterotylenchus autumnalis* parasitizes *Musca autumnalis* resulting in sterile female flies as nematode development occurs at the expense of egg production. Groups of predatory nematodes such as mononchids, dorylaimids, aphelenchids and diplogastrids are able to kill other nematodes by teeth, spears or stylets in their bucal cavity. The aphelenchids use a toxin to paralyze the prey during the battle. Their biology is unknown and it is open question if they may be of practical use in biocontrol in field conditions. Earthworm populations consume large volumes of soil and organic matter such as animal faeces. During feeding, they consume nematodes present in soil and faeces. The indirect beneficial effects of earthworms on the development of the free living stages by aerating deeper layers of the pats may be counterbalanced or even obliterated by more direct effects i.e. when earthworms start eating the dung. Dung beetles may significantly reduce infective larvae of gastrointestinal trichostrongyle nematodes when they erode cow pats, bury fresh dung in the soil and partially dispersevthe reminder. It must be concluded that in different parts of the world earthworms are responsible for natural biological control of trichostrongyle nematodes. Because of the beneficial effects of earthworms, it is important to protect these organisms in the areas where they live.

2.3 Bacteria

Strains of the entomopathogenic bacterium *Bacillus thuringiensis* are among the most widely used antagonists in biological control of insects. After ingestion, target insects are killed by a gut toxin which is released from crystal proteins in the bacterial spores. The first symptom is cessation of feeding, follow by a rapid breakdown of the gut epithelium. Because of the insect-killing abilities of *B. thuringiensis* depend to a large extent based on a toxin; the use of this bacterium is probably comparable in many ways to using pure toxin chemical compounds. Another bacterium, *Streptomyces avermitilis*, produces toxins collectively called "avermectins" which are highly effective against several invertebrates from the classes Insecta, Arachnida and Nematodes. Important anti-parasitic drugs, e.g. Ivermectin are produced by chemical modifications of the avermectins. Although according to our definition from biocontrol, use of avermectins is not in this category. In some countries, *B. thuringiensis* var. *israelensis* is available for control of mosquito larvae (Ravensberg 1994). The black fly *Simulium damnosum* which is an important vector of *Onchocerca volvulus*, causative agent of river blindness, is susceptible to *B. thuringiensis* var. *israelensis*. *Pasteuria (Bacillus) penetrans* is a well known nematopathogenic bacterium of plant parasitic root-knot nematodes. Bacteria spores adhere by adhesive microfibers to the cuticle of juvenile nematodes. As a consequence, the spores germinate and penetrate cuticle, filamentous microcolonies created inside the host body will destroy the reproductive capacity of the infected female host. Eventually, thousands of endospores release to the soel from the dead decomposing nematodes. Based on present knowledge, it is doubtful if *P. penetrance* can be applied in biocontrol of nematodes of veterinary importance.

2.4 Rickettsiae

Most known species of rickettsiae family are parasites of warm-blooded animals, but some of them also parasitize arthropods (Hsiao and Hsiao., 1985). For example, ticks become adapted as vectors, reservoirs and/or propagation sites of rickettsiae (Raoult and Roux., 1997) and often harbor generalized asymptomatic infections. Reckettsial infection may lead to alterations in tick behavior, interfere with their development and cause pathological changes in salivary glands and in ovarian tissues. In sever cases, depending on the degree of infection and the rapidity of generalized infection and other circumstances, this infection may lead to death (Sidorov., 1979).

Rickettsiae like organisms are obligatory intracellular organisms confined in most cases to the malpighian tubes and ovaries of the host (Nodaet et al., 1997). Some parasites ingest bacteria with the blood of their hosts or become contaminated for their skin. High humidity and temperature increase bacterial contamination of the many pathogenic bacteria against insects. Some are also pathogenic to useful insects, men and domestic animals, but they do not usually share the same ecological niches.

2.5 Protozoa

Entomopathogenic protozoans have received little consideration as antagonists in biological control of insects. One problem is that most protozoans have a narrow host range combined with a low virulence, so it must be expected that they cannot be used alone. Some protozoa such as *Haemogregarina, Nosema, Babesia* and *Theileria* are pathogenic for some parasites like "ticks". Successful insect biocontrol pathogens have not been tested against insect and ticks. Biological control of ticks with *Babesia* or *Theileria* is not promising because of their pathogenic effects to vertebrates. Although there are no examples of effective direct biological control of protozoans in veterinary science, however indirectly, some protozoans, e.g. *Plasmodium* spp., may be controlled by their intermediate hosts or vectors. The predatory soil amoeba *Theratromyxa weberi* is capable of ingesting nematodes. It flows over the nematode body and assimilates it within 24h. This and other amoeba can be expected to have limited biocontrol capacities because they are slow-moving compared with nematodes. Also they are sensitive to low soil water potentials, conditions under which nematodes may thrive. One genus of ciliated turbellarians flatworms, *Adenoplea,* prey exclusively on living nematodes and it is unknown if they may be of potential use in biological control of parasites of domestic animals.

2.6 Virus and virus-like particles

More than thousands of entomopathogenic viruses active against insect have been described but still only very few are commercially available. Viruses either do not play an important role in reducing parasites populations or else our knowledge is too limited to determine their effects.

3. Predators and their potential in biological control

Predators can be vertebrates or invertebrates, some of which are arachnids, but deployment of insects is most common. The efficiency of predators in controlling populations of some parasites in different habitats varies and may reach up to 100% (Wilkinson., 1970 a,b). For example, predation is lower in tall grass areas than in short grass areas (Mwangi et al., 1991). Likewise, predation was two to eight times higher in open areas than in a ticked pasture area and none in intensive pasture or agricultural areas (Krivolutsky., 1963).

3.1 Arthropods

Occasionally, female arthropods are eaten by males. As an example, cannibalism of engorged females by males is reported mainly for argasid ticks (Oliver et al., 1986). In ticks all unfed stages may parasitize engorged nymphs or females. Cannibalism is often found during overcrowding on a host, in laboratory colonies when there is a lack of host animals. In ticks this behavior leaves typical scars in the integument. Biological control of insects may include predators (e.g. spider) parasites, parasitoids, (insect parasites of insects) or pathogens like viruses, bacteria, fungi, protozoans, and nematodes. Spiders have defined habitats. A change in the habitat, such as mulching may increase the spider population by as much as 60%. (Jackson and Pollard., 1996; Riechert and Bishop., 1990). Nine genera of spiders from six families were reported to pray on five hard tick and two soft ticks' genera. (Carroll., 1995; Krivolutsky., 1963; Mwangi et al., 1991; Spielman., 1988; Verissimo., 1995 and Wilkinson., 1970). Genus *Teutana triangulosa* spiders prefer *Rhipiocephalus sanguinus* to flies.

3.1.1 Mites

Some mites are nematode predators and the role as nematodes predators played by some micro- arthropods like mites has yet to be defined. Some mites are capable of consuming *Ascaris* eggs.

3.1.2 Flies (Diptera)

A breakthrough in the indoor control of the house fly has been the use of the predatory fly *Hydrotaea (Ophyra) aenescens*. In several countries of northern Europe *H. aenescens* is commercially available for biological control of *Musca domestica*. The predatory fly was introduced from America to Europe in this century. Wild predatory flies were observed in Denmark for the first time in 1972 and a commercial product was released to the market 20 years later. In 1994, *H. aenescens* was used for biological control in 5-6% of Danish pig farms.

3.1.3 Ants: (Hymenoptera) and beetles

Around 27 species of ants from 16 genera mainly *Aphaenogaster*, *Iridomyrmex*, *Monomorium*, *Pheidol* and *Solenopsis* are known to be tick predators. Ants are known to pray on most tick genera. Application of S. *invicta* in the United States markedly reduced the number of anaplasmosis in seropositive cattle in Louisiana (Jemal and Hugh-Jones., 1993). The predation in open areas was two to eight times higher than in woody ones. (Mwangi et al., 1991) Wild rabbits living in *Formica polyctena* infested plots had far fewer ticks than those in ant-free plots and rabbits sprayed with formic acid were free of ticks for at least 5 days (Buttner., 1987).

Beetles (Coleoptera) pasture livestock flies breed primarily in cow pats. There have been many attempts to control these flies biologically by means of natural enemies and scavengers which consume and bury the dung. In this connection, dung beetles of the family Scarabaeidae (Scarabaeinae, Geotrupinae, and Aphodiinae) are relevant. Dung beetles such as *Onthophagus gazelle* and *Euoniticellus intermedius*, introduced from Africa to Australia are regarded as useful in biological control of *Musca vetustissima* and the buffalo fly *Haematobia exigua* pest flies. The African dung beetles are well adapted to cattle faeces and compete with fly larvae for food. The rapid burial of dung by the beetles reduces the breeding habitats for the flies. Dang beetles can play a role in natural biological control of bovine gastrointestinal nematodes (Trichostrongylidae).

Cattle infected with gastrointestinal trichostrongyle nematodes excrete parasite eggs in their faeces. After hatching, free living larvae develop in the cow pat to the infective stage which is spread to the surrounding herbage. In many tropical and subtropical areas, dung beetles of the family Scarabaeidae are the most important organisms responsible for the disappearance of fresh cow pats. They produce tunnels and break up the pats, thereby enhancing the drying-up of the dung. The result may be an increased mortality among the free living stage of trichostrongyle parasites, especially during dry spells. In this way at least some animals attracted to cattle dung may indirectly be involved in natural biological control of trichostrongylosis of cattle.

3.2 Amphibians and fishes

The water-tortoise *Pelomedusa subrufa* was reported to able to remove ticks from black rhinos in a streambed (Mwangi et al., 1991). Also in some areas the mosquito larvae may be controlled biologically by predatory fish such as *Gambusia affinis* and the *Guppy poecilia*. Snails are prey by fishes as well.

3.3 Reptilians

Some lizards can eat arthropods. The lizard stomachs may contain 2.4-15 ticks/stomach. However because there are few lizards near the bird nest, their effect on the tick population is limited. Insecticides suppress arthropods that prey on ticks. Thus using less insecticide that is more specific to the target and minimizing the area of its distribution to tick infested areas, would contribute to the preservation of these predators.

3.4 Avian and domestic fowl

Bird is generally thought to be the main predators of insects. This impression is based mainly on sporadic observations. Bird species pick the ticks off the host during flight or collected them from the ground. One of potential for biocontrol of trematodes is control of their intermediate hosts (snail). Domestic fowls and birds are predators of snails, although potential candidates for biological control of snails may be found among predators, parasites such as leeches, egg pathogenic fungi, and pathogenic bacteria.

The value of birds as suppressors of ticks' populations in nature is difficult to evaluate. It appears that the motionless insects are an easy and they prey too many birds, which thus help to reduce the insect populations. Scrub jays were observed to spend 89% of their time searching deer for ectoparasites (Isenhart and DeSante., 1985). In Africa, chickens are natural predators of ticks and actually pick ticks from the bodies of cattle as well as from the vegetation. Preliminary experiment has indicated that chickens may become viable biological control factors for tick control in Africa.

3.5 Rodents and mammals

Some mammals are insectivorous. As an example, *Sorex araneus* prey on ticks and at times preferred them to alternative foods. (Mwangi et al., 1991; Short and Norval., 1982). Shrews seem to locate hidden ticks by their smell. Mice and rats are often cited as preying on ticks. Also natural biological control of cestodes by destruction of cestode eggs when they are ingested by various animals may occur in nature. In this way vertebrates that are not suitable hosts may destroy cestode eggs, it is also possible that invertebrates like ants, earthworms and beetles may destroy eggs or take them down into the soil, like wise no practical or successful cases of biocontrol of cestodes are known.

4. Concluding remarks and future prospective

Few promising examples of biological control of insects and parasitic nematodes are found in veterinary science. This lack of success has left the industry skeptical and only few companies have been interested in developing biological control products. The lack of success may arise from lack of enough knowledge about complex natural biological systems and the antagonists which may be found in nature. So, research is essential for developing primary antagonists for biological control programs. However, the large number of potential antagonists that occur in nature presents a formidable interdisciplinary challenge to the scientists working on biological control. Moreover, they have to shown, in small-scale experimental models, that the selected antagonists are effective in biological control. It is estimated that to date only 15% of existing natural enemies of insects have been discovered. Yet for some insect species, over 100 enemies are known (De Bach and Rosen., 1991) In each case, they should be able to select one or more natural antagonists virulent to the different important pest organisms. Even less information exists about tick enemies than that of insect enemies. However to bring biological control candidates from experimental to commercial success, scientists obviously need practical supports from industry. We hope it will encourage scientists and policy makers to turn this neglected important field into an active branch of research and develop it as a component of integrated insect management. As yet only a few experimental data exist on the impact of parasite enemies under field condition, such studies are essential for the development of an effective biocontrol program. So it is necessary that industry be willing to develop technology and breeding media for large-scale industrial production of antagonists and mass production of the antagonists should be reasonably cheap. As antagonists often are used in huge amounts in biocontrol, it must be expected that selection for antagonists with high performance in production system is needed. The effect and the price of the biological control products should be similar to that of existing drugs. The handling and application of biological control products should fit in with standard farm practice. Finally, as an alternative to chemical control, the final product should be safe to users and consumers, to treated animals and to the environment.

5. Acknowledgment

I would like to appreciate Professor Mehdi Razzaghi-Abyaneh, Head of Mycology Department, Pasteur Institute of Iran for the critical reading, valuable advises, and useful comments and corrections throughout the chapter.

6. References

Barron G.L, 1977. The nematode-destroying fungi. Canadian Biological Publications, Guelph, Ont., 140 pp.

Berbee M. Land Taylor, J.W. 1999. Fungal phylogeny in molecular fungal biology (Oliver,R.&Schweizer,M., Eds), Cambridge University Press, Cambridge,UK,pp.21-77

Buttner K. 1987. Studies on the effects of forest ants on tick infestation of mammals, especially rabbits. *Waldhygiene* 17:3–14.

Cole MM. 1965. Biological control of ticks by the use of hymenopterous parasites-a review. World Health Organ. Publ. WHO/ebl /43 65:1–12.

Connole MD. 1969. Effect of fungal extracts on the cattle tick, *Boophilus microplus. Aust. Vet. J.* 45:207.

Carroll JF. 1995. Laboratory evaluation of predatory capabilities of a common wolf spider (Araneae: Lycosidae) against two species of ticks (Acari: Ixodidae). *Proc. Entomol. Soc.* 97:746–49.

Campbell W.C. and Benz G.W. 1984. Ivermectine : A review of efficacy and safety. *J. Vet. Pharmacol Therap.* 7:1-16.

Chandler D., Davidson G., Pell J.K., Ball B.V., Shaw K and Sunderland KD. 2000. Fungal biocontrol of acari. *Biocont. Sci. Tech.* 10, 357- 384.

DeBach P. and Rosen D. 1991. Biological Control by Natural Enemies. New York: Cambridge Univ. Press. 440 pp.

Eslami A., Ranjbar-Bahadori Sh., Zare R. and Razzaghi-Abyaneh M. 2005. The predatory capability of *Arthrobotrys cladodes* var. *macroides* in the control of *Haemonchus contortus* infective larvae. *Vet. Parasitol.* 130:263-266.

Gronvold G, Henriksen S.A, Larsen M, Nansen P. and Wolstrup J. 1996. Biological control aspects of biological control with special reference to arthropods, protozoans and helminthes of domesticated animals. *Vet. Parasitol.* 64:47-64.

Hall RA. and Papierok B. 1982. Fungi as biological control agents of arthropods of agricultural and medical importance. *Parasitology* 84:205-240.

Hassan SM, Dipeolu O.O, Amoo A.O and Odhiambo T.R. 1991. Predation on livestock by chickens. *Vet. Parasitol.* 38: 199-204.

Hsiao C. and Hsiao TH. 1985. Rickettsia as the cause of cytoplasmic incompatibility in the alfalfa weevil, Hypera postica. *J. Invertbr. Pathol.* 45:244-246

Henderson G, Manweiler SA, Lawrence WJ, Templeman RJ. and Foil LD. 1995. The effects of *Steinernema carpocapsae* (Weiser) application to different life stages on adult emergence of the cat flea *Ctenocephalides felis* (Bouche). *Vet. Dermatol.* 6:159-163.

Henry J. E, 1981. Natural and applied control of Insects by protozoa. *Annu. Rev. Entomol.* 26: 49-73.

Hom A, 1994. Current status of entomopathogenic nematodes. *IPM Practitioner*, 16: 1-12.

Isenhart FR. and DeSante DF. 1985. Observations of scrub jays cleaning ectoparasites from black-tailed deer. *Condor* 87:145-147.

Jackson RR, Pollard SD. 1996. Predatory behavior of jumping spiders. *Annu. Rev. Entomol.* 41:287–308

Jemal A and Hugh-Jones M. 1993. A review of the red imported fire ant (*Solenopsis invicta* Buren) and its impacts on plant, animal, and human health. *Prev. Vet. Med.* 17:19–32.

Kaaya GP, Mwangi EN and Ouna EA. 1996. Prospects for biological control of livestock ticks, *Rhipicephalus appendiculatus and Amblyomma variegatum,* using the entomogenous fungi *Beauveria bassiana* and *Metarhizium anisopliae. J. Invertebr. Pathol.* 67:15–20.

Kocan KM, Pidherney MS, Blouin EF, Claypool PL, Samish M, et al. 1998. Interaction of entomopathogenic nematodes (Steinernematidae) with selected species of ixodid ticks (Acari: Ixodidae). *J. Med. Entomol.* 35:514-520.

Krivolutsky DA. 1963. Eradication of larvae and nymphs of the tick *Ixodes persulcatus* by predators. *Proc. Conf. Ticks Encephalitis Hemoragic Fever Viruses, Omsk, Dec.* pp. 187-188.

Lacey L.A, Frutos R, Kaya H.K and Vail P. 2001. Insect patliogem, as biological control agents: do they have a future? *Biological Control* 21: 210-248.

Lipa JJ, Eilenberg J, Bresciani J and Frandsen F. 1997. Some observations on a newly recorded mermitid parasite of *Ixodes ricinus* L. (Acarina: Ixodidae). *Acta Parasitol.* 42:109-114.

Luthy p, 1986. Insect pathogenic bacteria as pest control agents. *Fortschr. Zool.* 32: 201-216.

McCoy C.W., Samson R.A and Boucias D.G. 1988. Entomogenous fungi, in CRC Handbook of natural pesticides , volume V(Microbial insecticides,part A; Entomogenous protozoa and fungi_) (Ignoffo,C.M., Ed.), CRCPress , Florida, USA,pp.151-236.

Martin WRJ. 1997. Using entomopathogenic nematodes to control insects during stand establishment. *Hortic. Sci.* 32:196–200

Mwangi EN, Newson RM and Kaaya GP. 1991. Predation of free-living engorged female *Rhipicephalus appendiculatus. Exp. Appl. Acarol.* 12:153–162.

Mwangi EN, Dipeolu OO, Newson RM, Kaaya GP and Hassan SM. 1991. Predators, parasitoids and pathogens of ticks: a review. *Biocont. Sci. Tech.* 1:147-156.

Mwangi EN, Newson RM, Kaaya GP. 1991. Predation of free-living engorged female Rhipicephalus appendiculatus. *Exp. Appl. Acarol.* 12:153–162.

Noda H, Munderloh UG and Kurtti TJ. 1997. Endosymbionts of ticks and their relationship to *Wolbachia* spp. and tickborne pathogens of humans and animals. *Appl. Environ. Microbiol.* 63:3926–3932.

Oliver JHJ, McKeever S and Pound JM. 1986. Parasitism of larval Ixodid ticks by chigger mites and fed female *Ornithodoros* ticks by *Ornithodoros* males. *J. Parasitol.* 72:811–812.

Pirali-kheirabadi, K.H, Haddadzadeh, H.R., Razzaghi-Abyaneh, M., Zare, R., Ranjbar-Bahadori, SH., Rahbari, S., Nabian, S and Rezaeian, M. 2007. Priliminary study on virulence of some isolates of of entomopathogenic fungi in different developmental stage of *Boophilus annulatus* in Iran: *Iranian J. Vet. Res.* 62: 113-118.

Pirali-kheirabadi, K.H., Haddadzadeh, H.R., Razzaghi-Abyaneh, M. Bokaie, S., Zare, R., Quazavi, M., Shams-Ghahfarokhi, M. 2007. Biological control of Rhipicephalus (Boophilus) annulatus by different strains of *Metarhizium anisopliae* , *Beauveria bassiana* and *Lecanicillium psalliotae* fungi. *Parasitol. Res.* 100: 1297-1302.

Pirali-kheirabadi K.H, Teixeira da Silva J. A, Razzaghi-Abyaneh, M. Nazemnia M 2011. A Field Experiment to Assess the Pathogenicity of *Metarhizium anisopliae* to *Varroa destructor* (Acari: Mesostigmata) (Un published data).

Poinar G.O. 1986. Entomophagus nematodes. *Fortschr. Zool.* 32:95-121.

Ranjbar Bahadori SH, Razzaghi Abyaneh M, Bayat M, Eslami A, Pirali-Kheirabadi Kh, Shams - Ghahfarokhi M and Lotfollahzadeh S. 2010. Studies on the effect of temperature, incubation time and in vivo gut passage on survival and nematophagous activity *Arthrobotrys oligospora* var. *oligospora* and *A. cladodes* var. *macroides* .*Global Veterinaria* 4: 112-117.

Raoult D and Roux V. 1997. Rickettsioses as paradigms of newer emerging infectious diseases. *Clin. Microbiol. Rev.* 10:694-719.

Riechert SE, Bishop L. 1990. *Prey control by an assemblage of generalist predators: spiders in garden test systems. Ecology* 71:1441-1450.

Sayre R.M and Wergin W.P, 1979. The use of SEM to classify and evaluate the parasites and predators of pest nematodes. *Scan Electron Micros.* 3:89-96.

Sutherst RW, Wharton RH, UtechKBW. 1978. Guide to studies on the tick ecology. Div. Entomol. Tech. Pap. No. 14, Commonw. Sci. Ind. Res. Org., Aust., pp. 1–59

Sidorov VE. 1979. Some features of *Coxiella burnetii* interaction with argasid ticks (experimental morphological study). In *Razvitie Parazitologicheskoi Nauki v Turkmenistane*, ed. IM Grochovskaia, MA Melejaeva, pp. 112-128. Ashchabad: Yilim.

Samish M, Glazer I and Alekseev EA. 1996. The susceptibility of the development stages of ticks (Ixodidae) to entomopathogenic nematodes. Anonymous pp. 121-123. Columbus, Ohio: Ohio Biological Survey

Samish M and Glazer I. 1992. Infectivity of entomopathogenic nematodes (Steinernematidae and Heterorhabditidae) to female ticks of *Boophilus annulatus* (Arachnida: Ixodidae). *J. Med. Entomol.* 29:614–618.

Samish M, Alekseev EA and Glazer I. 1998. The effect of soil composition on antitick activity of entomopathogenic nematodes. *Ann. NY Acad. Sci.* 849:398–399.

Short NJ and Norval RAI. 1982. Tick predation by shrews in Zimbabwe. *J. Parasitol.* 68:1052.

Spielman A. 1988. Prospects for suppressing transmission of Lyme disease. *Ann. NY Acad. Sci.* 539: 212-220.

Sayre R.M., 1986. Pathogens for biological control of nematodes. *Crop. Prot.* 5: 268-279.

Tanada , Y. and kaaya ,H.K.(1993)Insect patology , Academic Press , San Diego ,USA, 666 PP.

Verissimo CJ. 1995. Natural enemies of the cattle tick. *Agropecu. Catarin.* 8: 35-37.

Wilkinson PR. 1970. A preliminary note on predation on free-living engorged female rocky mountainwood ticks. *J. Med. Entomol.* 7:493–496.

Wilkinson PR. 1970. Factors affecting the distribution and abundance of the cattle tick in Australia: observations and hypotheses. *Acarologia* 12: 492–507.

Zhioua E, Lebrun RA, Ginsberg HS, Aeschlimann A. 1995. Pathogenicity of *Steinernema carpocapsae* and *S. glaseri* (Nematoda: Steinernematidae) to *Ixodes scapularis* (Acari: Ixodidae). *J. Med. Entomol.* 32: 900–905.

4

Genotyping of *Giardia Intestinalis* Isolates from Dogs by Analysis of *gdh*, *tpi*, and *bg* Genes

Enedina Jiménez-Cardoso, Leticia Eligio-García,
Adrian Cortés-Campos and Apolinar Cano-Estrada
Laboratorio de Investigación en Parasitología
Hospital Infantil de México Federico Gómez, México, D.F.
Mexico

1. Introduction

Giardia intestinalis, a flagellated protozoan parasite, is the most prevalent human intestinal protozoan worldwide (Adam, 2001). About 200 million people in the world are infected with giardiasis and each individual eliminates up to 900 million cysts per day (Minivielle , 2008). Higher prevalence is found in tropical and subtropical areas, where *Giardia* affects up to 30% of the population. In epidemiological studies carried out in Mexico and other sudamerican countries, prevalence between of 10-16% has been found in urban areas and 34% in shantytowns (Gamboa "et al", 2003; Giraldo-Gomez, 2005; Sulaiman, 2004). *G. intestinalis* is a cosmopolitan pathogen with a very wide host range, including humans, domestic animals, and wild animal species (Caccio, 2008; Thompson, et al 1993). The most common cause of infection with *Giardia* is the consumption of contaminated food or water (Ortega, 1997), although zoonotic transmission is also possible. Once a person is infected, the parasite lives in the intestines and is passed in the stool of the infected person. Animals such as cats, dogs and cattle can also be infected and spread the disease to humans.

Infections may be asymptomatic or include symptoms of chronic diarrhea, weight loss, and malabsorption. When children infected with *Giardia* have no symptoms of giardiasis, the parasite is present in their feces and they can pass the infection to others. Other symptoms of chronic giardiasis include: Loose, soft, greasy stools, discomfort in the abdomen, general feeling of discomfort or illness, weakness and fatigue.

The parasite has two interchangeable forms that guarantee a simple and efficient life cycle. The cyst that contaminate the environment and the trophozoite, which attach to the intestinal villi via a specialized microtubule structure, the ventral disc.

There are at least seven major genotypes referred to as assemblages (A-G) including 2 (A and B) known to infect humans (Mcpherson, 2005; Monis, 2009).

Assemblages A and B, of clinical significance to humans, differ from each other by as much as 20% at the DNA sequence level (Caccio, 2008). There is also evidence that genetic exchange has resulted in hybrids, or mixed types, based on assemblage-specific PCR of Giardia isolates from cases of human infection (Monis, 1999).

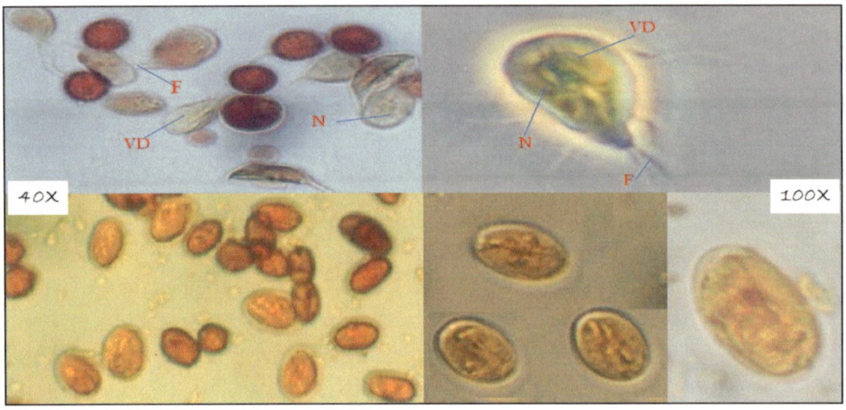

Fig. 1. Trophozoite (top) and Cyst (bottom) of *Giardia intestinalis* lugol´s stained. Ventral disc (VD), Flagella (F) and Nuclei (N). Olympus Bh2 microscopy. Laboratorio de Investigacion en Parasitologia. Hospital Infantil de Mexico.

Clinically, *G. intestinalis* assemblage A appears to be less prevalent than assemblage B and other mixed types worldwide (Tungtrongchitr, 2010; Singh A, 2009). However, infections with assemblage A appear to be more symptomatic. Although assemblages A and B are the only ones that infect humans, they also can infect other mammals (Volotao, et al. 2007). Interestingly, assemblage A is more frequently associated with animal hosts that may serve as reservoirs of infection for humans (Ballweber, 2010).

Although *Giardia* isolated from dogs typically belong to assemblages C or D, assemblages A and B have been identified in dogs in regions of high endemicity (Cooper, 2010). Genotypes E, F, and G have been isolated from pigs and other farm mammals (Jerlström-Hultqvist J, 2010), cats (Ballweber, 2010), and rodents (Monis, 1999), respectively.

The ability to genetically characterize *Giardia* strains isolated from clinical and animal samples should contribute to the understanding of the epidemiology and pathogenesis of *Giardia* infection and the relative contributions of distinct genotypes to the severity of clinical infection and zoonotic potential. Here we report our attempts to develop assays for the characterization of *Giardia* genomic DNA extracted from dog stool samples and from *Giardia* trophozoites Portland I, based on the Polymerase Chain Reaction amplification of multiple loci. We targeted the *G. intestinalis tpi*, *gdh*, and *bg* genes that encode the enzyme *triose-phosphate isomerase*, the enzyme *glutamate dehydrogenase*, and *β-giardin*, respectively.

2. Methodology

2.1 Biological samples

The 9 fecal specimens from dogs included gala1, gala2, gala3, croquetilla1, croquetilla2, croquetilla3, mila1, mila2, and mila3. One *Giardia* containing human fecal specimen was named 454LP. The Portland1 strain of *Giardia* served as a control representing the sub-genotype assemblage AI.

2.2 Coproparasitoscopic analysis

Fecal specimens were stained with Lugol's iodine (Faust, 1938) and examined by microscopy to find cysts of *Giardia intestinalis*. Cysts were concentrated from dog feces by repeated washing in distilled water and stored at 4 °C until use.

2.3 DNA extraction

DNA was extracted from the fecal samples by use of the QIAamp DNA Stool Mini Kit (Qiagen Inc., Valencia, CA) according to the manufacturer's instructions. All DNA concentrations were determined by using an Epoch spectrophotometer (Biotek, Winooski, VT).

2.4 PCR amplification

The *gdh* gene encoding *glutamate dehydrogenase*, the *tpi* gene encoding *triose phosphate isomerase*, and the *bg* gene encoding *β-giardin* were each amplified using the Polymerase Chain Reaction (PCR) as follows.

2.5 *gdh* gene amplification

The *gdh* gene was amplified by using 0.8 μM of each primer (578: 5′-GAGAGGATCCTTGARCCNGAGCGCGTNATC-3′ and 579:5′-CCGCGNTTGTADCGNCCNAAGATCTTCCA-3′) in 50 μL reactions containing 10 mM Tris-HCl, 50 mM KCl, 4 mM $MgCl_2$, 0.2 mM each dNTP, 1 U Taq DNA Polymerase and 200 ng of genomic DNA. Samples were subjected to 30 cycles of [94 °C for 30 s, 56 °C for 30 s, and 72 °C for 2 min], with an initial denaturation step at 94 °C for 4 min, and a final extension step at 72 °C for 6 min (Monis, 1996).

2.6 *bg* gene amplification

The *bg* gene was amplified in two steps via nested-PCR. The first round of PCR was conducted in a 25-μL reaction containing 200 pmol each primer (G7: 5′-AAGCCCGACGACCTCACCCGCACTGC-3′ and G759: 5′-GAGGCCGCCCTGGATCTTCGAGACGAC-3′), 10 mM Tris-HCl, 50 mM KCl, 1 mM $MgCl_2$, 0.2 mM each dNTP, 2.5 U Taq DNA Polymerase and 200 ng of genomic DNA. This was amplified for 45 cycles of [95 °C 30 s, 65 °C 30 s and 72 °C 1 min]. The second round of PCR, using the product of the first reaction as template, was performed in a 50-μL reaction with 200 pmol each primer (F: 5′-GAACGAGATCGAGGTCCG-3′; R: 5′-CTCGACGAGCTTCGTT-3′), 10 mM Tris-HCl, 50 mM KCl, 1 mM $MgCl_2$, 0.2 mM dNTPs, 2.5 U of Taq DNA Polymerase and 3 μL of template. Amplification was for 35 cycles of [94°C 30 s, 53°C 30 s and 72°C 1 min] (Lalle, 2005).

2.7 *tpi* gene amplification

The tpi gene was amplified by nested-PCR in which the first round was a duplex reaction to amplify two fragments corresponding to genotypes A and B simultaneously using four primers (TPIAF 5′-CGAGACAAGTGTTGAGATGC-3′, TPIAR 5′-GGTCAAGAGCTTACAACACG-3′ and TPIBF 5′-GTTGCTCCCTCCTTTGTGC-3′, TPIBR

5´-CTCTGCTCATTGGTCTCGC-3´). PCR amplification was performed in a volume of 50-µL with 500 ng of DNA in 1X PCR buffer, 2 mM $MgCl_2$, 0.25 mM of dNTP and 1 U of Taq DNA Polymerase. Amplification was achieved with 25 cycles of [94 °C for 20 s, 50 °C for 30 s and 72 °C for 1 min]. The second round of PCR comprised two separate hemi-nested PCRs to amplify internal fragments of 476 bp and 140 bp corresponding to the A and B genotypes respectively.

To amplify genotype A, primers TPIAIF: 5´-CCAAGAAGGCTAAGCGTGC-3´ and TPIAR were used using 3 µL of the first round amplicon as template in a 50-µL volume reaction. The amplification step used 33 cycles of [94 °C for 20 s, 56 °C for 30 s, and 72 °C for 1 min]. Alternatively, the 140 bp fragment corresponding to genotype B was amplified with primers TPIBIF: 5´-GCACAGAACGTGTATCTGG-3´ and TPIBR. Amplification was performed under the same conditions used for A except that the $MgCl_2$ concentration in the PCR mixture was 1.5 mM. (Amar, 2003. Molina, 2005)

2.8 Restriction analysis

The amplicons generated by PCR were digested with restriction enzymes for the purpose of subtyping. The *tpi* gene amplicons were digested with restriction enzyme *RsaI*, the *bg* gene amplicons were digested with *HaeIII*, and the *gdh* amplicons were digested with *BspHI*. The products of restriction enzyme digestion were separated by 2% agarose gel electrophoresis, using 100bp DNA ladder (Promega, Madison,Wi. USA) as a size standard, and visualized by staining with ethidium bromide.

3. Results

We developed a molecular method to test stool samples for the presence of *G. intestinalis* genotypes that are of clinical significance to human infection possibly by zoonotic transmission from dogs. *Giardia* infection of dog stool samples was confirmed by coproparasitoscópico analysis (data not shown). *Giardia* cysts isolated from feces was genotyped by a combination of multi-locus (*gdh, bg, tpi*) PCR followed by restriction analysis of the PCR amplicons. We analyzed nine samples of dog stool, one sample of human stool, and *G. intestinalis* cysts from the Portland-1 control strain. The Portland-1 standard is a control for the A-I assemblage.

3.1 Figure 2

Illustrates genotyping based on amplification and subsequent *BspHI* enzyme digestion of the *gdh* locus encoding *glutamate dehydrogenase*. All of the dog and human samples tested in this way yielded the same 1200 bp fragment as the Portland-1 control and after digestion they yielded two fragments of 900 and 300 bp respectively indicative of assemblage A.

3.2 Figure 3

Illustrates genotyping based on amplification and *HaeIII* enzyme digestion of the *bg* locus encoding *β-giardin*. Three fragments ranging from 100 to 200 bp are indicative of assemblage A-I. All 9 dog samples and 1 human sample were classified as assemblage A-I, the same as the Portland-1 control.

3.3 Figures 4

Illustrate genotyping based on amplification and *RsaI* enzyme digestion of the *tpi* locus encoding *triose-phosphate isomerase.* Again, all samples yielded products consistent with their identification as belonging to *G. intestinalis* genotype AI.

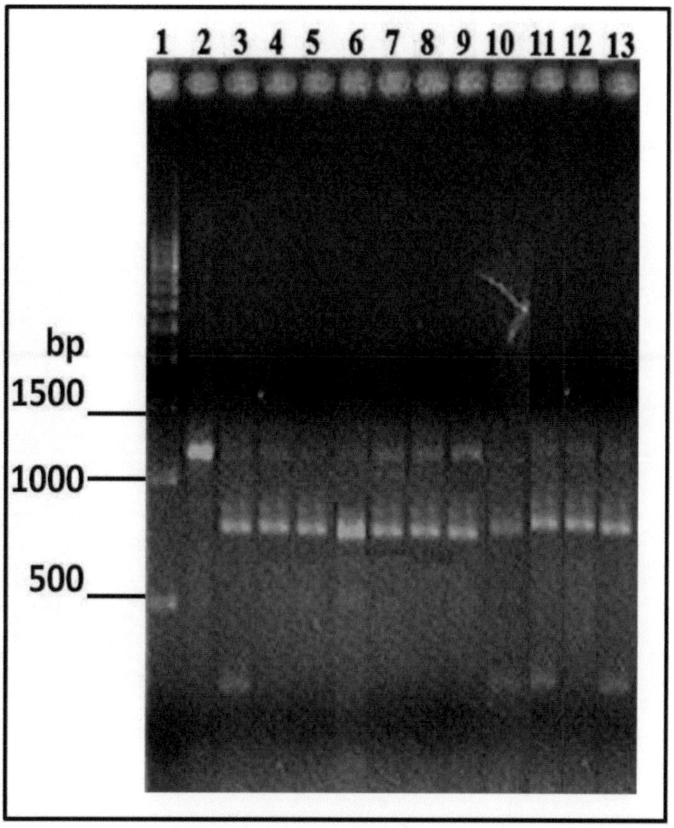

Fig. 2. Genotyping by *gdh*-specific PCR and restricted analyzed by agarose gel electrophoresis. The 900 bp band corresponds to the *BspHI*-digested *gdh*-specific PCR product. 1) Molecular weight marker (500 bp ladder), 2) Portland-1 control without digestion, 3) Portland-1 control restricted, 4) gala1, 5)gala2, 6)gala3, 7)croquetilla1, 8)croquetilla2, 9)croquetilla3, 10)mila1, 11) mila2, 12) mila3, 13) 454 LP.

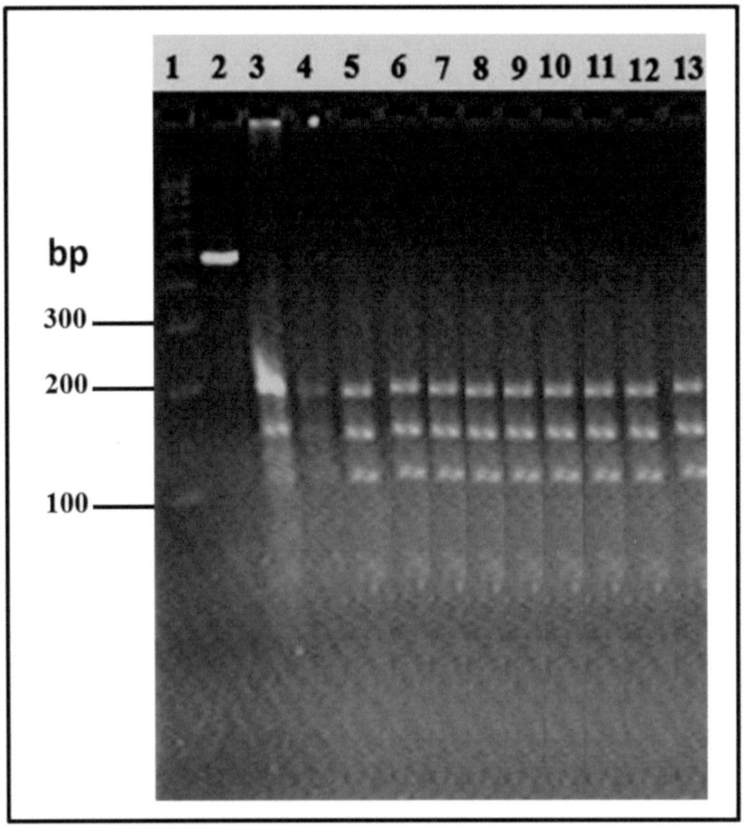

Fig. 3. Genotyping by *bg*-specific PCR and restriction analyzed by agarose gel electrophoresis. The fragments ranging from 100 to 200bp corresponding to the *HaeIII*-digested bg-specific nested-PCR product. 1) Molecular weight marker (500 bp ladder), 2) Portland-1 control without digestion, 3) Portland-1 control restricted, 4) gala1, 5)gala2, 6)gala3, 7)croquetilla1, 8)croquetilla2, 9)croquetilla3, 10)mila1, 11) mila2, 12) mila3, 13)454 LP.

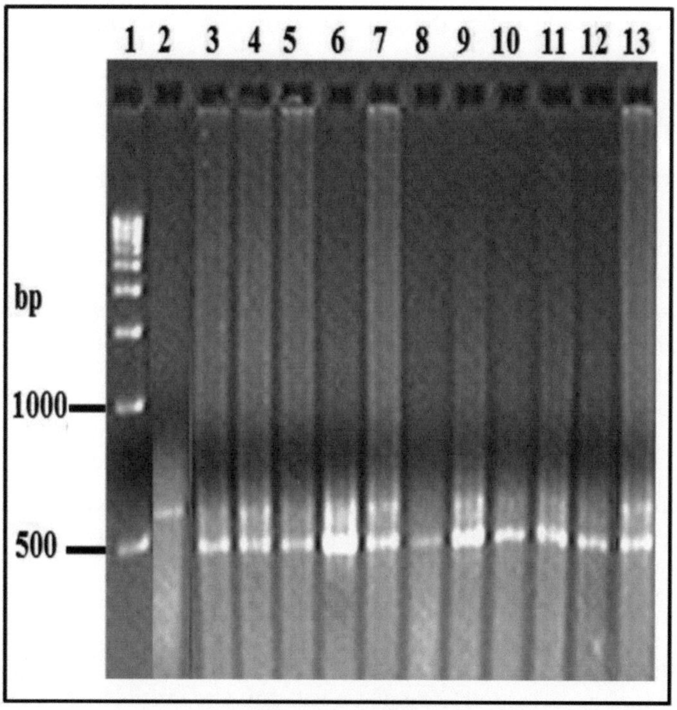

Fig. 4. Genotyping by *tpi*-specific PCR and restriction analyzed by agarose gel electrophoresis. The 437 bp band corresponds to the *RsaI*-digested amplicon representative of assemblage A-I. 1) Molecular weight marker (500 bp ladder), 2) Portland-1 control without digestion, 3) Portland-1 control restricted, 4) gala1, 5)gala2, 6)gala3, 7)croquetilla1, 8)croquetilla2, 9)croquetilla3, 10)mila1, 11) mila2, 12) mila3 13) 454 LP.

4. Discussion

Human giardiasis is caused by two genetically distinct assemblages (A and B) of *G. intestinalis*. A number of molecular assays have been developed for their specific detection in stool and environmental samples (Caccio, 2008).

We have developed a method to detect *Giardia* based on the PCR amplification of three genes (*gdh, bg, tpi*) used in prior genotyping studies.

Although DNA-based methods reported in the literature have been used with success to genotype *Giardia*, we did not have observed differences among the analysis of different genes in studied samples. Some researchers had found frequent mismatches, intra-assemblage discordances and mixed positions, in *tpi* and in *bg* sequences, especially in assemblage B (Bonhomme, 2011).

All of the fecal samples analyzed in this report (9 from dogs, 1 from humans) were determined to belong to the sub-genotype A-I assemblage. This predominance of assemblage A-I probably reflects the mechanism that led to infection of the animals from which the fecal samples came. The dogs might have drunk from water that had been contaminated by livestock rather than by humans. This has important epidemiological ramifications.

5. References

Adam RD. (2001). Biology of *Giardia lamblia. Clinical Microbiology Review.* ; 14 (3), pp.447-75.

Adam RD, Nigam A, Seshadri V, Martens CA, Farneth GA, Morrison HG, Nash TE, Porcella SF, Patel R. (2010). The *Giardia lamblia* vsp gene repertoire: characteristics, genomic organization, and evolution. *BMC Genomics*, 11 (9), pp. 424.

Almeida A, Pozio E, Cacciò SM. (2010). Genotyping of *Giardia duodenalis* cysts by new Real-Time PCR assays for detection of mixed infections in human samples. *Applied and Environmental Microbiology*, 76(6), pp. 1895–1901.

Almeida A, Moreira MJ, Soares S, Delgado ML, Figueiredo J, Silva Magalhães E, Castro A, Da Costa AV, Correia da Costa JM. (2010). Biological and genetic characterization of *Cryptosporidium spp.* and *Giardia duodenalis* isolates from five hydrographical basins in northern Portugal. *Korean Journal of Parasitology*, 48(2) pp. 105–111.

Ballweber LR, Xiao L, Bowman DD, Kahn G, Cama VA. (2010). Giardiasis in dogs and cats: update on epidemiology and public health significance. *Trends in Parasitology*, 26(4), pp. 180-9.

Bonhomme J, Le Goff L, Lemée V, Gargala G, Ballet JJ, Favennec L. (2011). Limitations of tpi and bg genes sub-genotyping for characterization of human *Giardia duodenalis* isolates. *Parasitology International*, 60(3), pp. 327-30.

Cacciò SM, Ryan U. (2008). Molecular epidemiology of giardiasis. *Molecular and Biochemical Parasitology*, 160(2), pp.75-80.

Cooper MA, Sterling CR, Gilman RH, Cama V, Ortega Y, Adam RD. (2010). Molecular analysis of household transmission of *Giardia lamblia* in a region of high endemicity in Peru. *The Journal of Infectious Diseases*, 202(11), pp. 1713-21.

Amar CF, Dear PH, McLauchlin J. (2003). Detection and genotyping by real-time PCR/RFLP analyses of *Giardia duodenalis* from human feces. *Journal of Medical Microbiology*, 52, pp. 681-683.

De Boer RF, Ott A, Kesztyüs B, Kooistra-Smid AMD. (2010). Improved Detection of Five Major Gastrointestinal Pathogens by Use of a Molecular Screening Approach. *Journal of Clinical Microbiology*, 48(11), pp. 4140–4146.

Faust EC, D´antonio JS, Odom V, Miller MJ, Peres C, Sawitz W, Thomen LF, Tobie J, Walker JH . (1938). A critical study of clinical laboratory techniques for the diagnosis of the protozoan cysts and helminthes egg in feces. *The American Journal of Tropical Medicine and Hygiene*, 18, pp. 169-83.

Jerlström-Hultqvist J, Franzén O, Ankarklev J, Xu F, Nohýnková E, Andersson JO, Svärd SG, Andersson B. (2010). Genome analysis and comparative genomics of a *Giardia intestinalis* assemblage E isolate. *BMC Genomics*, 11, pp.543.

Lalle M, Jimenez-Cardosa E, Cacciò SM, Pozio E. (2005). Genotyping of *Giardia duodenalis* from humans and dogs from Mexico using a beta-giardin nested polymerase chain reaction assay. *The Journal of Parasitology*, 91(1), pp. 203-5.

Macpherson CN. (2005). Human behaviour and the epidemiology of parasitic zoonoses. *International Journal of Parasitology*, 35(11-12), pp.1319-31.

Minvielle MC, Molina NB, Polverino D, Basualdo JA. (2008). First genotyping of *Giardia lamblia* from human and animal feces in Argentina, South America. Memorias do Instituto Oswaldo Cruz, 103(1), pp. 98-103.

Molina N, Polverino D, Minvielle M, Basualdo J. (2007). PCR amplification of triosephosphate isomerase gene of *Giardia lamblia* in formalin-fixed feces. *Revista Latinoamericana de Microbiología*, 49(1-2), pp. 6-11.

Monis PT, Mayrhofer G, Andrews RH, Homan WL, Limper L, Ey PL. (1996). Molecular genetic analysis of *Giardia intestinalis* isolates at the glutamate dehydrogenase locus. *Parasitology*, 112 (Pt 1), pp. 1-12.

Monis PT, Andrews RH, Mayrhofer G, Ey PL. (1999). Molecular systematics of the parasitic protozoan *Giardia intestinalis. Molecular Biology and Evolution*, 16(9), pp. 1135-44.

Ortega YR, Adam RD. (1997). Giardia: overview and update. *Clinical of Infectious Diseases*, 25, pp. 545-550.

Plutzer J, Ongerth J, Karanis P. (2010). *Giardia* taxonomy, phylogeny and epidemiology: Facts and open questions. *International Journal of Hygiene and Environmental Health*, 15(5), pp. 321-33.

Singh A, Janaki L, Petri WA Jr, Houpt ER. (2009). *Giardia intestinalis* assemblages A and B infections in Nepal. *The American Journal of Tropical Medicine and Hygiene*, 81(3), pp. 538-9.

Sulaiman IM, Jiang J, Singh A, Xiao L. (2004). Distribution of *Giardia duodenalis* genotypes and subgenotypes in raw Urban Wastewater in Milwaukee, Wisconsin. *Applied Environmental Microbiology*, 70(6), pp. 3776–3780.

Ten Hove RJ, van Esbroeck M, Vervoort T, van den Ende J, van Lieshout L, Verweij JJ. (2009) Molecular diagnostics of intestinal parasites in returning travelers. *European Journal of Clinical Microbiology and Infectious Diseases*, 28(9), pp. 1045–1053.

Thompson RC, Reynoldson JA, Mendis AH. (1993). *Giardia* and giardiasis. *Advances in Parasitology*, 32, pp. 71-160.

Tungtrongchitr A, Sookrung N, Indrawattana N, Kwangsi S, Ongrotchanakun J, Chaicumpa W. (2010). *Giardia intestinalis* in Thailand: identification of genotypes. *Journal of Health, Population and Nutrition*, 28(1), pp. 42-52.

van Keulen H, Macechko PT, Wade S, Schaaf S, Wallis PM, Erlandsen SL.(2002). Presence of human Giardia in domestic, farm and wild animals, and environmental samples suggests a zoonotic potential for giardiasis. *Veterinary Parasitology*, 108(2), pp.97-107.

Volotão AC, Costa-Macedo LM, Haddad FS, Brandão A, Peralta JM, Fernandes O. (2007). Genotyping of *Giardia duodenalis* from human and animal samples from Brazil using beta-giardin gene: a phylogenetic analysis. *Acta Tropica*, 102(1), pp.10-9.

Gamboa M, Basualdo J, Córdoba M, Pezzani B, Minvielle M, Lahitte H. (2003). Distribution of intestinal parasitoses in relation to environmental and sociocultural parameters in La Plata, Argentina. Journal of Helminthology, 77, pp. 15-20.

Giraldo-GómezI J; LoraII F; Henao LH; Mejía S, Gómez-Marín J. (2005) Prevalence of giardiasis and intestinal parasites in pre-school children from homes being attended as part of a state programme in Armenia, Colombia. *Revista de Salud Pública*, 7(3), pp. 327-338.

5

Electrocardiography as a Diagnostic Method for Chagas Disease in Patients and Experimental Models

Patricia Paglini-Oliva, Silvina M. Lo Presti and H. Walter Rivarola
Cátedra de Física Biomédica, Facultad de Ciencias Médicas,
Universidad Nacional de Córdoba
Argentina

1. Introduction

The electrocardiogram (ECG) is a simple test that detects and records the electrical activity of the heart that is externally recorded by skin electrodes. It is a noninvasive recording produced by an electrocardiographic device. The etymology of the word is derived from the Greek *electro*, because it is related to electrical activity, *cardio*, Greek for heart, and *graph*, a Greek root meaning "to write".It is used to detect and locate the source of heart problems.

The electric activity of the heart is produced by the depolarization and repolarization of the cardiac cells and in each heart beat a healthy heart will have an orderly progression of a wave of depolarization that is triggered by the cells in the sinoatrial node, spreads out through the atrium, passes through intrinsic conduction pathways and then spreads all over the ventricles. This electric activity will be responsible of an ordered contraction first of the atria and then of the ventricles.

The recording of an electrocardiogram is using usually more than 2 electrodes that can be combined into a number of pairs (Left arm (LA), right arm (RA) and left leg (LL) electrodes form the pairs: LA+RA, LA+LL, RA+LL). The output from each pair is known as a lead. Each lead registers the electric activity of the heart from a different angle.

The electrocardiogram is one of the best and easy way to measure and diagnose abnormal rhythms of the heart, particularly abnormal rhythms caused by damage to the conductive tissue that carries electrical signals, or abnormal rhythms caused by electrolyte imbalances. In a myocardial infarction , the ECG can identify if the heart muscle has been damaged in specific areas, though not all areas of the heart are covered. The ECG cannot reliably measure the pumping ability of the heart, for which ultrasound-based (echocardiography) or nuclear medicine tests are used.

Heart failure is a highly prevalent chronic disease that results in varying degrees of functional alteration. One of the most important determinants of congestive heart failure and sudden death in Latin America is Chagas disease provoked by the infection with the intracellular protozoan *Trypanosoma cruzi.* It affects approximately 20 million people (WHO 2007; Moncayo and Silveira 2009) and represents a serious public health problem in Central and South America (Biolo et al 2010)

Among the different aetiologies, chagasic cardiopathy appears to carry the worst prognosis (Pereyra et al 2008) and has become the most frequent cause of heart failure and sudden death, as well as the most common cause of cardioembolic stroke in Latin America.

In Chagas-endemic areas, the main mode of transmission is through an insect vector called a triatomine bug that becomes infected with *T. cruzi* by feeding on the blood of an infected person or animal. During the day, triatomines hide in crevices in the walls and roofs. The bugs appears at night and bite the sleeping people to ingest blood, after that they defecate and by scratching the host favors the *T. cruzi* (trypomastigotes) entrance that are in the bug feces . Once inside the host, the trypomastigotes invade cells (amastigotes) The amastigotes multiply and differentiate again into trypomastigotes, which are then released into the bloodstream. This cycle is repeated in each newly infected cell and every time a triatomine bites an infected people.

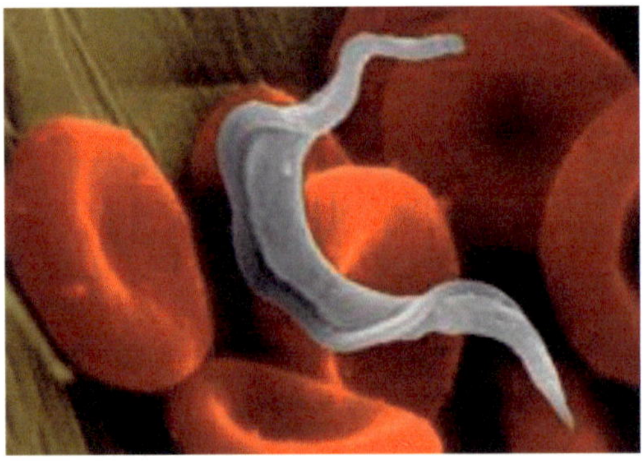

Fig. 1. Trypomastigote of *Trypanosoma cruzi* between red blood cells.

T. cruzi can also be transmitted through blood transfusions; this form is not common because in endemic areas the blood control is exhaustive and in EEUU and Europe are now paying attention to this matter. Other modes of transmission include organ transplantation, accidental laboratory exposure and congenitally through the placenta.

There are 3 stages in Chagas disease: the **acute** one with a local inflammatory lesion that appears at the site where the metacyclic trypomastigotes enter, and the parasite spreads throughout the host organism (Prata 2001, Umezawa et al 2000); the **chronic phase** in which the diversity and severity of the symptoms range from a mild electrocardiographic alteration to sudden death due to cardiac dysrhythmias, varing in different patients and in different regions (Storino & Milei 1994). In this disease the heart is the organ most commonly involved and the dysrhythmias , branch blocks and cardiac heart failure are symptoms of the 30% of patients that develop chagasic cardiomiopathy (Storino & Milei, 1994; Andrade, 1999). but may evolve into the digestive forms, or both cardiac and digestive forms together. Between the **acute** and the **chronic phases** exists a period called the **chronic indeterminate** stage, which is generally symptomless and may last 10±20 years (Macedo 1999; Ribero and Rocha 1998).

Electrocardiographic studies give important information about aspects of cardiac function and are a useful tool for measuring the severity of this and others cardiopathies and also helps in the prognosis.

During the clinical course of Chagas disease electrocardiographic alterations are usually the first clinical evidence of disease progression, but the onset of this abnormality is rarely detected, since it tends to be asymptomatic at the beginning and heart involvement is usually clinically detected in the chronic phase.

The normality or abnormality of the ECG in a chagasic patient is one of the factors that is used to determine the evolution and risk of the cardiopathy (Cuneo et al 1989).

The first human patient infected with *T. cruzi* to be identified by Carlos Chagas' died of apparently unrelated causes when she was an adult. She had no cardiac, digestive or other clinical manifestations of the disease, and thus constitutes one of the best examples of the indeterminate stage of this disease. This form is seen in 60-70% of chronic patients, and 2-5% of patients in the indeterminate phase convert to a cardiac or digestive form each year, for reasons that are not yet clear (Umezawa et al 2000)

This form was thought to be symptomless, but more sensitive tests have demonstrated that patients in this stage may present significant abnormalities (Ribeiro and Rocha 1998). According to cardiologists, this period is the most important to study because could be key in knowing which patient develops the cardiac form of infection (Elizari 1999).

This variable progression from a clinically silent period to another more severe phase is probably the consequence of many factors. One of these could be parasite strain, as it has been suggested that genetically different stocks may produce different clinical symptoms (Miles et al 1981; Montamat et al 1996).Another possible factors are the health of the host and the possible exposure to re-infections (Prata 2001; Revelli et al 1990; Bustamante et al 2002; 2003; 2004; 2005; 2007).

The cardiac chronic form is the most expressive manifestation of Chagas disease, both because of its frequency and because of its severity. It generally appears between the second and fourth decades of life, 5–15 years after the initial infection. The most common signs and symptoms of chronic Chagas cardiopathy are arrhythmia, cardiac failure, atrioventricular and branch blocks, and thromboembolism (Coura 2007). The chronic chagasic cardiomyopathy is an often fatal outcome of this infection, with a worse prognosis than other cardiomyopathies (Bestetti and Muccillo, 1997; Freitas et al 2005). A diffuse myocarditis, intense myocardial hypertrophy, damage and fibrosis, in the presence of very few circulating T. cruzi forms, are the histopathological hallmarks (Higuchi et al 1987). It is also common to find dilatation of the cavities, with the presence of thrombi, fibrosis, and thinning of the ventricular apices, particularly in the left ventricle (Coura 2007). Serious alterations in the sympathetic and parasympathetic nervous systems have also been described (Sterin-Borda and Borda, 1994).

Different researches demonstrates that Chagas' disease continues to be a major cause of heart failure from Mexico to all South America (Capps and Abad 2004; Rigou et al 2001).

Besides Chagas disease also represents an increasing challenge for clinicians in the United States (Bern et al 2007) and some European countries (Reesink 2005) due to the continuous immigration of people from disease-endemic countries (Polo Romero et al 2011)

The entrance of the parasite in the target cells provokes a focal mononuclear inflammation and the cell lysis (Andrade, 1999; Texeira et al., 2006); these pathological lesions are detected in every chagasic patient, present in the heart of 94.5% of the deaths, and directly related to the persistence of the parasite and the pathogenesis of the disease (Texeira et al., 2006).

The development of different diagnostic methods with great capacity to evaluate anatomy and cardiac functions-multi planal echodopplercardiography, scintigraphy and radioisotopic angiography-or to identify in long registers the presence of arrhythmias dynamic electrocardiography can create the impression that conventional electrocardiography (ECG) might be an exam of secondary importance for chagasic patients.

But today the ECG is still of great value due to its simplicity to do it by a medical doctor or a technician , low cost and its high sensitivity in detecting, most of the manifestations of chagasic cardiopathy (Garzon et al 1995). Having in mind the epidemiology and distribution of chagasic or potential chagasic patients the use of a simple technology is absolutely relevant.

It has great epidemiological value and is the method of choice in longitudinal population studies in endemic areas; besides the advantages mentioned, its register does not require great qualification or training of the operator. It is known that in the natural history of Chagas disease, the precocity and prevalence of electrocardiographic alterations are related to the survival curves. For all of these reasons it has great diagnostic value.

2. Electrocardiogram in the acute phase of Chagas disease

The acute phase of Chagas' disease is the consequence of a generalized infection by *T. cruzi,* and is characterized by the finding of the parasite in the peripheral blood. It generally takes a benign course with fever and the symptoms are compatible with other pathologies. The mortality of 5% and 10% described in this phase is due to myocarditis or meningoencephallitis, and occurs mainly in the first years of life (Garzon et al 1995).

The myocarditis can show variable severity; it may present only with tachycardia or as cardiac insufficiency and hypotension.

The ECG are normal in 63% of the acute cases (Porto 1964). Sometimes it can show transitory alterations: the most frequent findings are non-specific and common to any myocarditis such as: sinus tachycardia and primary alteration of the ventricular repolarization , low QRS voltage, left ventricular overload and atrioventricular block of first degree.

If the acute chagasic infection goes on with a severe myocarditis, atrioventricular blocks and bundle-branch block can appear. Electrocardiographic characteristics such as inactive areas, ST segment changes, complex ventricular arrhythmia and atrial fibrillation indicate a worse prognosis. The compromise of the ECG in the acute phase could be indicative of the late prognosis of the disease.

Many authors (Macedo 1999; Rassi et al. 2000; Bustamante et al. 2007; Elizari 1999; Storino and Milei 1994) propose that among patients with a normal ECG in this phase only 30% will have an altered electrocardiogram in the chronic phases; this is the average of infected people that will develop the cardiopathy ; on the other hand, among those showing some abnormality, 60.9% will show an altered ECG. After the clinical symptoms disappear in the acute phase the electrocardiographic alterations do the same.

One year later 75% of the cases show a normal ECG. Some (10%-20%) alternate normal tracings and abnormal tracings with intermittent first degree atrioventricular block and alteration of the ventricular repolarization.

3. Electrocardiogram in the chronic indeterminate phase of Chagas disease

A positive serological reactions for *T. cruzi,* a normal thoracic radiography and a normal electrocardiographic tracing are the elements used for the characterization of the chronic indeterminate form of Chagas' disease. This electrocardiographic normality varies in diverse endemic regions: 83% in Argentina (Rigou et al 2001) 91.6% in the Brazilian state of Rio Grande do Sul and 68% in the state of Goias (Garzon et al 1995). It is more common in the first 20 years after the acute form, with the posterior appearance of some type of electrocardiographic alteration at a frequency of 2% to 5% per year.

But the study of this silent and long period of the disease, with more sensitive diagnostic methods, either invasive or non-invasive, demonstrates that most chagasic patients with normal ECG have some type of anatomical or functional alteration.

Between 10 and 20 % of patients in the chronic indeterminate stage present electrocardiographic alterations, almost 40% of them show abnormal echocardiogram and Doppler studies, such as alterations in ventricular relaxation were found in 27.6%, enlargement of cavities in 31%, both phenomena in 31% and alteration of the parietal motility in 10.3%.(Rigau et al 2001).

Carrasco et al. 1982, followed up patients for 12 year showing that 100% of them survived this time when they belong to the group with normal ECG, or with minor ventriculographic alterations, against only 42% of the group with abnormal ECG without cardiac insufficiency. Other authors (Garzon et al. 1993) studied 109 seropositives patients with normal ECG , 91% of them presented normal left ventricular ejection fractions, but 43.1 % showed some abnormalities on the cineangiography of the left ventricle.

Table 1 summarizes the most frequent findings on electrocardiograms from 1010 patients with positive serology , in the chronic indeterminate phase of Chagas disease, and that were analyzed by cineangioventriculography or other clinical and hemodynamic-cineangiocardiographic evaluation,

	N° of cases	Age	minor left ventricle ejection fraction (%)	Abnormal left ventricle(%)
Normal ECG	109	**39.3 ± 9.1**	8.5	43
Ventricular extrasystoles	40	**47.5± 9.9**	50	20
Right branch block	39	**46.1± 13**	23.1	30.8
Left anterior hemiblock	18	**45.3± 9.8**	33.3	27.8
Anteroseptal fibrosis	5	**58.5 ±12**	60	20

Table 1. Isolated findings on the electrocardiogram of 1010 chagasic patients submitted to cineangioventriculography or other clinical and hemodynamic evaluation (Garzon et al 1995).

According with Manzullo et al. 2001, in endemic areas, the right branch block is a strong indicator for probable Chagas etiology, with a probability of 7 to 1 for this disease. However, among 902 young men they have studied, they detected 19 right branch block from which 13 had not positive Chagas serology, and must be necessarily attributed to other causes (Manzullo et al. 2001).

It is important to conclude that in chagasic patients that are coursing this long and generally asymptomatic period of the disease a normal ECG does not mean absence of functional or anatomical alterations, but all the authors agree that a normal ECG in chagasic patients, symptomatic or not, even coinciding with anatomical or functional alterations indicates a favorable prognosis with less myocardial dysfunction, than in patients with isolated ECG alterations (Garzon et al.1995; Manzullo and Chuit 1999)

4. Electrocardiogram in the chronic phase of Chagas disease

The cardiac chronic form is the most expressive manifestation of Chagas disease, both because of its frequency and because of its severity. It generally appears between the second and fourth decades of life, 5-15 years after the initial infection. The most common signs and symptoms of chronic Chagas cardiopathy are arrhythmia, cardiac failure, atrioventricular and branch blocks, and thromboembolism (Coura, 2007). The chronic chagasic cardiomyopathy is an often fatal outcome of this infection, with a worse prognosis than other cardiomyopathies (Bestetti and Muccillo, 1997; Freitas et al. 2005). A diffuse myocarditis, intense myocardial hypertrophy, damage and fibrosis, in the presence of very few circulating T. cruzi forms, are the histopathological hallmarks (Higuchi et al. 1987). It is also common to find dilatation of the cavities, with the presence of thrombi, fibrosis, and thinning of the ventricular apices, particularly in the left ventricle (Coura, 2007). Serious alterations in the sympathetic and parasympathetic nervous systems have also been described (Sterin-Borda and Borda, 1994; Lo Presti et al 2009).

The prevalence of abnormal ECG is described by some authors (Garzon et al. 1995; Manzullo et al. 1995) as 4.3 times greater in seropositive men than in seronegative men, while seropositive women are 2.6 times greater. This means that an important number of patients do not have ECG alterations in the chronic phase of Chagas disease and these are the patients with low risk of death (Manzullo et al. 1995; Rassi et al. 1995) showing that the electrocardiographical studies done periodically are a good prediction indicator of evolution of the cardiac disease.

Table 2 shows a mean of the findings of different authors as the most frequent electrocardiographic abnormalities found in the chronic phase from different regions (Garzon et al. 1995; Manzullo and Chuit 1999; Prata et al. 1993)

Ventricular extrasystoles	40%
Right branch block	35%
Left anterior hemiblock	31%
Left branch block	5%
Alterations of the ST-T segment	27%
Low voltage of the QRS	5%
First degree auricular-ventricular block	3%
Ventricular tachycardia	8%
Atrial fibrillation	10%
Anteroseptal fibrosis;	10%
Presence of inactive electrical area.	15%

Table 2. Mean of the findings of different authors as the most frequent electrocardiographic abnormalities found in the chronic phase from different regions.

If the analysis is done over dead people by Chagas disease 100% of them presented cardiomegaly and abnormal ECG. The most frequent ECG abnormalities are summarized in Table 3 (Manzullo and Chuit 1999; Garzon et al 1995)

Right bundle branch block	96.8%
Repolarization primary alterations	80%
Areas of inactivation	72%
Polifocal ventricular arrithmia	100%

Table 3. Most frequent ECG abnormalities in patients dead by cardiac insufficiency provoked by Chagas disease.

In the study of 5710 patients carried out by Manzullo and Chuit (1999), they also analyzed the ECG alterations in 15 people that died by sudden death with chagasic cardiopathy. Their results showed that only 1 patient presented normal ECG, 1 with indication of pace maker and the last 13 presented associated the following ECG alterations: right bundle branch block, left anterior hemiblock, repolarization primary alterations, ventricular inactivated areas, ventricular arrithmia.

The Argentinean people with an age between 20 and 60 years die 2.6 per/1000 yearly while chagasic people of the same age die 4 per/1000, demonstrating that chagasic patient have 53. % higher risk of death than the rest of the population.

5. Experimental model for Chagas disease

The mice model for Chagas' disease was described by Laguens et al. (1980), from a pathological, immunological and electrocardiographic point of view, demonstrating that they reproduce in a short time the three phases of Chagas disease in a similar manner that in patients. The vantages is that 10 to 30 year are reduced to 365 days; in one year post infection this experimental model reproduces the chronic chagasic cardiopathy allowing studies that produce findings to understand the pathophysiology of the disease and consequently the prevention of it. Mover, electrophysiology of normal mice and infected mice have been profusely reviewed (Berut et al. 1996; Wehrens et al. 2000) and have been largely studied in our lab (Bustamante et al. 2004; 2005; Lo Presti et al. 2006; 2008; 2009) .

6. Electrocardiograms in the experimental model

Electrocardiogram (ECG) tracings can be obtained with a digital electrocardiographic unit or any other electrocardiographic unit, under Ketamine CLH, anaesthesia (10 mg/kg). Electrocardiographic recording of non infected and infected with *T. cruzi* mice are obtained under anesthesia. The electrocardiographic tracings can be obtained with 6 standard leads (contact electrode) (dipolar leads DI, DII, DIII and unipolar leads aVR, aVL, aVF), as shows Figure 2 , recording at 50 mm/s with amplitude set to give 1 mV/10 mm. The electrocardiographic parameters analysed are: cardiac frequency, length of the PR segment and duration of the Q-T interval. Data were then transferred to a computer for further analysis. Wave durations (in sec) can be calculated automatically by the software (CardioCom) after cursor placement or can be read by the operator as usually.

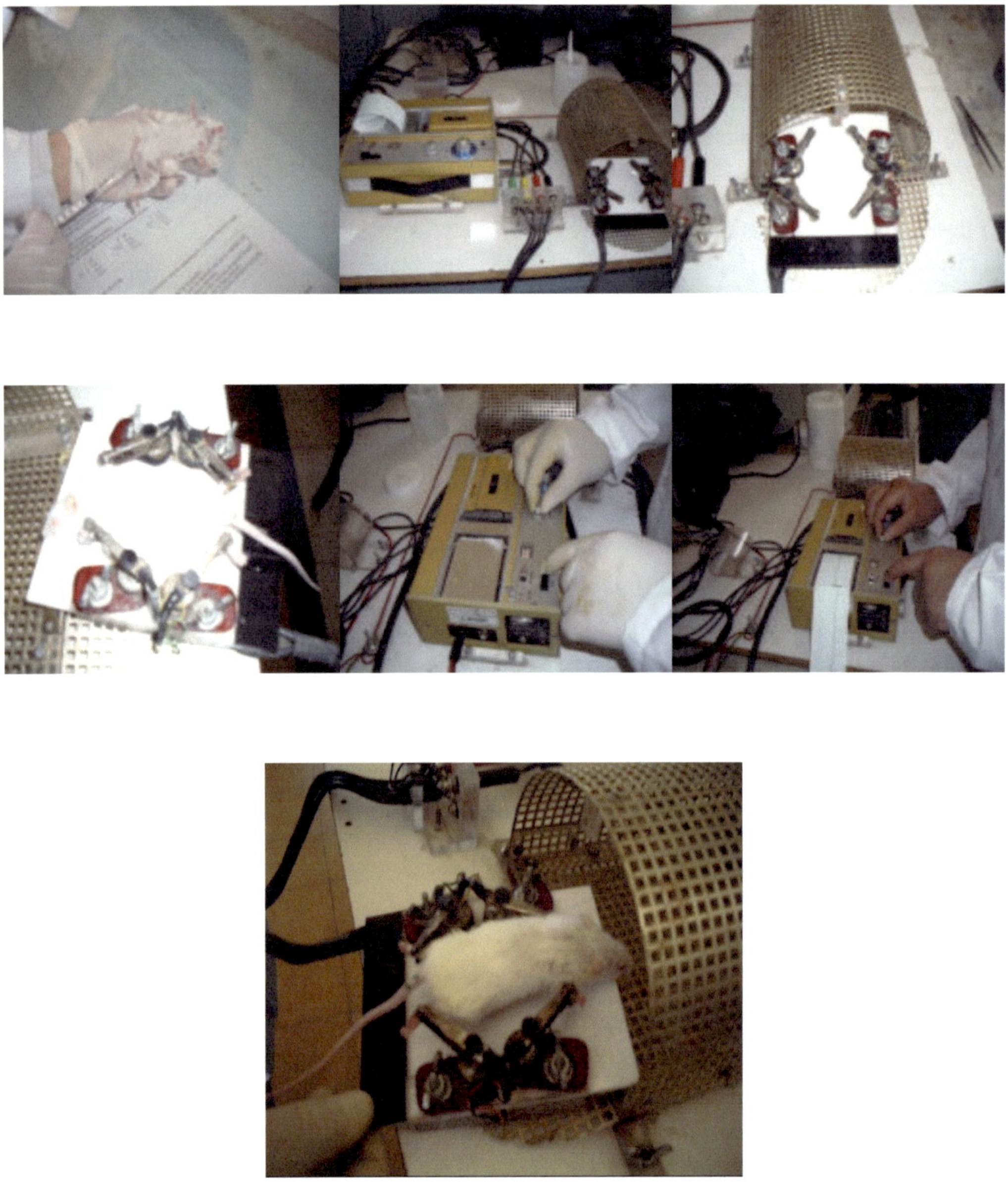

Fig. 2. Mouse placed for the ECG recording under Kethamine CLH anaesthesia The mouse is introduced in a Faraday cage to avoid electrical interferences.

The main electrocardiographic alterations obtained in this experimental model are summarized in Table 4 and were: modifications in auricle-ventricle conduction (prolonged PQ segment) and in intraventricular conduction (prolonged QRS complex), alteration in auricle-ventricle conduction associated to intraventricular conduction and arrhythmia. Results shown in Table 4 were obtained from several works carried out in our lab (Rivarola et al. 1999; 2001; Bustamante et al. 2002; Rivarola and Paglini-Oliva 2002;Bustamante et al. 2003)

Figure 3 shows the electrocardiographic alterations provoked by the infection of mice with two different *T cuzi* strain: Tulahuen strain (Taliafero and Pizzi 1955) and with the SGO Z12 isolate (Montamat et al. 1996; Bustamante et al 2003). This isolate was obtained from a chronic patient who lived in an endemic area of Argentina and it was demonstrated, through its electrophoretic pattern (Montamat et al. 1996), that it belongs to zymodeme 12 from Argentina (Bustamante et al 2003).

	Uninfected	Infected (35 dpi, acute phase)	Infected (75 dpi,chronic indeterminate phase	Infected (135 dpi,early chronic phase)	Infected (365 dpi, late chronic phase)
Mean(SE)pulse rate (beats/m)	446(13.5)	468 (12.1)	575 (4.8)	526(16.9)	646.19(22.08)
Mean(SE)axes (grades)	66 (4.7)	51(4.7)	44(2.3)	55(2.9)	57(3)
PQ intervals (s)	0.02	0.02-0.04	0.03-0.04	0.02-0.05	0.02-0.05
QRS intervals (s)	0.02-0.03	0.02-0.03	0.02-0.04	0.02-0.06	0.02-0.06
% of mice showing some ECG abnormalities	2	12.5	60	66	60

Dpi : days post infection. Mean (SE)

Table 4. Mean results of the electrocardiographic studies carried out in 100 uninfected mice and in 100 mice during the acute, chronic indeterminate and chronic stage of the *T. cruzi* infection.

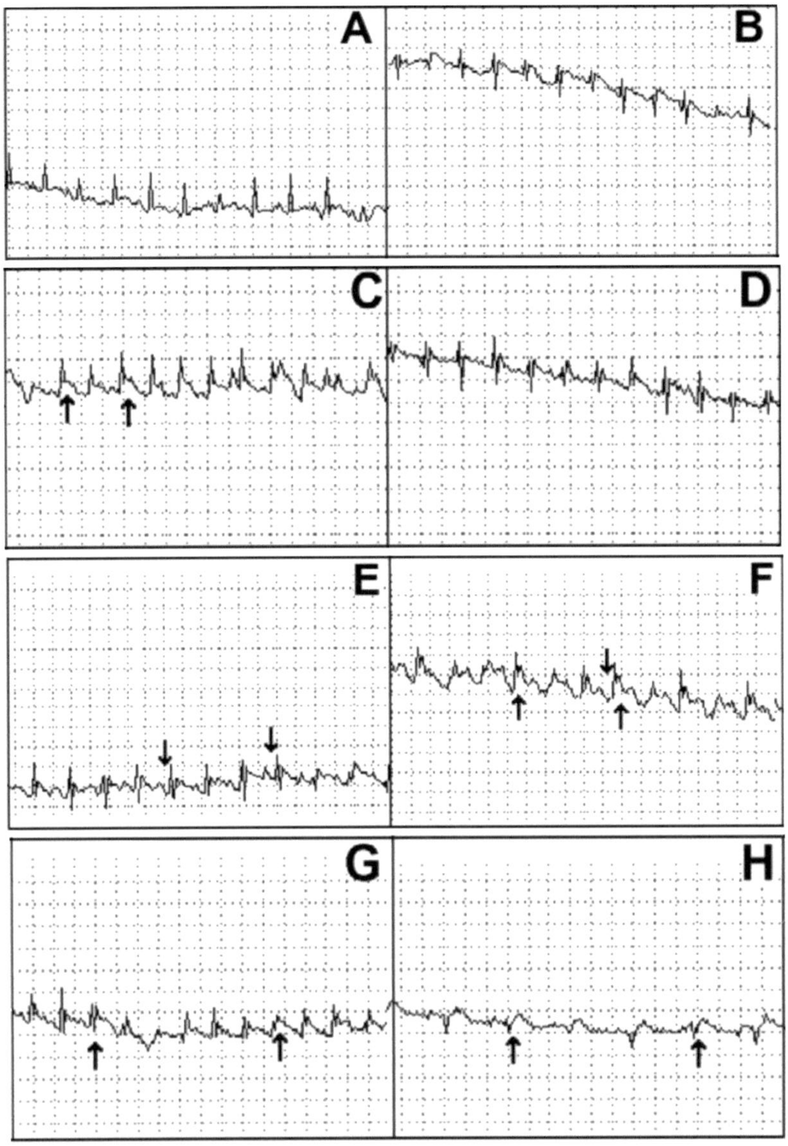

Fig. 3. Electrocardiograms in DIII dipolar lead obtained from: (A) uninfected mice showing no electrocardiographic alterations; (B) Tulahuen strain infected mice 75 days p.i.(post-infection) with no conductive alterations (50% of the mice); (C) Tulahuen strain-infected mice 75 days p.i. showing intra-ventricular blockade (IVB) (arrows) (19% of the mice from this group); (D) SGO-Z12 isolate-infected mice 90 days p.i. with no electrocardiographic alterations (65% of the mice); (E) SGO-Z12 isolate-infected mice 90 days p.i. showing auricle-ventricle blockade (AVB) (arrows) (19% of the mice); (F) SGO-Z12 isolate infected mice 90 days p.i. showing IVB associated with AVB (arrows) (8% of the mice); (G) Tulahuen strain-infected mice 135 days p.i. (cardiac chronic phase) showing IVB associated with AVB (arrows) (38% of the mice); (H) SGO-Z12 isolate-infected mice 135 days p.i. (cardiac chronic phase) showing IVB associated with AVB (arrows) (56% of the mice).

There is another important aspect to analyze in endemic countries for Chagas disease and is that people living in endemic areas are exposed not only to infections but also to reinfections at any time, therefore we concentrated our efforts on studying this factor as a matter that increases the electrocardiographic abnormalities and the severity of the cardiac damage (Bustamante et al . 2002; 2003; 2004; 2005).

Figure 4 shows the importance of the reinfections to increase the number of ECG abnormalities found in infected mice.

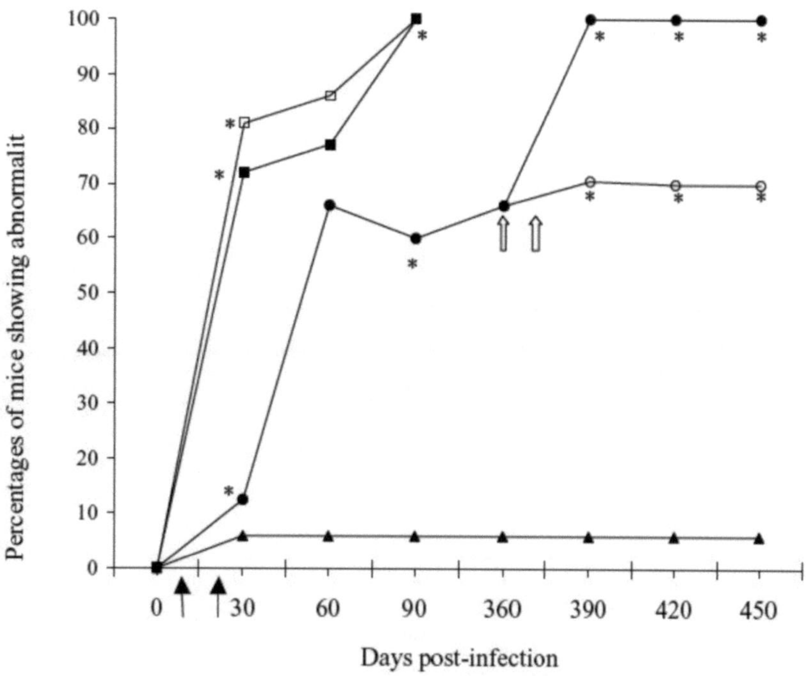

Fig. 4. Evolution of the percentages of non-infected (▲ , infected without reinfections (○), acutely reinfected with 50 trypomastigotes (□) or with 500 trypomastigotes (■) and chronically reinfected (●) mice showing at least 1 kind of electrocardiographic abnormality along the 3 phases of experimental Chagas' disease. Dark arrows indicate acute reinfection time and white arrow indicates chronic reinfection time. *P<0.01 when compared between groups at the same time.

Table 5 shows the most important ECG alterations found in the reinfected models along the evolution of the chagasic infection in a long term study of 450 days post infection (Bustamante et al. 2004).

Groups	Auricle–ventricle blockade (prolonged PQ segment)	IVB: intraventricular blockade (prolonged QRS complex)	Auricle-venticular blockade associated with intraventricular	Arrhythmias
30 dpi				
Infected n:32	9.4	3.1	NF	NF
Reinfected in the acute satage n:21	61.9	NF	9.5	9.5
Reinfected in the chronic stage n:18	11.1	38.9	16.5	5
Non Infected n:50	2	NF	NF	4
60 dpi				
Infected n:15	46.7	NF	20	NF
Reinfected in the acute satage n:14	50	14.3	7	14.3
Reinfected in the chronic stage n:15	15.4	30.8	23.1	7.7
Non Infected n: 50	2	NF	NF	4.3
90 dpi				
Infected n:15	26.7	13.3	NF	13.3
Reinfected in the acute satage n:9	67	NF	33.3	NF
Reinfected in the chronic stage n:9	71.4	NF	28.6	NF
Non Infected n:50	2	NF	NF	4
360 dpi				
Infected n:29	48.3	3.4	6.9	6.9
Reinfected in the chronic stage n:29	65	5	20	4
Non Infected n:50	2	NF	NF	10
390 dpi				
Infected n:30	50	NF	10	10
Reinfected in the chronic stage n:30	65	5	20	10
Non Infected n:50	2	NF	NF	4
420 dpi				
Infected n:24	40	NF	15	15
Reinfected in the chronic stage n:30	90	NF	8	5
Non Infected n:50	2	NF	NF	4
450 dpi				
Infected n:24	50	NF	NF	20
Reinfected in the chronic stage n:24	91.6	NF	8.4	NF
Non Infected n:50	2	NF	NF	4

NF: not found

Table 5. Percentage of the most frequent ECG alterations in infected and reinfected with *T. cuzi* mice.

Results shown in the previous Table demonstrate that when the host is reinfected in the acute phase of experimental Chagas'disease, present significantly more serious electrocardiographic alterations than those developed when the reinfections occur in the chronic stage. Reinfections increased the number of electrocardiographic abnormalities

Thus sudden death described in some chagasic patients, might be related to some of these results.

7. Final considerations

Chagas disease affects nearly 16 million people in Latin America and causes 75 to 90 million people to be at risk of infection predominantly in poor regions of Latin America. This disease is also urbanizing and globalizing due to frequent migrations. The electrocardiogram is one of the best and easy way to measure and diagnose Chagas disease. Because of its low cost, easy use and interpretation, it has epidemiological value in endemic areas with difficulties to get access to more sensitive diagnosis methods.

The prevalence of certain alterations such as right bundle branch block associate with left bundle branch and/or ventricular extrasystoles with a positive serological reaction are very simple methods and available any where to make a clear diagnosis of Chagas disease. More sensitive diagnostic methods that allow a better evaluation of the structure and cardiac functions and many different professionals dedicated to the study of Chagas disease from different points of views, have significantly increased the knowledge of this cardiopathy. But the correlation of these findings with characteristics ECG alterations has made this simple method of great valuable to follow patients and make a prognosis of the evolution of the chagasic cardiopathy.

8. References

Andrade Z. Immunopathology of Chagas' disease. Mem do Instituto Oswaldo Cruz 94: 71-80; 1999.

Bern, C., Montgomery, S.P., Herwaldt, B.L., Rassi Jr., A., Marin-Neto, J.A., Dantas, R.O., Maguirre, J.H., Acquatella, H., Morillo, C., Kirchhoff, L.V., Gilman, R.H., Reyes,

Berul CI, Aronovitz MJ, Wang PJ, Mendelsohn ME. In vivo cardiac electrophysiology studies in mouse. Circulation 94:2641- 2648; 1996.

Bestetti, R. B. and Muccillo, G. Clinical course of Chagas' heart disease: a comparison with dilated cardiomyopathy. Internat J Cardiol 60,: 187-193; 1997.

Biolo A, Ribeiro AL, Clausell N. Chagas cardiomyopathy--where do we stand after a hundred years? Prog Cardiovasc Dis.52:300-316; 2010.

Bustamante JM , Rivarola HW , Fernández AR , Enders JE , Fretes R, Palma JA and Paglini-Oliva P. *Trypanosoma cruzi* reinfections in mice determine the severity of cardiac damage.Int J Parasitol 32: 889-896; 2002.

Bustamante JM, Novarese M, Rivarola HW, Lo Presti MS, Fernández AR, Enders JE, Fretes R, Paglini-Oliva PA. Reinfections and Trypanosoma cruzi strains can determine the variability and the prognosis of the chronic Chagas disease. Parasitol Res 100: 1407-1410; 2007 .

Bustamante JM, Rivarola HW, Ferna´ndez AR, et al. Trypanosoma cruzi reinfections provoke synergistic effect and cardiac h-adrenergic receptors' dysfunction in the acute phase of experimental Chagas' disease. Exp Parasitol 103:136- 142; 2003.

Bustamante JM, Rivarola HW, Fretes R, Paglini-Oliva PA. Weekly electrocardiographic pattern in mice infected with two different Trypanosoma cruzi strains .Internat J Cardiol Int J Cardiol. 102:211-217; 2005.

Bustamante JM, Rivarola HW Palma JA, Paglini-Oliva P. Electrocardiographic characterization in Trypanosoma cruzi reinfected mice. Parasitology 128:415–419; 2004.

Capps L and Abad B. Chagas cardiomyopathy and serologic testing in a small rural hospital in Chiapas, Mexico. Pan Am J Public Health 15: 337-340; 2004.

Carrasco H.A.; Barbosa, J.S.; Inglessis, G.; Fuenmayor, A. & Molina, C. -Left ventricular cineangiography in Chagas' disease: detection of early myocardial damage. Am Heart J 104: 595-602; 1982.

Coura, J. R. . Chagas disease: what is known and what is needed . A background article. Mem do Instituto Oswaldo Cruz 102:113–122; 2007.

Cuneo CA, Molina de Raspi E, Basombrio MA. Prevention of electrocardiographic and histopathological alterations in the murine model of Chagas' disease by preinoculation of an attenuated Trypanosoma cruzi strain. Rev Inst Med Trop Sao Paulo 31: 248- 55; 1989.

Elizari, M.B.. Chagasic myocardiopathy. Historical prospective. Medicina (Buenos Aires) 59: 25–40; 1999.

Freitas, H. F., Chizzola, P. R., Paes, A. T., Lima, A. C. Mansur, A. J. Risk stratification in a Brazilian hospital-based cohort of 1220 outpatients with heart failure : role of Chagas' heart disease. Internat J Cardiol 102: 239–247; 2005.

Garzon SAC, Lorga AM, Nicolau JC. Electrocardiography in Chagas' heart disease. Sao Paulo Med J 113:802-813; 1995.

Higuchi, M. L., De Morais, C. F., Pereira Barreto, A. C., Lopes, E. A., Stolf, N., Bellotti, G. and Pileggi, F. . The role of active myocarditis in the development of heart failure in chronic Chagas' disease: a study based on endomyocardial biopsies. Clin Cardiol 10: 665–670; 1987.

Laguens RP, Cabeza Meckert P, Basombrio M A, Chambó M A, Cossio P, Arana A R. & Gelpi R J. Infección crónica del ratón con Trypanosoma cruzi. Modelo experimental de enfermedad de Chagas. Medicina 40: 33; 1980.

Lo Presti S, Bustamante JM, Rivarola HW, Fernández AR, Enders J, Fretes R, Levin G, Paglini-Oliva P. Changes in the cardiac β adrenergic system provoked by different T. cruzi strains. Internat J Cardiol 111: 104-112; 2006.

Lo Presti S, Bustamante JM, Rivarola HW, Fernández AR, Enders J, Fretes R, Levin G, Paglini-Oliva P. Some components of the cardiac beta adrenergic system are altered in the chronic indeterminate form of the experimental *Trypanosoma cruzi* infection. I J Parasitol 38:1481-92; 2008.

Lo Presti S, Rivarola W, Levin G, Cerban F, Fretes R, Paglini-Oliva P. Involvment of the cardiac beta adrenergic system in the chronic phase of Chagas disease. Parasitology. 136: 905-918; 2009.

Lo Presti, Rivarola HW, Fernández AR, Enders JE,Levin G,Fretes R, Cerbán FM, Garrido VV and Paglini-Oliva P Involvement of the b-adrenergic system in the cardiac chronic form of experimental Trypanosoma cruzi infection. Parasitology 136:905-918; 2009.

Macedo, V. Indeterminate form of Chagas disease. Mem. Inst. Oswaldo Cruz. 94: 311-316; 1999.

Manzullo E,Boggero HB; Andrade J, Foglia L, Masaúti A .Electrocardiographic Alterations in Young People Seemingly .www.fac.org.ar/scvc; 2001.

Manzullo EC and Chuit R. Risk of Death Due to Chronic Chagasic Cardiopathy . Mem Inst Oswaldo Cruz 94: 317-320; 1999 .

Miles, M. A., Cedillos, R. A., Povoa, M., Souza, A. A., de Prata, A. and Macedo, V. Do radically dissimilar *Trypanosoma cruzi* strains (zymodemes) causeVenezuelan and Brazilian forms of Chagas' disease? Lancet i:1338-1340; 1981.

Moncayo A, Silveira AC.Current epidemiological trends for Chagas disease in Latin America and future challenges in epidemiology, surveillance and health policy. Mem Inst Oswaldo Cruz. 104 :17-30; 2009.

Montamat EE, De Luca D'Oro GM, Galerano RH, Sosa R, Blanco A. Characterization of Trypanosoma cruzi population by zymodemes: correlation with clinical picture. Am J Trop Med Hyg 55:625-628; 1996.

Montamat, E. E., De Luca D'oro, G. M., Galerano, R. H., Sosa, R. and Blanco, A. Characterization of *Trypanosoma cruzi* population by zymodemes: correlation with clinical picture. Am. J. Trop. Med. Hyg. 55: 625-628; 1996.

P.A., Salvatella, R., Moore, A.C. Evaluation and treatment of Chagas disease in the United States: a systematic review. JAMA 298: 2171-2181; 2007.

Pereira Silva C, Del Carlo CH, Tavares de Oliveira Jr M, Scipioni A, Strunz Cassaro C, Franchini Ramírez JA, et al. Why do patients with chagasic cardiomyopathy have worse outcomes than those with non chagasic cardiomyopathy? Arq Bras Cardiol 91:358-362; 2009.

Polo-Romero FJ, Beato-Pérez JL, Romero-Portilla C. Chagas: an emergent and unknown disease. Rev Clin Esp.211:165-166; 2011.

Porto,C. 0 eletrocardiograma no progn6stico e evoluaoda Doenca de Chagas. Arq Bras Cardiol 17:3 13-46; 1964.

Prata A. Clinical and epidemiological aspects of Chagas' disease. Lancet, Infect Dis 1:92-100; 2001.

Prata SP, da Cunha DF, da Cunha SF, Prata SC, Nogueira N. Prevalence of electrocardiographic abnormalities in 2,000 aged and non-aged chagasic patients. Arq Bras Cardiol. 60:369-372; 1993.

Rassi, A., Jr., Rassi, W. C. and Little, W. C. Chagas heart disease. Clin Cardiol 23: 883-889; 2000.

Rassi, Jr A, Rassi A, Little WC, Xavier SS, Rassi SG, Rassi AG, Rassi GG, Hasslocher-Moreno A, Sousa AS, Sacanavacca M. Development and Validation of a Risk Score for Predicting Death in Chagas' Heart Disease Sao Paulo Med J 113:802-813; 1995.

Reesink, H.W. European strategies against the parasite transfusion risk. Transf Cliniq et Biol 12: 1–4; 2005.

Revelli, S., Berra, H., Valenti, J. et al. Effect of reinfection on the development of rats infected with *Trypanosoma cruzi*. Rev. Inst. Med. Trop. Sao Paulo 32: 260-268; 1990.

Ribeiro, A.L., Rocha, M.O., Indeterminate form of Chagas disease:considerations about diagnosis and prognosis. Rev.Soc. Bras. Med.Trop. 31: 301–314; 1998.

Rigou DG, Gullone N, Carnevali L, De Rosa AF. Symptomatic Chagas disease. Electrocardiographic and echocardiographic findings. Medicina (Bs Aires).61 :541-544; 2001.

Sterin-Borda, L. J. and Borda, E. S. Participation of autonomic nervous system in the pathogenesis of Chagas' disease. Acta Physiol Pharmacol et Ther Lat 44: 109–123; 1994.

Storino, R. & Milei, J.Enfermedad de Chagas. Mosby, Doyma Argentina, Buenos Aires.1994.

Strino RA and Milei J. Enfermedad de Chagas. Ed Mosby Doyma Argentina; 1994.

Taliaferro WH, Pizzi T. Connective tissue reactions in normal and immunized mice to a reticulotropic strain of Trypanosoma cruzi. .J Infect Dis 96:199–226: 1955.

Texeira, A.R.L., Nascimento, R.J., Sturm, N.R. Evolution and pathology in Chagas disease. Mem do Instituto Oswaldo Cruz 101: 463–491; 2006..

Umezawa E, Stalf AMS, Corbett CEP, Shikanai-Yasuda MA. Chagas' disease. Lancet 357:797- 799; 2000.

Wehrens XHT, Kirchhoff S, Doevendans PA. Mouse electrocardiography: an interval of thirty years. Cardiovasc Res 45:231-237; 2000.

WHO Report on Chagas Disease. World Health Organization on behalf of the Special Programme for Research and Training in Tropical Diseases. 2007.

Part 2

Parasite Ecology, Evolution, Morphology, Epidemiology and Biodiversiy

6

Cestode Development Research in China: A Review

Gonghuang Cheng
Fisheries College, Guangdong Ocean University, Zhanjiang, Guangdong China

1. Introduction

Adult cestode is parasitic in the intestine of the vertebrate and/or Human being. It contains a series of parasites in the world. The taxonomy position of the parasites is as follows: Platyhelminthes, Cestoda. Cestodes parasitic in human and vertebrates can cause parasitic diseases. Chinese ancestors in Tang dynasty had already concerned about this. Chao Yuanfang recorded that "... the worm is an inch in length with white colour..." ["Discussion of disesase origins", 610 A.D. From Zhao,1983] and it is infected by eating the beef that roasted by porking with mulberry twigs. So we can see that the Chinese ancestors had cestode knowledge very earlier. The little problem is that ancestors took the gravid proglottids as the whole worm and had no complete idea about this worm, nor had the life-history recognition. The report and research work of cestodes are just modern history and the work is a little later than foreign scientists.

Taenia saginata and *Taenia solium* are parasites of the human intestine, they may cause diseases. The more serious condition is that the cestode larvae parasitic in the liver, brain and other important organs, especially the *Echinococcus* which contain *Echinococcus granulosus* and *E. multilocularis.* These parasites take human and sheep as the intermediate host but cat and dog as the final host. The development of *E. multilocularis* larva in the host liver can cause serious result as a cancer. *Echinococcus* cause the disease called Echinococcosis and it was spreaded broadly in pasturing area of China. So we need to propagandize to those people that they cannot feed the dogs and cats with the bowels of the goats and cattles so that they may cut the mechanisms for transmission of the disease.

The studies of cestode is mainly with taxonomy level before 1960 but there are some other research of them as the life-cycle (Liao & Shi, 1956; Tang, 1982; Li, 1962a; Lin, 1962b,etc) and ultrastructure (Li & Arai,1991) as well as molecular biology (Liao & Lu, 1998).

According to Professor Lin Yuguang, cestodes species found in China was 213 in 1979 and it reached about 400 recorded by Cheng Gonghuang (2002).

Here we mainly discuss the life-history researches of cestode in China. These research works can be mainly divided into the following 4 aspects: Cestodes of Fishes (Liao & Shi, 1956; Tang, 1982.); Cestodes of Snakes (Cheng, Wu et Lin, 2008) ; Cestodes of chicken and ducks (Lin, 1959; Su et Lin, 1987); Cestodes of mammals (Lin, 1962a; Lin, 1962b; Lin & He,1975). It is to say common species of cestodes from fishes, snakes, birds, and mammals in China have all been studied with their life-history and it takes long time and hard work to finish these jobs.

2. Brief introduction to the works done by scientists in China

2.1 Life cycle of *Polyonchobothrium ophiocephalina* Dubinina (Tang C. C.,1982)

The cestode was collected from *Monopterus albus* (Zuiew), but ever collected by Tseng Shen from *Ophiocephalus agrus* and named as *Anchistrocephalus ophiocephalina*. And it was transferred to Genus *Polyonchobothrium* by Dubinina (1962).

Description for the adult (Plate 1: Fig 1-4): worm length is 15.5 cm, scolex, 1.2x0.6 mm. Scolex rectangular. Bothria shallow in both ventral and dorsal; apical disc present, armed with 48-62 hooks arranged in 2 and a half cycles. External segmentation present but feebly demarcated. Mature proglottid, 1x1.6 mm. Genital pore median, dorsal, pre-equatorial. Testes medullary, in two lateral fields. Ovary posterior, bilobed, 0.14x0.44 mm, transversed, elongated. Vitelline follicles cortical, in lateral bands dorsaly and ventrally, occasionally continuous around lateral margins of proglottid. Uterus loops forward, forms small uterine sac which opens midventrally when laid. In freshwater teleosts.

Development: the eggs were obtained from uterus of the cestode and put in a culture dish with fresh water for 3 days at temperature of 22-29°C. The coracidium turned out to swim. It measured 65μm in diameter with a cilia membrane 5-16μm outside. There is a spherical hexacanth in it, 60-64μm. In the development the front part of the worm is more active while old tissue is left in late part. Hexacanth had 2 granula unicellular penetrated glands with ducts to edge at the front of it. Reid ever reported hexacanth of *Raillitina cesticillus* also has the same glands.

Infection experiments show that *Mesocyclops leuckartii* Claus and *Thermocyclops hyalinus* (Rehberg) can serve as intermediate host of the cestodes. These 2 species of cyclops were put in the dish with the coracidium and coracidium were eaten. The hexacanth pierced into the body cavity of the cyclops and developed into a spherical larva then become narrow. 15 days later there comes a tail of the worm, 18 days later it turned to procercoid (Plate 1: Fig 7-8) as the mature larva of the worm at the temperature of 21-23°C. Procercoid larva measured 0.40x0.18 mm in the body, and 0.24x0.07 mm for tail. The front of the body swollened with a pit, following part is narrow and slender, penetrated glands are spherical with bulbed neucleus.

After 18 days of development the procercoid become mature, measured 067×0.16 mm for the body, 0.34×0.08 mm for tail. At this time the excretory system is much more obvious. collecting pipes were 4 longitudinal ducts with small cross discharging ducts at the first 1/5 of the body. It may become the discharge ducts of the adult cestode scolex. Ducts of the tail is not clear, only 4 flamming cells. 8 pairs of granula glands and buddles of tunnels are still there. Procercoid can survive for 30 days in a cyclops by experiment observation.

Final host infection: 15 *M. albus* from a negative area were used as infection plan. They were fed with cyclops infected with cestode for 18 day, dissected the M. albus after 3 days of infection and a 0.53 mm worm were found with 2 and a half cycles of hooks, but it is just a little for each hook. 7 days after infection, 3 mature worms with 50 more hooks in the scolex were found. The whole life cycle is now completed.

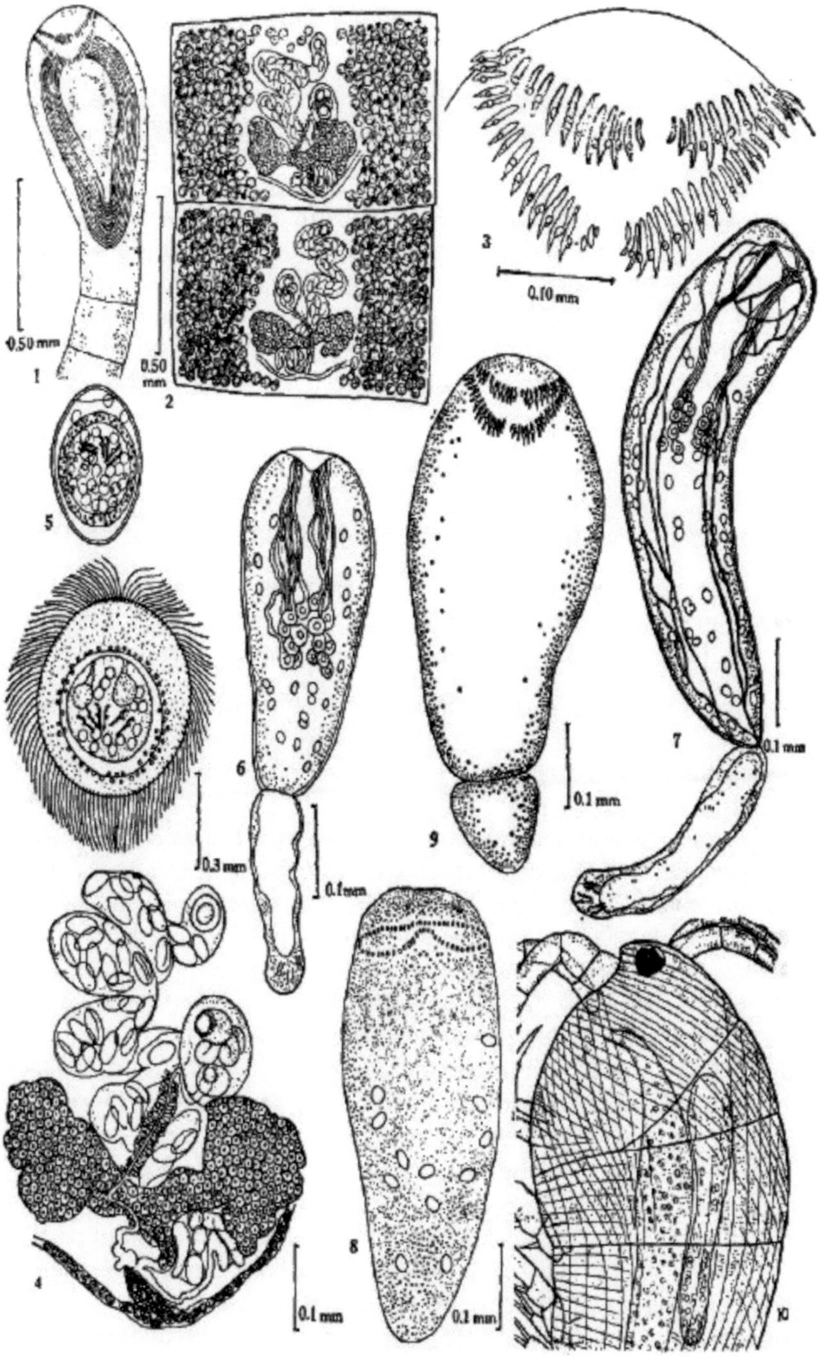

Explanation to Plate 1. 1. Scolex of *Polyonchobothrium ophiocephalina* 2. Mature proglottid of *P. ophiocephalina* 3. Hooks on top of the scolex 4. Genital systems of mature proglottid 5. Eggs and coracidium 6. Procercoid 7. A mature procercoid 8. Early stages of procecoid developed in a intestine of *M. albus* 9. Scolex in a intestine of *M. albus* 10. a cyclops with a procercoid in it.

2.2 The development process of *Ophiotaenia monnigi* in the copepods is as follows (Cheng, Wu et Lin, 2008)

Experimental animals: Copepods (*C. leuckarti* and *C. prasinus*) were obtained from ponds and ditches in Fuzhou with dredging nets. Snakes, *Enhydris plumbae,* were bought from Markets. The research was carried out in the laboratory on September in southern China.

The freshwater snakes, *E. plumbae,* were dissected. After the cestodes were collected, their gravid proglottids were torn into very small pieces to release the eggs if mature tapeworms were found. Then, the pieces of the gravid proglottids were cultivated with water for 4–10 days and fed to the copepods. In the cultivation processes, water should be changed everyday, otherwise the eggs would be poisoned by their metabolites. To make the copepods take in more eggs, it is necessary to stop feeding the copepods for 24 h before they were fed with the pieces of the tapeworm.

Copepods were dissected after they were fed with eggs 1, 3, 6, 8, and 11 days according to the development speed of the tapeworm's larvae, the procercoid, in their host. Shapes of the larva of different stages were drawn under the microscope (Olympus) (measurement unit is μm).

The tapeworms obtained by the authors were identified as *O. monnigi* Fuhrmann, 1924. Furthermore, no more species of cestodes parasitizing the same host, the water snake (*E. plumbae*), were found. During the experiment the temperature is around 28°C.

1. One day after infection: Hexacanths with a diameter of 0.020 μm in the eggs developed into procercoid larvae with a size of 0.027 x 0.039, and the hooks became dispersing. Embryonic cells increased apparently and were larger than those in the hexacanths (Plate 2: Figs. 1, 2).
2. Three days after infection: There appeared two parts in the procercoids. Hooks were in the larger part, which became the cercomere (tail) gradually and came off in the future. Embryonic cells luxuriantly developed, where the larger ones measured 0.010 x 0.008 and the smaller only 0.005 in diameter. The procercoid measured 0.024 x 0.020 and 0.037 x 0.029 in *C. prasinus* and *C. leuckarti* respectively, and the embryonic cells developed slower in the former host. The following description is based on the development of procercoid larvae in *C. leuckarti* (Plate 2: Fig. 3).
3. Five days after infection: Procercoids measured 0.041–0.082 x 0.059–0.100. An embryonic coelom, which measured as 0.019–0.063 x 0.011–0.045, appeared. In front of the coelom, embryonic cells were densely gathered; of the cells, there were four that contain a lot of granules looking like glands. Hooks were around the later edge of the embryonic coelom (Plate 2: Fig. 4).
4. Six days after infection: Procercoids were divided into body and tail parts, measuring 0.085 x 0.137 and 0.056 x 0.059, respectively. In the body part of the procercoid larvae, there was a primary apical sucker of the tapeworm (Plate 2: Fig. 5).
5. Eight days after infection: Procercoids were the same shape as that described above. Two pairs of gland cells, whose tubules reach the front edge of the worm through the apical sucker, appeared behind the sucker. Large dark cells could be seen in the center of the body. About ten calcareous granules were in the body. The tail part was spherical and had a transparent coelom. Cells in the tail were soft and transparent. The sizes of the worm were: the body 0.096 x 0.241, the cercomere, 0.059 x 0.052 (Plate 2: Fig. 6).

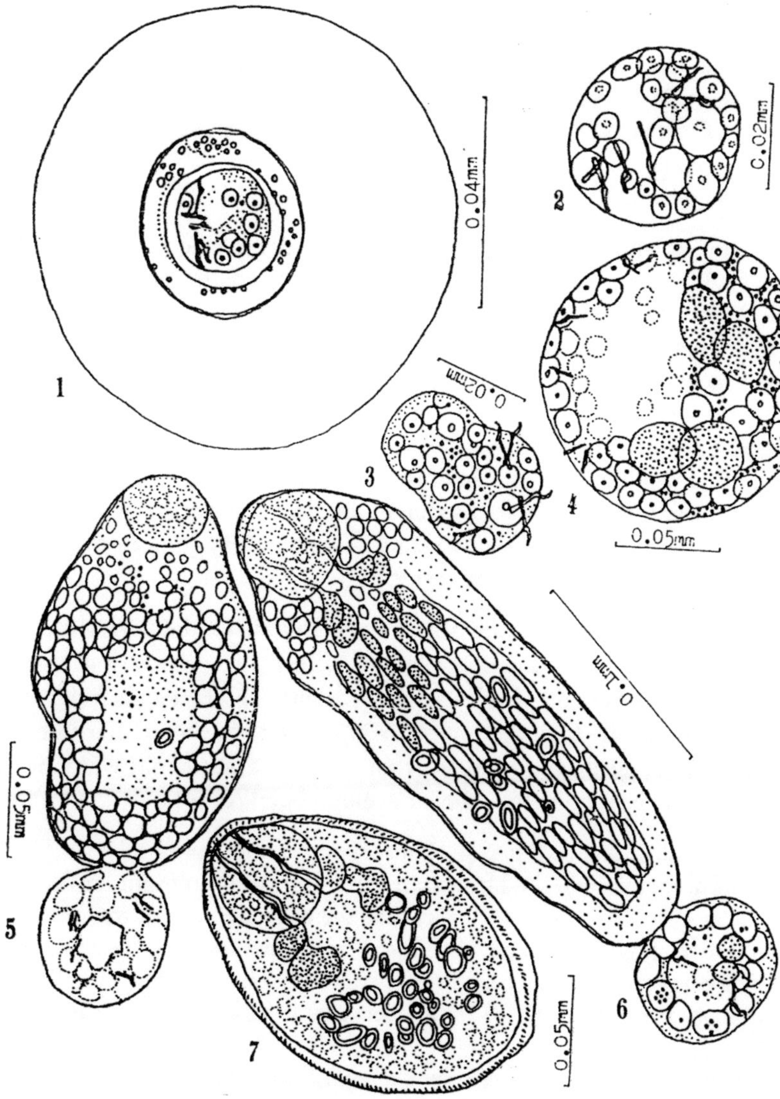

Explanation to Plate 2. 1. Mature egg with a hexacanth 2. Procercoid developed after 1 day in *Cyclops leuckarti* 3. Procercoid of 3 days after infection 4. Procercoid of 5 days after infection 5. Procercoid of 6 days after infection 6. Procercoid of 8 days after infection 7. A mature procercoid in the copepod, *Cyclops leuckarti*; the cercmere had come off.

6. Eleven days after infection: Most procercoids became oval mature larvae whose cercomere dropped in the copepods. There were crowded fibers on the surface of the worm. An apical sucker was in front of the procercoid. Two pairs of gland cells were behind the sucker. Some cell might be the primitive embryonic cells that will develop in the next host. The worm measured 0.195 × 0.112, while the apical sucker is 0.091 in diameter. In a high density of infected copepods, ten mature and one immature larvae with a cercomere were found. In general, three to four procercoids were parasitizing in one copepod (Plate 2: Fig. 7).

2.3 Chicken and duckcestode lifecycle (Su et Lin, 1987)

During 1981~1984,a total of 250 ducks and geese were examined in Xiamen,Fujian. It was found that 92 out of 228 ducks(40.4%) and 6 out of 22 geese(27.3%) were foud to be infected with 9 species of cestodes,such as (1) *Hymenolepis paramicrosoma,* (2) *H.gracilis,*(3) *H. venussa,*(4) *H. setigera,* (5) *H. przewalskii,*(6) *Drepanidotaenia lanceolata,* (7) *Diorchis stefanskii,* (8) *Dicranotaenia coronuna* and (9) *Fimbriaria fasciolaris.*

The development of larval stages within the hemocoele of intermediate hosts of five species of cestodes, namely *Hymenolepis vensusta, H. setigera, Fimbriaria fasciolaris, Drepanidotaenia lanceolata* and *Diochis stefanskii* were also studied, and the specific characters of each stage of larvae, especially their cysticercoids, were carefully studied and compared. It was revealed that they had a general pattern in the course of their oncogenesis. The process of larval growth can be divided into five stages: a.oncosphere stage,b.lacuna stage, c. cysticavity stage, d.scolex formation stage,and e.cysticercoid stage. Based on their observations, the features of these hymenolepidae cysticercoids, including the shape and size of cysticercoid, the cystic wall and fibrous membrane, the shape, size and number of rostellar hooks etc. can be identified as the specific diagnostic characters of species.Take *H. venusta* as an example to explain the development process of these cestodes.

Egg of *H. venusta* is with a feeble, transparent shell, roundish, 51-61x39-46µm, with a oval out embryomembrane, then innermembrane which enclosed the hexacanth.The intermediate host of the cestode is freshwater *Heterocypris* sp.The egg can developed into a cysticercoid in 11 days at the temperature of 26-30°C (average, 28°C) after infected with its host. At least 15 days is needed to become whole mature cysticercoid which is infective. 5 development stages can be seen in the whole developmental course.

1. stage of hexacanth (Plate 3: Fig 2-4). After 24 hours the egg is taken by its host (it is called infection, thereafter), the hexacanth can get through the gut and enter the body cavity of *Heterocypris* sp. It takes 2-3 days for the development of this stage. The worm is roundish or oval, with a diameter of 20-50µm. Sometimes the worms moved like an amoeba. The measurement for cells in it is variously changed but the cells' membrane and nucleus are very clear. The 6 hooks become to leave their position and arranged irregularly.
2. Lacunna stage (Plate 3: Fig 5-8). 4-6 days after infection hexacanth becomes bigger, 60-180µm. A transparent cavity comes out in the center of the worm and it is the primitive cavity. It increased with the growth of the worm, and become a ball body with empty center. The 6 hooks arranged in surface of the cavity, arranged irregularly. The characteristics of the stage are the worm growing fast and the primitive cavity formation.
3. cysticcavity stage (Plate 3: Fig 9). From 5 to 8 days after infection, the growth of the worm toward to 2 ends. The first part of the worm grows more fast with quite often cell division and become sturdy tissue then comes a cavity called cysticavity. Another part of the worm with little growth and showed sag states, the hooks and the primitive cavity stay there. So the worm can be divided into 2 parts, and 2 cavities at this time. In the beginning the two cavities are communicating with each other, after development, the primitive cavity with hooks is blocked with cells and it becomes the tail part of the worm. The first part of the worm developed well with fast cell division and form the organs of suckers, and rostellum etc. The length of worm is 250-330µm.

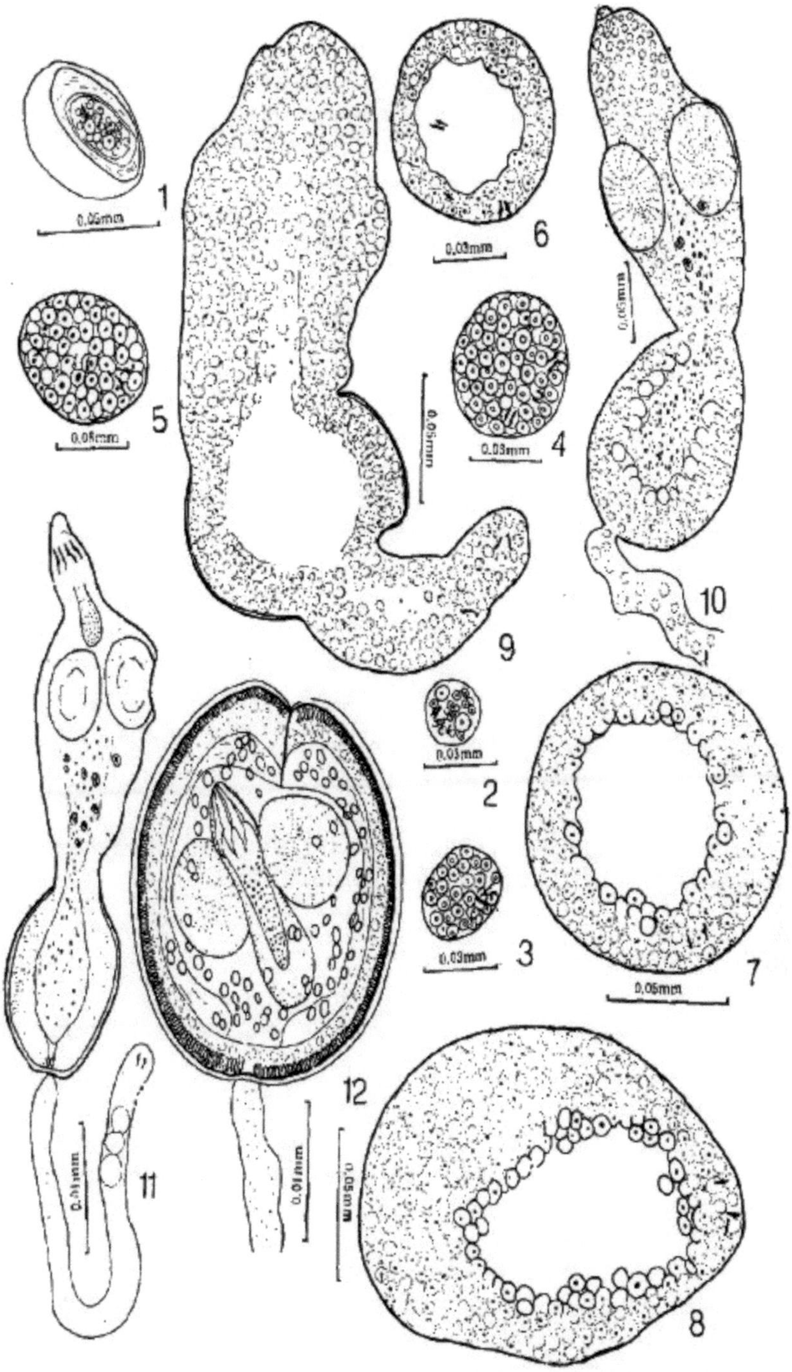

Explanation to Plate 3. Larva development of *H. venusta* 1. Egg 2. Oncosphere 2 days after infection 3 and 4. 3th day oncosphere 5 and 6. 4th day oncosphere 7. 5th day lacuna stage 8. 7th day lacuna 9.8th day cysticavity stage. 10. 9th day scolex formation stage 11. 10th day scolex formation stage 12. 12th day cysticercoid

4. Scolex formation stage (Plate 3: Fig 10-11). 9 days after infection the worm comes to this stage. In front of the worm there comes the scolex, then in the middle there is the roundish or oval cavity body, after then there is a slender tail part. 4 oval suckers can be seen in the scolex, then rostellum come into being, then hooks come at the top of the rostellum. After the scolex the neck present, there are many calcium carbonate granules. At the center of the cavity body part there is the cavity and it connected with the neck at the front. The cavity wall is composed of several layer of cells arranged tidily. The tail part is slender and with 6 hooks. Sometimes the primitive cavity still can be seen in the tail. The measurement of the worm at the time is as follows: scolex width,90-110μm; suckers, 40-50x70-72μm; cavity body width, 130-200μm; tail length, 300-400μm; rostellum 50-60μm; hooks, 14-15μm.
5. cysticercoid stage (Plate 3: Fig 12). After 11 days of infection the scolex of the worm retracted into the cavity body part and the cysticercoid is formed. It is not infective unless after 15 day of infection it becomes mature enough. The mature cysticercoid 210-237x187-205μm, is composed of three layers of body wall. Outside it is transparent cuticle, 3-5μm; the middle layer is composed of soft cells with one line of mast cells and several lines of round cells, 3.5-18μm; inner layer is with fibers, 9-15μm. The scolex is retracted in the cavity, 4 suckers, 62-64x77-81μm. Outside the rostellum there is a rostellum sac. At the top of rostellum there are 8 hooks, 39-42μm. Calcium carbonate granules ever at the neck is now around the scolex. The tail, 300-400μm. With the developedment of the worm to mature calcium carbonate granules increased with those fibers and the cysticercoid become more and more infective.

Other 4 species of cestode developed in the same course mainly but with different host, egg, development time as well as characteristics.

2.4 Studies on the developmental cycle of *Paranoplocephala ryjikovi* Spassky,1950 in the intermediate hosts (Lin, Guan, Wang et. al.,1982)

From Aug to Nov 1980 21 *Marmorta himalayana* Hodgson were dissected in Amuke River and Longriba pastures of Hongyuan County, Sichuan Province and found 3 of them infected with *Paranoplocephala ryjikovi* 95 worms (4-78). The mature segments of the worm were fed the soil mites and various stages of cysticercoids of the worm were obtained. The results are as follows:

1. Materials and Method:
a. Selection of the pregnant segments: take few of the pregnant proglottids to dissect and release the eggs and observe under microscopes. To prove them is full mature by that the embryo is developed enough with quite active hexacanth. And take 5-10 pregnant proglottids to do the experiment. The pregnant segments from feces of *Marmorta himalayana* can also be used to infect the mites.
b. Collection, isolation and feed with soil mites. Same as Lin Yuguang (1962,1975). The soil mites were taken from the local place.
2. The results of study for the life cycles
a. Adult (measurement unit is mm)
The adult worm is 12-451 in length with a width of 4.5-23, and 133-184 segments. Genital pores irregularly alternate at the late 1/3 of both sites with spherical genital atrium which can turn out of the body. The scolex is square and/or spherical,0.214-

0.386×0.171-0.329. Testes 122-144, distributed around the uterus and opposite site of the genital pore, without the sperm reservoir. Cirrus sac is oval, 1.128×0.233 (1.014-1.289×0.204-0.263). Inner sperm reservoir take take the most part of the cirrus sac, 0.526×0.263. There are thorns on the cirrus surface. Ovary is fan shaped, with many lobes, 1.368×0.395. Vitelline glands are rseshoe,0.696×0.175. spermatheca is fusiform, 0.683×0.309. Early stage of uterus is a transverse tube then it becomes to enlarge with 20-30 branches in both sites. The adult worms are quite similar with the description of Spassky (1950,1951). But Spassky only got 3 specimen with the biggest worm of 190×10, and the scientists in China got 95 worms with the biggest one of 450×23.

b. The eggs

The fresh Hexacanth eggs are white, spherical with thin wall, 70.9×74.16, easy to be broken. Egg shell is transparent, 51.48×51.12, the membrane Outside embryo is transparent, ruffled, 72.12×41.04. There are many vitelline granule between the outside embryo membrane and the egg shell. Inner embryo membrane is specialized as pyriform organ, 34.2×25.2. Hexacanth, oval, 18.0×23.4.

c. Various stages of systicercoid (measurement unit is μm).

In Sep. 5-8,1980, three batches of soil mites were infected with *P. ryjikovi* but the temperature in Longriba is too low to continue the research so specimen were taken to Chengdu and put in the incubator at 29-30°C to continue the experimental study. So all the following experimental results were under this temperature condition and the development processs were observed under the fit constant temperature.

1. Hexacanth stage: after one day of infection the soil mites can be dissected and the hexacanth was found to be 21.6x28.8, with 8-12 embryo cells, the location of hooks are the same as that in eggs. Since the temperature is so low that the embryo stopped to develop without any changes from 8-16 Sep. (Plate 4: 5-6)
2. Lacuna stage: from 16 to 23 Sep, after 5 days in incubator the hexacanths are in different stages, the smallest one—36x25.5, then 43.2x32.4, the biggest one, roundish, 43.2x39.6, the lacuna is appeared in the central, with big embryo cells 6-8, small embryo cells 12-14. (Plate 4: 7)

   23-26 Sep. (8 days after incubator culture), all hexacanths developed into lacuna stage, spherical. The hexacanth is 46.8×46.8, lacuna is 18.0×28.8. hooks are changed the location to the outside of lacunna. (Plate 4: 8)

   27-30 Sep. (12 days after incubator culture): hexacanth oval,104.4×122.4, lacuna is decreased. Hexacanth developed to pear shaped, 158.4×115.2. Lacuna is locted at the narrow part of the worm, hooks are outside of lacuna. (Plate 4: 9,10,11)

   1-4 Oct. (16 days after incubator culture): An extended worm or lacuna, 162×115.2 were found in *Parakalumma lydia,* front part is blunt, with small and crowded cells, late part with the lacuna, cells are incompact around it, hooks are irregularly arranged around the lacuna. (Fig 1:12)
3. blastula stage: 4-5 Oct. (17-18 days after incubator culture): All worms are at blastula stage, the larvae are now divided into two parts—the front body and the tail. The small worm with a body of 144.0x86.4, early stage of blastula was at the center of the late half, boundary irregular. The tail, 90×28.8, has no distinct boundary with the body, more transparent. The developed ones were splitting head part,115.2x118.8, apart the body. The suckers are faintly seen. The blastula tail, 108.0x115.2. Blastula cavity is bottle shaped with irregularly boundary. Tail, slender, biggest width 64.8. (Plate 4: 13)

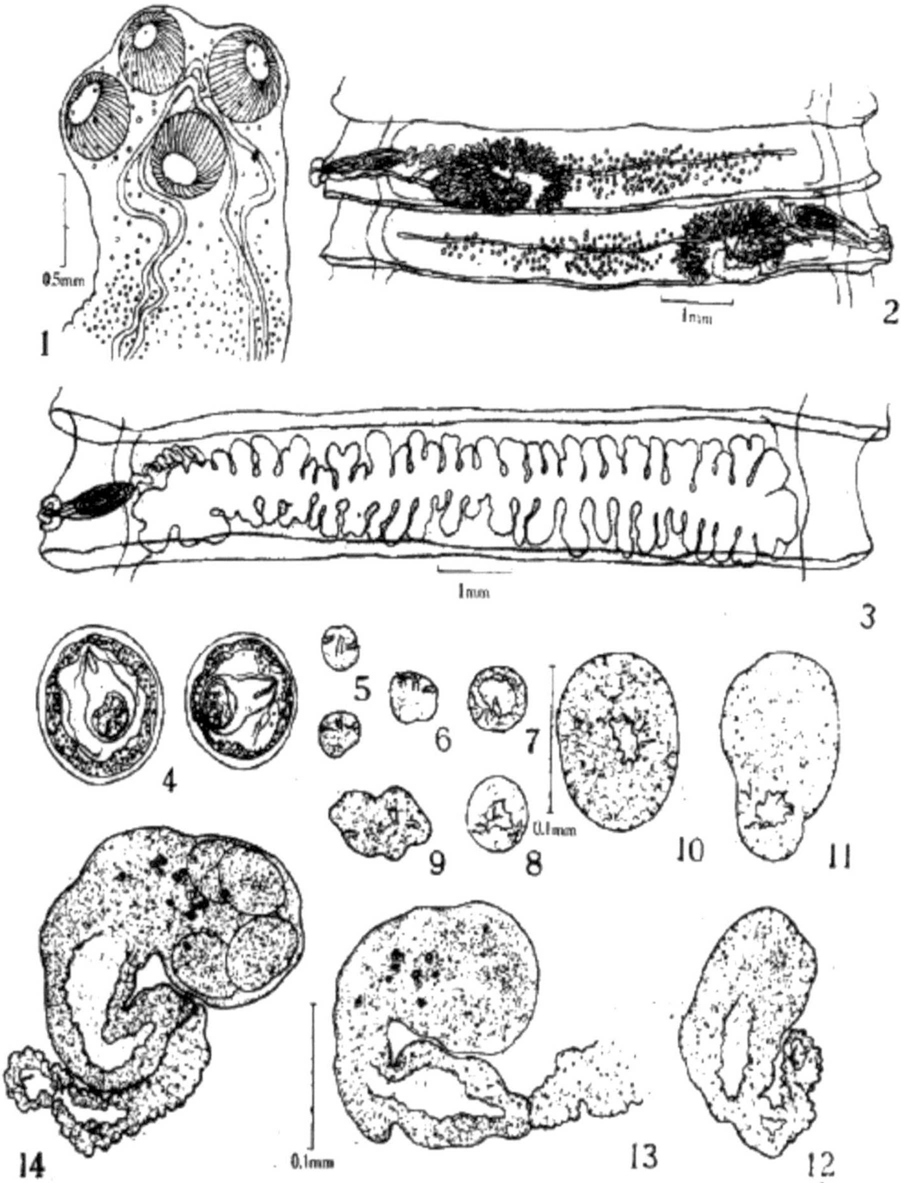

Explanation to Plate 4: 1. Scolex 2. mature proglottid 3. gravid proglottid 4. egg 5. Hexacanth of 24 h after infection to soil mite 6. Hexacanth of 8 days after infection 7.hexacanth of 5 days after incubator culture; 8. Lacuna stage larva of 7 days after incubator culture. 9-11 Lacuna stage larva of 12 days after incubator culture 12. Blastula stage larva of 16 days after incubator culture 13. Blastula stage larva of 17 days after incubator culture 14. Scolex formation stage larva of 20 days after incubator culture

4. Scolex formation stage:
   6-7 Oct. (20 days after incubator culture) in a *Scheloribates* sp. a worm of scolex formation stage were found. Front part of the worm are developed into a

scolex,118.8×122.4. 4 suckers are seen, 32.4×43.2. blastula cavity, 90.0×165.0, front of the blastula connected with scolex, with no distinct boundary between them. Tail part stripped,216.0×36.0. Lacuna and hooks are still at the end, there are 10 more calcium carbonate granules between scolex and the blastula cavity (Plate 4: 14). Another worm of the stage were found: scolex 108.0×116.6. Blastula cavity, 72.0×97.2, with distinct cavity in it, blastula wall 4-5 lines of cells, the cavity is fusiformis but the tail is stripped,187×46.5. (Plate 5: 15).

8 Oct. (21 days after incubator culture): the scolex extended and become active, 118.8×198.0. Suckers can be stretched, there are 11 calcium carbonate granules at the end of the tail. The blastula cavity developed mature as a bottle, 162×104.4. The balstula wall with 3-5 line of cells. There is a cuticular around the scolex and the blastula cavity. The tail are decreased to degenerate: 74.4×50.4. Hooks are arranged at the late part of the tail.

19-13 Oct. (26 days after incubator culture): early stage of cysticercoid, the scolex retracted to the blastula cavity. The blastula cavity, 205.2×216.0. There is a cuticular around it, a big hole at the front can be seen, Scolex,162.0×172.8. The suckers are much active, 64.8×46.8. 42 calcium carbonate granules are at the base, and they are in different sizes. Blastula wall is constructed by 2-3 column epithelial cells. The tail is connected with the base of blastula cavity and there is distinct boundary. The tail is stripped with a width of 54.0, the hooks are there. (Plate 5: 17).

14-15 Oct. (28 days after incubator culture): cysticercoid developed almost the same. Blastula body is quite sturdy, 140.4×160.5. Scolex are separated with blastula wall, 104.4×11.6. Blastula wall are divided two layers, out layer are one line cells. Inner wall are soft cells, and with fibrosis. The calcium carbonate granules are distributed at the base of the scolex and around the inner layer of the blastula wall. The tail is apparently decreased to as a stick, 54.0×28.8. (Plate 5: 18)

16-19 Oct. (32 days after incubator culture): cysticercoids are almost mature. The blastula is spherical, 133.2×187.2. Scolex oval, 108.0×126.0, suckers, 79.2×39.6. Cuticular layer with deep colour, become thick, the edge of the blastula sac it is corrugation. The wall is with two layers, out layer is with epithelial cells arranged very tidy, thickness is 7.2, inner layer is fibrosis, 18.0-21.6. More calcium carbonate granules are appeared, most of them are distributed late part of the scolex and front part of the blastula sac. Tail like a small sac, 43.2×28.8. (Plate 5: 19)

20-26 Oct. (39 days after incubator culture), whole mauture cysticercoids are found, oval body, 198.0×172.8. The cuticule is black, with compactness fiber lines,out side with irregular undulance protuberance, with a thickness of 3.6-10.8. The bastula wall is two layer, out part with 1-2 lines of epithelial cells, transparent, thickness, 10.8-18.0. Number of calcium carbonate granules is 63-70, maily distributed at base of scolex and fiber layer. Tail degenarated to a small sac, transparent, 50.4×36, hooks are still there. After then all the cysticercoids are almost the same, changed quite few (Plate 5: Fig 20,21;Plate 4:Fig 1-5)

2 rabbits were used as host to infect the cysticercoids, adult worms were not found after 58 days of infection. 2 Guinea pigs were also used to infect with 4 and 6 mature cysticercoids, after 28 days adult worms were still not found. Maybe they are not suitable normal hosts.

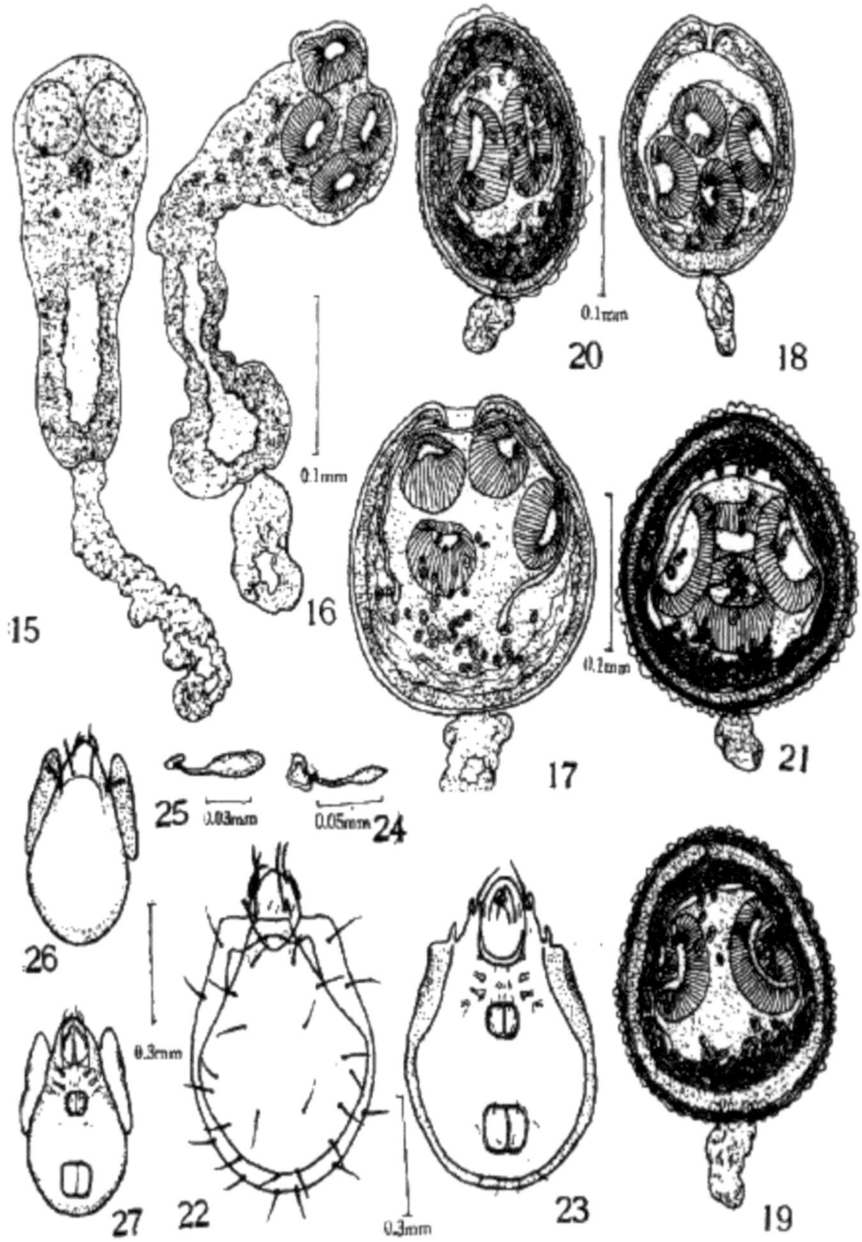

Explanation to Plate 5: 15. Scolex formation stage larva of 20 days after incubator culture 16. formation stage larva of 21 days after incubator culture Scolex 17. Early stage of cysticercoid, 26 days after incubator culture 18. cysticercoid, 28 days after incubator culture 19 cysticercoid, 32 days after incubator culture (near to mature). 20. and 21. cysticercoid, 39 and 70 days after incubator culture. 22. Dorsal view of *Scheloribates* sp. I. 23. Ventral view of *Scheloribates* sp. I. 24. Pseudostomatal apparatus of *Parakalumma lydia* 25. Pseudostomatal apparatus of *Scheloribates* sp. I. 26. Dorsal view of *Parakalumma lydia* 27. Ventral view of *Parakalumma lydia*.

3. Afterwords

These are the maily representative works, but there are still very good jobs done by many other scientists in China: The life-cycle,ecology and prevention of *Bothriocephalus gowkongensi*(Liao et Shi, 1956); Sudies on the development and intermediate hosts of *Moniezia expansa* (Rudolphi, 1810)(Lin, 1962a); Comparative studies on the procercoid development in their intermediate hosts for *Hymenolepis diminuta* and *H. nana* (Lin, 1962b); Studies on the lifecycle of *Moniezia benedeni* (Cai et Jin, 1984); Studies on the life cycle of *Ctenotaenia citelli* (Kirshenblat) and *Mosgovoyia pectinata* (Goeze) (Lin et Hong,1986), etc. But it is limited pages to put everything here so the author can just take those papers mainly introduced as above.

4. Appendix

A Catalogue of Cestodes in China

A. Proteocephalidea Mola,1928
I.Proteocephalidae La Rue,1911

1 *Proteocephalus* Weinland,1853
(1)*P. fima*(Meggitt,1927)
(2)*P. fixus*(Meggitt,1927)
(3)*P. exiguus* La Rue,1911
(4)*P. longicollis*(Zeder,1800)
(5)*P. torulosus*(Butsch,1786)
(6)*P. parasiluri* Yamaguti,1934
2. *Ophiotaenia* La Rue,1911
(7)*O. nankingensis* Hsü,1935
(8)*O. fixa* Meggitt,1927
(9)*O. sinensis* Cheng et Lin,2002
(10)*O. akgistrodontis* Harwood,1933
(11)*O. mönnigi* Fuhrmann,1924
(12) *Ophiotaenia wuyiensis* n. sp.

3. *Gangesia* Woodland,1924
(13)*G. oligorchis* Roylman et Frece,1964
(14)*G. parasiluri* Yamaguti,1934
(15) *G. pseudobagre* Chen,1984

4. *Silurotaenia* Nybelin,1924
(16)*S. spinula* Chen,1984
(17)*S. siluri*(Batsch,1786)

5. *Paraproteocephalus* Chen,1984
(18)*P. parasiluri* Chen,1962

6. *Corallotaenia* Freze,1965
(19)*C. nanfengensis* Cheng,1997

7. *Corallobothrium* Fritsch,1886
(20)*C. parasiluri* Zmeev,1936

B. Cyclophyllidea van Beneden in Braun,1900

II Dilepididae (Railliet et Henry,1909) Lincicome,1939

8. *Ophiovalipora* Hsü,1935
(21)*O. houdemeri* Hsü,1935
(22)*O. lintonis* Yamaguti,1959
9. *Paradilepis* Hsü,1935
(23)*P. duboisi* Hsü,1935

10. *Amoebotaenia* Cohn,1900
(24)*A. cuneata* Linstow,1872
(25)*A. oligorchis* Yamaguti,1935
(26)*A. brevicollis* Fuhrmann,1907
(27)*A. vanelli* Fuhrmann,1907
(28) *A. pekingensis* Tseng,1932
(29)*A. fuhrmanni* Tseng,1932
(30)*A. lingi* Li et. al,1994
(31) *A. scolopax* Li et. al,1994
(32) *A. lumbrici*(Villot,1883)
(33)*Amoebotaenia* sp.
(34)*A. tropica* Xu,1959

11. *Unciunia* Skrjabin,1914
(35)*U. ciliata*(Fuhrmann,1913)
(36)*U. sinensis* Lin,1976
(37)*U. falconis* Lin,1976
(38)*U. hypsipetis* Lin,1976

12. *Anomotaenia* Cohn,1900 ·
(39) *A. hoepplii* Tseng,1933
(40) *A. microhyncha*(Krabbe,1869)
(41) *A. citrus*(Krabbe,1869)
(42) *A. nymphaea*(Schrank,1790)
(43) *A. stentorea*(Frölich,1802)

(44)*Anomotaenia* sp. Tseng,1932
(45)*A. nycticoracis* Yamaguti,1935
(46)*A. ciliata* Fuhrmann,1913
(47)*A. erolia* Li et.al.,1994
(48) *A. hypoleucus* Li et.al.,1994
(49)*A. passerum* Joyeux et Timon-David,1934
(50) *A. rustica* Neslobinsky,1911

(51) *A. arionis*(Siebold,1850)
(52)*A. garrulax* Li et. al.,1994
(53)*A. amaurornisus* Cheng et Lin,2002

13. *Choanotaenia* Railliet,1896
(54)*C. infundibulum*(Bloch,1779)
(55)*C. quiarti* Tseng,1932
(56)*C. macracantha* (Fuhrmann,1907)
(57)*C. joyeuxi* Tseng,1932
(58)*C. cingulifera*(Krabbe,1869)
(59)*C. porosa*(Rudolphi,1810)
(60)*C. coromandus* Li et. al.,1994
(61)*C. merula* Li et. al.,1994
(62)*C. stenura* Li et. al.,1994
(63)*C. joyexibaeri* López -Neyra,1952
(64)*C. decacantha*(Fuhrmann,1913)
(65)*C. slesvicensis*(Krabbe,1882)
(66)*C. stellifera*(Krabbe,1869)
(67)*C. rotunda*(Clerc,1913)

14. *Anonchotaenia* Cohn,1900
(68)*A. globata*(Linstow,1819)
(69) *A. oriolina* Cholodkovsky,1906
(70)*A. dendrocitta*(Woodland,1929)

15. *Paricterotaenia* Fuhrmann,1932
(71)*P. paradoxa*(Rudolphi,1802)
(72)*P. arquata*(Clerc,1906)

16. *Dilepis* Weinland,1858
(73)*Dilepis* sp.1 Tseng,1932
(74)*Dilepis* sp.2
(75)*D. undula*(Schrank,1788)
(76)*D. unilateralis*(Rudolphi,1819)

17. *Dipylidium* Leuckart,1863
(77)*D. caninum*(Linnaeus,1758)
18. *Diplopylidium* Beddard,1913
(78)*D. nölleri* Skrjabin,1914

19. *Paruterina* Fuhrmann,1906
(79)*Paruterina* sp. 1
(80) *Paruterina* sp.2

20. *Biuterina* Fuhrmann,1902

(81)*B. passerina* Fuhrmann,1908

21. *Cyclorchida* Fuhrmann,1907
(82)*C. omalancristrota* Wedl,1855

22. *Kowalewskiella* Baczynska,1914
(83)*K. buzzardia* Tubangui et Masilungan,1937

23. *Vitta* Burt,1938
(84)*V. wulingensis* Yun et Tang,1993
(85)*V. magniuncinata*(Burt,1938)

24. *Lateriporus* Fuhrmann,1907
(86)*L. exiensis* Yun et Tang,1992

25. *Deltokeras* Meggitt,1927
(87)*D. delachauxi* Hsü,1935

26. *Angularella* Strand,1928
(88)*A. ripariae* Yamaguti,1940

27. *Parvirostrum* Fuhrmann,1908
(89)*P. magisomum* Southwell,1930

III.Nematotaeniidae Lühe,1910

28. *Nematotaenia* Lühe,1910
(90)*N. dispar*(Goeze,1782)

29. *Baerietta* Hsü,1935
(91)*B. baeri* Hsü,1935

IV. Diploposthidae (Poche ,1926) Southwell, 1929

30. *Diploposthe* Jacobi,1896
(92)*D. skrjabini* Mathevossian,1942
(93) *D. laevis*(Bloch,1782)

V. Anoplocephalidae Cholodkovsky,1902

31. *Oochoristica* Lühe,1898
(94)*O. hainanensis* Hsü,1935
(95)*O. crassiceps* Baylis,1920
(96)*Oochoristica* sp.
(97)*O. ratti* Yamaguti et Miyata,1937

32. *Schizorchis* Hanson,1948
(98)*S. tibetana* Wa-cheih,1965
(99)*S. changduensis* Wa-cheih,1965
(100)*S. altaica* Gvozdev,1951
(101)*S. tangi* Guan et. al.,1986

33. *Anoplocephala* Blanchard,1848
(102)*A. magna*(Abildgaard,1789)
(103)*A. perfoliata*(Goeze,1782)

34. *Paranoplocephala* Lühe,1910
(104)*P. mamillana*(Mehlis,1831)
(105)*P. ryjikovi* Spassky,1950
(106)*P. transversaria* Krabbe,1879

35. *Moniezia* Blanchard,1891
(107)*M. benedeni* Moniez,1879
(108)*M. expansa* Rudolphi,1810
(109)*M. denticulata* (Rudolphi,1810)
(110)*M. planissima* Stiles et Hassall,1892
(111)*M. sichuanensis* Wu,1982

36. *Cittotaenia* Riehm,1881
(112)*C. denticulata* Rudolphi,1804
(113)*C. citelli*(Kirschenblat,1939)

37. *Bertiella* Stiles et Hassal,1902
(114)*B. studeri* Blanchard,1891
(115)*Bertiella* sp.

38. *Paronia*.Diamare,1700
(116)*P. pycnonoti*.Yamaguti,1935
(117)*P. corvi* Guan et Lin,1987
(118)*P. calcauterina* Burt,1939

39. *Avitellina* Gough,1911
(119)*A. minuta* Yang et. al.,1977
(120)*A. tatia* Bhalerao,1936
(121)*A. magavesiculata* Yang et. al., 1977
(122) *A. centripunctata* Rivolta,1874

40. *Stilesia* Railliet,1893
(123)*S. globipunctata*(Rivolta,1874)

41. *Pseudanoplocephala* Baylis,1927
(124)*P. crowfordi* Baylis,1927

42. *Aprostatandrya*(Kirschenblat,1938)
(125)*A. macrocephala* Douthitt,1915
(126)*A.(S.)cricetuli* Lin et. al,1984

43. *Mosgovoyia* Spassky,1951
(127)*M. pectinata*(Goeze,1782)

44. *Killigrewia* Meggitt,1927
(128)*K. orientalis*(Yun et Tang,1992)
(129)*K. delafondi*(Railliet,1892)

45. *Thysaniezia* Skrjabin,1926 ·
(130)*T. giardi* Moniez,1879
(131)*T. ovilla* (Rivolta,1878)

46. *Diuterinotaenia* Gvosdev,1961
(132)*D. daofuensis* Guan et Lin,1992
(133)*D. polyclada* Yun et Lin,2000
VI.Amabilliidae Fuhrmann,1908

47. *Schistotaenia* Cohn,1900
(134)*S. indica* Johr,1959
(135)*S. macrorhycha*(Rudolphi,1810)

48. *Tatria* Kowalewski,1904
(136)*T. acanthorhyncha*(Wedl,1855)

VII. Dioecocestidae (Southwell, 1930) Burt, 1939

49. *Gyrocoelia* Fuhrmann,1900
(137)*G. fausti* Tseng,1933
(138) *Gyrocoelia* sp.

50. *Dioecocestus* Fuhrmann,1900
(139)*Dioecocestus* sp.

VIII.Taeniidae Ludwig,1866

51. *Echinococcus* Rudolphi,1801
(140)*E. granulosus*(Batsch,1786)
(141) *E. multilocularis*.Leuckart,1863
(142)*Echinococcus russicensis* Tang et al.,2007
52. *Multiceps* Goeze,1782
(143)*M. multiceps*(Leske,1780)
(144)*M. serialis*(Gervais,1847)
(145)*M. skrjabini* Popov,1937

53. *Taeniarhynchus* Weinland,1858
(146) *T. saginata*(Goeze,1782)

54. *Hydatigera* Lamarck,1816
(147)*H. taeniaeformis*(Batsch,1780)

55. *Taenia* Linnaeus,1758
(148)*T. hydatigera* Pallas,1766
(149)*T. solium* Linnaeus,1758
(150) *T. pisiformis* Bloch,1780
(151)*T. tenuicollis* Rudolphi,1819
(152)*T. ovis* Cobbold,1860

56. *Cladotaenia* Cohn,1901
(153)*C. cylindracea*(Bloch,1782)
(154)*Cladotaenia* sp.

(155)*C. circi* Yamaguti,1935

IX.Catenotaeniidae Wardle et McLeod, 1952

57. *Catenotaenia* Janicki,1904
(156)*C. pusilla*(Goeze,1782)
(157)*Catenotaenia* sp.
(158)*C. linsdalei* McIntosh,1941

X.Mesocestoididae Perrier, 1897

58. *Mesocestoides* Vaillant,1863
(159)*M. lineatus* Goeze,1782
(160)*Mesocestoides* sp.

XI. Davaineidae Fuhrmann, 1907

59. *Cotugnia* Diamare,1893
(161)*C. digonopora*(Pasquale,1890)
(162)*C. taiwanensis* Yamaguti,1935
(163)*C. seni* Meggitt,1926

60. *Davainea* Blanchard,1891
(164)*D. proglottina*(Davaine,1860)
(165)*D. himatopodis* Johnston,1911
(166)*Davainea* sp. Hoeppli,1920
(167) *D. anderi* Fuhrmann,1933

61. *Raillietina* Fuhrmann,1920
(168)*R. cesticillus*(Molin,1858)
(169)*R. echinobothrida*(Megnin,1881)
(170)*R. tetragona*(Molin,1858)
(171)*R. taiwanensis* Yamaguti,1935
(172)*R. shantungensis* Winfield et.al.,1936
(173)*R. tetragonoides* Baer,1926
(174)*R. huebscheri* Hsü,1935
(175)*Raillietina* (*Fuhrmannetta*)sp. Tseng,1933
(176)*R. garrisoni* Tubangui,1931
(177)*R. sinensis* Hsü,1935
(178)*Raillietina* sp. Chen,1933
(179)*R. celebensis* (Tanicki,1902)
(180)*R. madagascariensis*(Davaine,1870)
(181)*R. fragilis* Meggitt,1931
(182)*R. compacta* (Clerc,1906)
(183)*R. parviuncinata* Meggitt et Saw,1924
(184)*R. sartica*(Skrjabin,1914)
(185) *R. kantipura*(Sharma,1943)
(186)*R. pycnonoti*(Yamaguti et Mitunaga,1943)
(187) *R. torquata*(Meggitt,1924)
(188)*R. lini* Cheng et Lin,2002

62. *Ophryocotyle* Friis,1870
(189)*O. insignis* Lonnbery,1890

63. *Fernandezia* López-Neyra,1936
(190)*F. indicus*(Singh,1964)Artjuch,1964

XII.Hymenolepididae Railliet et Henry,1907

64. *Aploparaksis* Clerc,1903
(191)*A. sinensis* Tseng,1933
(192)*A. filum*(Goeze,1782)
(193)*A. parafilum* Joyeux et Bear,1939
(194)*A. crassirostris*(Krabbe,1869)
(195)*A. brachyphallos*(Krabbe,1869)
(196)*A. penetrans* Clerc,1902
(197)*A. fukienensis* Lin,1959
(198)*A. bubulcus* Li et. al.,1994
(199)*A. larina* Fuhrmann,1921

65. *Diorchis* Clerc,1903
(200)*D. flavescens*(Krefft,1871)
(201)*D. anatina* Ling,1959 ·
(202)*D. anomallus* Schmelz,1941

(203)*D. crassicollis* Sugimoto,1934
(204)*D. formosensis* Sugimoto,1934
(205)*D. nigrocae* Yamaguti,1935
(206)*D. wigginsi* Schultz,1940
(207)*Diorchis* sp.
(208)*D. ransomi* Schultz,1940
(209)*D. sobolevi* Spasskaja,1950
(210)*D. inflata* (Rudolphi,1891)
(211)*D. elisae* Skrjabin,1914
(212)*D. bulbodes* Mayhew,1929

66. *Fimbriaria* Froelich,1802
(213)*F. amurensis* Kotellnikov,1960
(214)*F. fasciolaris* (Pallas,1781)

67. *Drepanidotaenia*.Railliet,1892

(215)*D. nyrocae*.(Yamaguti,1935)
(216)*D. lanceolata*.(Bloch,1782)
(217)*D. przewalskii* (Skrjabin,1914) ·

68. *Hsuolepis*.Yang et al,1957
(218)*H. shengi*.Yang et al,1957 ·
(219)*H. shensiensis* (Liang et Cheng,1963)
(220)*H. crowfordi* (Baylis,1927)

69. *Echinocotyle*.Blanchard,1891
(221)*E. anatina* (Krabbe,1869)

(222)*E. echinocotyle* (Fuhrmann,1907)
(223)*E. nitida* (Krabbe,1869)

70. *Echinolepis* Spassky et Spasskaja,1954
(224)*E. carioca* (Magelhas,1898)
71. *Hymenosphenacanthus* López-Neyra,1958
(225)*H. exiguus* (Yoshida,1910)
(226)*H. fasciculata* (Ransom,1909)
(227)*H. giranensis* (Sugimoto,1934)
(228)*H. longicirosa* (Fuhrmann,1906)
(229)*H. oshincai* (Sugimoto,1934)
(230)*H. venusta* (Rosseter,1897)

72. *Anatinella* Spassky et spasskaja,1954
(231)*A. meggitti* (Tseng,1932)

(232)*A. spinulosa*

73. *Cloacotaenia* Wolffhügel,1938
(233)*C. megalops*(Creplin,1829)

74. *Dicranotaenia* Railliet,1892

(234) *D. coronula* (Dujardin,1845)
(235)*D. introversa* (Mayhew,1923)

(236)*D. pingi* (Tseng,1932)
(237)*D. mergi* (Yamaguti,1940)
(238)*D. querquedula* (Fuhrmann,1921)
(239) *D. simplex* (Fuhrmann,1926)
(240)*D. himantopodis* (Krabbe,1869)
(241)*D. aequabilis* (Rudolphi,1819)
(242)*Dicranotaenia* sp. (Li,1994)

75. *Abortilepis* Yamaguti,1959
(243)*A. abostiva* (Linstow,1904)

76. *Sobolevicanthus* Spassky et Spasskaja, 1954
(244)*S. fragilis* (Krabbe,1869)
(245)*S. gracilis* (Zeder,1903)
(246)*S. octacantha* (Krabbe,1869)
(247)*S. rugosas* (Clerc,1906)
(248)*S. krabbeella* (Krabbe,1869)

77. *Dubininolepis* Spassky et Spasskaja,1954
(249)*D. multistriata* (Rudolphi,1810)

78. *Nadejdolepis* Spassky et Spasskaja,1954
(250)*N. solowiowi* (Skrjabin,1914)
(251)*N. compressa* Linton,1892
(252)*N. longicirrosa* Fuhrmann,1906
(253)*N. nitidulans* (Krabbe,1882)

79. *Wardoides* Spassky et Spasskaja,1954
(254)*W. anasae* Yun,1973
(255)*W. nyrocae* Yamaguti,1935

80. *Tschertkovilepis* Spassky et Spasskaja,1954
(256)*T. setigera* (Froelich,1789)
(257)*Tschertkovilepis*.sp.

81. *Stylolepis* Yamaguti, 1959
(258)*S. longistylosa* (Tseng,1932)

82. *Microsomacanthus* López-Neyra,1942
(259)*M. collaris*(Batach,1786)
(260)*M. compressus*(Linton,1892)
(261)*M. microsoma*(Creplin,1829)
(262)*M. fausti*(Tseng,1932)
(263)*M. paramicrosoma*(Gasowska,1931)
(264)*M. tritesticulata* Fuhrmann,1907
(265)*M. mayhewi*(Tseng,1932)
(266)*M. teresoides*(Fuhrmann,1906)
(267) *M. clerci*(Tseng,1933)
(268)*M. styloides*(Fuhrmann,1906)
(269)*Microsomacanthus* sp.
(270)*M. arcuata*(Kowalewski,1904)
(271)*M. floreata*(Meggitt,1930)
(272)*M. paracompressa* Czaplinski,1956
(273)*M. carioca* Magalhaes,1898
(274)*M. parvula* (Kowalewski,1904)

83. *Rodentolepis* Spassky,1954
(275)*R. sinensis* (Oldhan,1929)
(276)*R. ximengsis* Yun et Tang,1999

84. *Hymenolepis* Weinland,1858
(277)*H. diminuta* (Rudolphi,1819)
(278)*H. nana* (Siebold,1852)
(279)*H. peipingensis* Hsü,1935
(280)*H. uralensis* Cleric,1902
(281)*H. parafola* Ling,1959
(282)*H. hipposidera* Ling,1962
(283)*Hymenolepis* sp.1 Tseng,1933
(284)*Hymenolepis* sp.2 Tseng,1933
(285)*Hymenolepis* sp.3 Tseng,1933
(286)*H. cantaniana* Polonio,1860
(287)*H. chibia* Li et. al.,1994
(288)*H. abundus* Li et. al.,1994
(289)*H. punctulata* Li et. al.,1994
(290)*H. fringillarum* Rudolphi,1809
(291)*H. recurvirostroides* Meggitt,1927
(292)*H. stylosa* Rudolphi,1809
(293)*H. amphitricha* Rudolphi,1819
(294)*H. clandestina* Krabbe,1869
(295)*H. brachycephala* Creplin,1829
(296)*H. variabile* Mayhew,1925
(297)*H. interrupta* Rudolphi,1809
(298)*H. fasciculata* Ranson,1909
(299)*H. parvula* Kowalewsky,1905
(300)*H. citelli* McLeod,1933

(301)*H. carioca* (Magalhaes,1898)
(302)*H. exigua* Yoshida,1910
(303)*H. rustica* (Meggitt,1926)

85. *Retinometra* Spassky,1955 ·
(304)*R. chinensis* Yun,1982
(305)*R. giranensis* (Sugimoto,1934)
(306)*R. venusta* (Rosseter,1897)

86. *Mayhewia* Yamaguti,1959
(307)*M. acridotheris* Cheng et Lin,1995
(308)*M. serpentulus* (Schrank,1788)

87. *Vampirolepis* Spasskii,1954
(309)*V. taiwanensis* Sawada,1984
(310)*V. copihamata* Sawada,1984
(311)*V. curvihamata* Sawada,1985
(312)*V. versihamata* Sawada,1985
(313)*V. longicollaris* Sawada,1985
(314) *V. chiangmaiensis* Sawada,1985
(315)*V. acollaris* Sawada,1985

XIII. Progynotaeniidae Burt, 1936

88. *rogynotaenia* Fuhrmann,1909
(316)*P. odhnei* Nybelin,1914

89. *Proterogynotaenia* Fuhrmann,1911
(317)*P. variabilis* Belopolskaya,1863

C. Caryophyllidea van Beneden in Carus, 1863

XIV.Lytocestidae Wardle et McLeod,1952
90. *Khawia* Hsü,1935
(318)*K. sinensis* Hsü,1935
(319)*K. tenuicollis* Li,1964
(320)*K. cyprini* Li,1964
(321)*K. japonensis* Yamaguti,1934
(322)*K. rosittensis* (Szidat,1937)

91. *Caryophyllaeides* Nybelin,1922
(*Tsengia* Li,1964)
(323)*C. neimongkuensis* (Li,1964)
(324)*C. tangi* Cheng et Lin,2002

(325)*C. xiamenensis*(Liu et.al.,1995)

92. *Lytocestus* Cohn,1908
(326)*L. adhaerens* Cohn,1908

XV. Caryophyllaeidae Leuckart, 1878
93. *Caryophyllaeus* Müeller,1787
(327)*C. parvus* Zmeev,1936
(328)*C. brachycollis* Janiszewska,1953
(329)*C. laticeps*(Pallas,1781)
(330)*C. minutus* Chen,1964

94. *Paracaryophyllaeus* Kulakovskaya,1961
(331)*P. dubininae* Kulakovskaya,1962

95. *Breviscolex* Kulakovskaya,1962
(332) *B. orientalis* Kulakovskaya,1962

D. Pseudophyllidea Carus,1863

XVI. Amphicotylidae Ariola,1899

96. *Eubothrium* Nybelin,1922
(333)*Eubothrium* sp.

XVII. Triaenophoridae (Loennberg,1889)

97. *Triaenophorus* Rudolphi,1793
(334)*T. nodulosus* (Pallas,1781)
(335)*T. crassus* Forel,1868

98. *Anchistrocephalus* Monticelli,1890
(336) *Anchistrocephalus* sp. Cheng et Liu, 2008
XVIII. Dibothriocephalidae Lühe,1902

99. *Digramma* Cholodkovsky,1915
(337)*D. interrupta*(Rudolphi,1809)
(338)*D. nemachili* Dubinina,1957

100. *Ligula*. Bloch,1782
(339) *L. intestinalis*(Goeze,1782)

101. *Bothridium* Blainville,1824
(340)*B. pythonis* Blainville,1824

102. *Diphyllobothrium* Cobbold,1858
(341)*D. fuhrmanni* Hsü,1935

103. *Spirometra* Mueller,1937
(342) *S. mansoni*(Cobbold,1883)
(343)*S. decipiens*(Diesing,1850)
(344)*S. erinacei* (Rudolphi,1819)

104. *Duthiersia* Perrier,1873
(345) *D. fimbriata* (Diesing,1850)

105. *Dibothriocephalus* Lühe,1899 ·
(346)*D. latus* (Linnaeus,1758)

XIX.Ptychobothriidae Lühe, 1902

106. *Senga* Dollfus,1934
(347)*Senga* sp.
(348)*S. ophiocephalina* (Tseng,1933)

107. *Polyonchobothrium* Diesing,1854
(349)*P. magnum* (Zmeev,1936)
(350)*P. ophiocephalina* (Tseng,1933) Dubinina,1962

XX.Bothriocephalidae (Rudolphi,1808) Lühe,1899

108. *Bothriocephalus* (Rudolphi,1808)Lühe,1899
(351) *B. scorpii* (Müeller,1776)
(352) *B. brachysoma* Wang,1977
(353)*B. gowkongensis* Yeh,1955
(354)*B. japonicus* Yamaguti,1934
(355)*B. opsariichthydis* Yammaguti,1934
(356)*B. sinensis* Chen,1964
(357)*Bothriocephalus* sp.

109. *Taphrobothrium* Lühe,1899
(358)*T. japonensis* Lühe,1899

110. *Oncodiscus* Yamaguti,1934
(359)*O. sauridae* Yamaguti,1934

XXI. Parabothriocephalidae Yamaguti, 1959

101. *Parabothriocephaloides* Yamaguti,1934
(360)*Parabothriocephaloides* sp. Wang et. al.,2001

112. *Parabothriocephalus* Yamaguti,1934
(361)*P. gracilis* Yamaguti,1934

XXII.Echinophallidae Schumacher, 1914

113. *Echinophallus* Schmacher,1914
(362)*E. japonicus*(Yamaguti,1934)

E. Tetraphyllidea Carus,1863

XXIII. Phyllobothridae Braun, 1900

114. *Phyllobothrium* Beneden,1849
(363)*P. lactuca* Beneden,1850
(364)*P. laciniatum*(Linton,1889)
(365)*P. loculatum* Yamaguti,1952
(366)*P. tumidum* Linton,1922
(367)*P. ptychocephalum* Wang,1984

115. *Dinobothrium* Beneden,1889
(368)*D. septaria* Beneden,1889

116. *Echeneibothrium* Benoden,1850
(369)*E. hui* Tseng,1933
(370)*E. variabile* Beneden,1850

117. *Anthobothrium* Beneden,1850
(371)*A. bifidum* Yamaguti,1952
(372)*A. parvum* Stossich,1895
(373)*A. pteroplateae* Yamaguti,1952

118. *Rhodobothrium* Linyon,1889
(374)*R. palvinatum* Linton,1889

119. *Rhinebothrium* Euzet,1953
(375)*R. xiamenensis* Wang et al.,2001

120. *Pithophorus* Southwell,1925
(376)*P. musculosus* Subhaparadha,1957

XXIV.Onchobothridae Braun, 1900

121. *Acanthobothrium* Beneden,1850
(377)*A. coronatum* (Rudolphi,1819)Beneden,1849
(378)*A. benedeni* Loennberg,1889
(379)*A. grandiceps* Yamaguti,1952

(380)*A. ijimai* Yoshida,1917
(381)*A. microcantha* Yamaguti,1952
(382)*A. tsingtaoensis* Tseng,1933
(383)*A. pingtanensis* Wang,1984
(384)*A. xiamenensis* Yang,1994
(385)*A. zugeimensis* Yang,1994
(386)*A. polytesticularis* Wang et al.,2001

F. Trypanorhyncha Diesing,1863

XXV. Otobothriidae Dollfus, 1942

122. *Otobothrium* Linton,1890
(387)*O. linstowi* Southwell,1912
(388)*Otobothrium* sp.

123. *Tetrarhynchus* Shipley et Hornell,1906
(389)*T. equidentata* Shipley et Hornell,1906

XXVI. Hornelliellidae Yamaguti,1954

124. *Hornelliella* Yamaguti,1954
(390)*H. musteli* Wang et al.,2001

XXVII. Gymnorhynchidae Dollfus,1935

125. *Gymnorhychus* Rudolphi,1819
(391)*Gymnorhychus* sp. Wang et al.,2001

XXVIII. Eutetrarhynchidae (Guiart,1927)

126. *Eutetrarhynchus* Pintner,1913
(392)*Eutetrarhynchus* sp. Wang et al.,2001

XXIX. Tentaculariidae Poch, 1926

127. *Nybelinia* Poch,1926
(393)*N. rhyncobatus* Yang et al,1995

XXX. Grillotiidae Dollfus, 1969

128. *Grillotia* Guiart,1927
(394)*G. dollfusi* Carvajal,1976

G. Lecanicephalidea Baylis,1920

XXXI. Lecanicephalidae Braun,1900

129. *Lecanicephalum* Linton,1890
(395)*L. xiamenensis* Liu et.al.,1995
(396)*L. peltatum* Linton,1890

130. *Cephalobothrium* Shipley et Hornell,1906
(397)*C. longisegmentum* Wang,1984

XXX. Tetragonocephalidae Yamaguti,1952

131. *Tetragonocephalum* Shipley et Hornell,1905
(398)*T. akajeienesis* Yang et. al.,1995

H. Spathebothriidea Wardle et McLeod, 1952

XXXII. Cyathocephalidae Nybelin, 1922

132. *Cyathocephalus* Kessler,1868
(399)*C.truncatus* (Pallas,1781)

133. *Schyzocotyle* Achmerov,1960
(400) *S. fluviatilies* Achmerov,1960

I. Nippotaeniidea Yamaguti,1939

XXXIII. Nippotaeniidae Yamaguti, 1939

134. *Amurotaenia* Achmerov,1941
(401)*N. percotti* Achmerov,1941

135. *Nippotaenia* Yamaguti,1939
(402) *N. mogurndae* Yamaguti et Miyata,1940

5. Reference

Cai XP and Jin JS. 1984. Studies on the lifecycle of *Moniezia benedeni*. *Chinese Journal of Veterinary Science and Technology*, 12,26-30

Cheng GH. 2002. *Studies on the cestodes in China*. China women publishing house. Beining:3~49

Cheng GH, Wu ZH and Lin Y. 2008. The experimental development of *Ophiotaenia monnigi* Fuhrmann, 1924 in Cyclops leuckarti. *Parasitol Res*:875~878

Li M. et Arai,H. P. 1991. On the ultrastructure of the scolex tegument, organelles and sensory receptors of *Gloridacris catostomi* Cooper (Cestoda: Caryophyllidea). *Acta Zoologica Sinica*, 37(2) : 113~122

Liao XH & Lun ZR. 1998. Taxonomy and relatives studies for *Bothriocephalus opsariichthydis* parasitic in grass carp, carp and opsariichthyd in China. *Science Bulletin*, 43(10): 1073~1076.

Liao XH et Shi LZ. 1956. A fry disease of Guangdong, the life-cycle,ecology and prevention of *Bothriocephalus gowkongensis*. *Bulletin of hydrobiology*. 2: 129~186.

Lin Yuguang,1979. Catalog of Cestodes in China, memoir of the meeting for Cestoda fauna in China

Lin Y. 1962a, Studies on the development of *Moniezia expansa* (Rudolphi,1810) and its intermediate host. *Journal of Fujian Normal College*. 2:45~68.

Lin Y. 1962b, Comparative studies on the development of cysticercoid for *Hymenolepis expansa* and *H. nana* within the intermediate hosts. *Journal of Fujian Normal College*. 2:263~283.

Lin Y., and Guan JZ, Wang PP and Yang WC.1982. Studies on the developmental cycle of *Paranoplocephala ryjikovi* Spassky,1950 in the intermediate host. *Acta Zoologica Sinica*,28(3): 262~271

Lin, Y. and Hong LX. 1986. Studies on the life cycle of Ctenotaenia citelli (Kirshenblat) and Mosgovoyia pectinata (Goeze). *Acta Zoologica Sinica*, 32 (2): 144-151

Su XZ & Lin Y. 1987. Studies on the developmental cycle of cestodes from domestic ducks and geese in Xiamen, China. *Acta Zoologica Sinica*,33(4) :334~340.

Tang C. C. (Tang Zhongzhang).1982. Developmental studies on Polyonchobothrium ophiocephalina (Tseng, 1933) and bothriocephalus opsariichthydis Yamaguti, 1934. *Acta Zoologica Sinica*,28(1): 53~59.

Zhao WX. editor in chief, 1983. *Human Parasitology*, People's medical publishing house. Beijing: 484~491.

7

Soft Ticks as Pathogen Vectors: Distribution, Surveillance and Control

Raúl Manzano-Román[1], Verónica Díaz-Martín[1], José de la Fuente[2,3] and Ricardo Pérez-Sánchez[1]
[1]*Instituto de Recursos Naturales y Agrobiología de Salamanca (IRNASA-CSIC)*
[2]*Instituto de Investigación en Recursos Cinegéticos IREC (CSIC-UCLM-JCCM)*
[3]*Veterinary Pathobiology Department, Oklahoma State University, Stillwater*
[1,2]*Spain*
[3]*USA*

1. Introduction

Ticks are highly specialized obligate haematophagous ectoparasites of mammals, birds and reptiles. Ticks are distributed worldwide and are of enormous medical and veterinary relevance owing to the direct damage they cause to their hosts and, especially, because they are vectors of a large variety of human and animal pathogens. In fact, ticks are second to mosquitoes as vectors of human pathogens and the most important vectors of pathogens affecting cattle worldwide (Peter et al., 2005). In humans, tick infestations typically involve few specimens and the greatest risk for people bitten by a tick lies in infection due to a tick-borne pathogen (Parola & Raoul, 2001). Such pathogens are diverse and include viruses, bacteria, and protozoa (Jongejan & Uilenberg, 2004; de la Fuente et al., 2008a). In animals, tick infestations are much more severe than in humans. Animals can be parasitized by hundreds or even thousands of ticks, which obviously multiplies the effect on the host, either by direct injuries or disease transmission. Direct injuries to animals can be very serious, especially in tropical climates, and are mainly observed in infestations with ixodid ticks but also in infestations with some argasid ticks as *Ornithodoros lahorensis* and *O. savignyi* (Hoogstraal, 1985). The most frequent of these direct forms of damage include: (i) tissue destruction caused by the tick mouth parts and by the local inflammatory reaction of host to tick saliva; (ii) loss of blood, which in massive infestations can cause acute anaemia; (iii) paralyses caused by salivary toxins, such as the holocyclotoxin from the Australian tick *Ixodes holocyclus*, a tick species that can paralyze and kill a young animal with only one female bite; (iv) toxicoses, such as the Sweating sickness caused by the African *Hyalomma truncatum;* in ruminants this disease elicits eczematous skin lesions, hyperexcretion of exudates and more than 75% mortality in young animals, and (v) immunosuppression, which renders animals more susceptible to pathogen transmission (Mans et al., 2008a). All these direct forms of damage together with tick-transmitted diseases (including Babesiosis, Theileriosis, Anaplasmosis and Cowdriosis) cause important economic losses to the livestock industry, mainly affecting tropical and subtropical countries, where ticks constitute one of the main difficulties for the development of the livestock breeding industry (Jongejan and Uilenberg, 2004; Rajput et al., 2006).

Tick species can be grouped in two main families, the Argasidae or soft ticks, and the Ixodidae or hard ticks. A third tick family, Nuttalliellidae, only has one species, *Nuttalliella namaqua*. These three families share common basic properties that are modified distinctively inside each family according to their particular behaviour patterns and life-style (Hoogstraal, 1985).

The family Argasidae includes some 193 species, but their phylogeny and taxonomy is as yet controversial, the genus-level classification of the family Argasidae being much less settled than that of the Ixodidae (Estrada-Peña et al., 2010), and most species of Argasidae can be assigned to more than one genus. A discussion of these issues is out of the scope of this review and the reader is referred to recent papers addressing them (Nava et al., 2009a; Guglielmone et al., 2010).

Argasid ticks differ from ixodids in a range of morphological and biological characteristics. Typically, argasids do not possess a dorsal shield or scutum; their capitulum is less prominent and ventrally -instead anteriorly- located; their coxae are unarmed (without spurs), and their spiracular plates are small. In Argasidae, there are more than four developmental stages in the life cycle: egg, larva, several nymphal stages, and adult. Nymphs have from two to eight separate instars. The exact number of instars varies according to the species and its future sex when adult. It is also influenced by the individual's state of nutrition. Argasids tend to be endophilic/nidicolous parasites that colonize the nests and burrows of their hosts and feed when the host arrives. In contrast, ixodids are mostly exophilic ticks that actively seek hosts when the seasons are suitable, although examples of nidicolous ixodid ticks also exist, especially among species of the genus *Ixodes*.

Some soft tick species exhibit extremely rigid host specificity. However, it has been suggested that most soft ticks show indiscriminate host feeding and such apparent variation in host preference probably reflects microhabitat preference and host availability within the microhabitat (Vial, 2009). Most argasids are fast feeders, ingesting a relatively small amount of blood per meal and adult specimens can feed and reproduce repeatedly. Argasids are very resistant to starvation and can survive for several years without feeding (Sonenshine, 1992). This, and their diapause periods, affords them great flexibility in their developmental cycles (Vial, 2009).

Argasid distribution can be considered cosmopolitan since they can be found throughout the world with the exception of places showing extreme conditions, although specimens have been found in Sub-Antarctic biogeographical regions (Estrada-Peña et al., 2003). The distribution of each particular species is more limited, but it may be very extensive, depending on factors such as the adaptability of each particular species to new ecological environments, the dissemination of immature phases by migratory birds, and the ability of adult specimens to infest different host species. It is therefore possible that species that have never been identified on one continent can be imported from different continents, and that new species can be identified in different parts of the world, contributing to a geographic distribution of soft tick species in constant evolution. Changes in argasid distribution are more difficult to predict than those of ixodids and currently no distribution models have yet been published for them. However, investigations are in progress, suggesting that soft tick distribution modelling is also possible. This modelling is based on the natural niche concept and takes into account the influence of climatic factors and the particularities of soft ticks, including their nidicolous lifestyle, indiscriminate host feeding, and a flexible developmental cycle along diapause periods (Vial, 2009). In this context, the development of new methods for systematic soft tick surveillance, i.e. serological methods, would help to monitor soft tick occurrence and the prediction of their distribution and its evolution. Table 1 offers information about the known distribution of a number of argasid species grouped by biogeographical regions (Udvardy, 1975). It should be noted that this table does not aim to be exhaustive but simply illustrative and that it might contain unconfirmed reports and some controversial species names.

Species	Localization	Hosts	References
Paleartic region			
Argas abdussalami	Pakistan	Birds	Ghosh et al. (2007)
Argas arboreus	Israel	Cattle, birds	Belozerov et al. (2003)
Argas assimilis	China	Livestock	Chen et al. (2010)
Argas beijingensis	China	Livestock	Chen et al. (2010)
Argas miniatus	Portugal	Poultry	Lisbôa et al. (2009),
Argas japonicus	China, Japan	Livestock, poultry	Chen et al. (2010), Yamaguti et al. (1968)
Argas persicus	Spain, Italy, Iran, Pakistan, China, Russian Federation	Birds, poultry, livestock	Cordero del Campillo et al. (1994), Pantaleoni et al. (2010), Ntiamoa-Baidu et al. (2004), Keirans & Durden (2001), Ghosh et al. (2007), Chen et al. (2010), Dikaev (1981)
Argas polonicus	Poland	Birds	Siuda (1996)
Argas pusillus	Tadzhikistan, Kyrgyzstan, Turkmenistan	Bats, humans	Gavrilovskaya (2001), de la Fuente et al. (2008a)
Argas reflexus	Poland, Italy, France, Spain, Iran, Pakistan, Russian Federation	Humans, birds	Karbowiak & Supergan (2007), Poggiato (2008), Gilot & Pautou (1982), Cordero del Campillo et al. (1994), Ntiamoa-Baidu et al. (2004), Siuda (1996), Ghosh et al. (2007), Dikaev (1981)
Argas robertsi	China	Birds	Chen et al. (2010)
Argas vespertilionis	Sweden, Portugal, Great Britain, Germany, Pakistan, Tadzhikistan, Kyrgyzstan, Turkmenistan, Russian Federation	Bats, humans, livestock	Jaenson et al. (1994), Caeiro (1999), Hubbard et al. (1998), Gavrilovskaya (2001), de la Fuente et al. (2008a), Cornely & Schultz (1992), Ghosh et al. (2007), Dikaev (1981)
Argas vulgaris	China, Russian Federation	Livestock	Chen et al. (2010), Dikaev (1981)
Carios capensis	Great Britain, Croatia, Spain, China, Torishima Island, Japan	Seabirds	Converse et al. (1975), Reeves et al. (2006), Ushijima et al. (2003), Chen et al. (2010)

Species	Localization	Hosts	References
Carios pusillus	China	Livestock	Chen et al. (2010)
Carios sinensis	China	Livestock	Chen et al. (2010)
Carios vespertilionis	China	Livestock	Chen et al. (2010)
Ornithodoros alactagalis	Armenia, Azerbaijan, Georgia, Iran, Northern Caucasus, Transcaucasia, Turkey	NR	Filippova (1966)
Ornithodoros asperus	Caucasus, Iraq	Humans, rodents	Assous and Wilamowski (2009), Parola & Raoult (2001)
Ornithodoros coniceps	Italy, France, Spain, Israel, Jordan, Egypt, Afghanistan, Ukraine,	Pigeons	Hoogstraal et al. (1979), Khoury et al. (2011), Ghosh et al. (2007)
Ornithodoros erraticus	Portugal, Spain, Greece, Italy, Cyprus, Algeria, Egypt, Tunisia, Morocco, Iraq, Iran	Humans, pigs	Caeiro (1999), Oleaga-Pérez et al (1990), Parola & Raoult (2001), EFSA (2010a)
Ornithodoros lahorensis	Armenia, Kazakhstan, Russian Federation, Kosovo, Syria, Turkey, Iran, China	Cattle	Moemenbellah-Fard et al (2009), Ahmed et al. (2007), Chen et al. (2010), Ghosh et al. (2007), Aydin & Bakirci (2007), EFSA (2010c), Dikaev (1981)
Ornithodoros maritimus	Portugal, Italy	Seabirds	Caeiro (1999), Manilla (1990)
Ornithodoros pavlovsky	Kazakhstan, Kirghizia, Tajikistan, Turkmenistan, Uzbekistan	Mammals	Filippova (1966)
Ornithodoros savignyi	Egypt	Camel, sheep, goat, cow, buffalo	Helmy (2000)
Ornithodoros sonrai	Morocco, Libya, Egypt, Turkey , Iran	Domestic and sylvatic pigs	Vial et al. (2006), Vial (2009)
Ornithodoros tartakowskyi	Iran, central Asia, China	Humans	Parola & Raoult (2001), Chen et al. (2010)
Ornithodoros tholozani	Cyprus, Daghestan, Egypt, Iraq, Iran, China, Israel, Jordan, Kazakhstan, Kyrgyzstan, Lebanon, Libya, Syria, Turkey, Ukraine, USSR	Humans, livestock	Moemenbellah-Fard et al. (2009), Assous et al. (2009), Chen et al. (2010)
Ornithodoros verrucosus	Armenia, Georgia, Russian Federation	NR	Maruashvili (1965), Gugushvili (1972), Dikaev (1981)

Species	Localization	Hosts	References
Afrotropical region			
Argas africolumbae	Kenya, Tanzania, South and South-West Africa	Birds	Hoogstraal et al. (1977)
Argas arboreus	South Africa	Cattle, birds	Mumcuoglu et al. (2005)
Argas persicus	Ghana	Poultry	Ntiamoa-Baidu et al. (2004), Jongejan & Uilenberg (2004)
Argas reflexus	Ghana	Humans, poultry	Ntiamoa-Baidu et al. (2004), Siuda (1996), Jongejan & Uilenberg (2004)
Argas walkerae	South Africa	Poultry	Nyangiwe et al. (2008)
Argas vespertilionis	Ghana	Bats	Ntiamoa-Baidu et al. (2004)
Carios capensis	Indic ocean islands	Seabirds	Converse et al. (1975)
Ornithodoros compactus	South Africa	Tortoises	Horak et al. (2006)
Ornithodoros coniceps	Kenya	Pigeons	Hoogstraal et al. (1979)
Ornithodoros coriaceus	Africa	Domestic and sylvatic pigs	Labuda & Nuttall (2004), de la Fuente et al. (2008a)
Ornithodoros graingeri	Africa	Humans	Parola & Raoult (2001)
Ornithodoros moubata	Central and South Africa	Humans, domestic and sylvatic pigs	Ntiamoa-Baidu et al. (2004), Parola & Raoult (2001)
Ornithodoros porcinus	Southern and East Africa	Humans, domestic and sylvatic pigs	Bastos et al. (2009), Mitani et al. (2004)
Ornithodoros savignyi	Kenya, Central and South Africa	Livestock, humans	Walton (1951), Howell (1966), Hoogstraal (1985)
Ornithodoros sonrai	Kenya, Mauritania, Senegal, Mali, Gambia	Domestic and sylvatic pigs	Vial et al. (2006), Vial (2009)
Ornithodoros turicata	Africa	Domestic and sylvatic pigs	Labuda & Nuttall (2004), de la Fuente et al. (2008a)
Ornithodoros zumpti	Africa	Humans	Rebaudet & Parola (2006)
Neartic region			
Argas cooleyi	USA	Humans	Calisher et al. (1988)
Argas monolakensis	Mono Lake (USA)	Humans	Schwan et al. (1992)
Argas persicus	USA	Poultry	Keirans et al. (2001)
Carios capensis	Hawaii, South Carolina, and Texas (USA)	Seabirds	Reeves et al. (2006), Rawlings (1995)
Ornithodoros coriaceus	California, Oregon and Nevada (USA)	Cattle	Teglas et al. (2006), Failing et al. (1972)

Species	Localization	Hosts	References
Ornithodoros hermsi	USA, Canada	Humans	Dana (2009), Schwan et al. (2007), Parola & Raoult (2001)
Ornithodoros kelleyi	USA	Bats, humans	Cilek & Knapp (1992)
Ornithodoros parkeri	USA, Canada	Human	Dana (2009), Dworkin et al. (2002)
Ornithodoros puertoricensis	USA	Reptiles	Venzal et al. (2006, 2008), Bermúdez et al. (2010)
Ornithodoros rossi	USA	Bats	Steinlein et al. (2001)
Ornithodoros talaje	USA	Rodents, domestic animals, humans	Parola & Raoult (2001)
Ornithodoros turicata	USA, Canada	Humans, dogs, tortoises	Dana (2009), Dworkin et al. (2008), Whitney et al. (2007), Adeyeye et al. (1989)
Otobius megnini	USA	Humans, cattle	Nava et al. (2006, 2009b)
Neotropical region			
Antricola delacruzi	Brazil	Bats	Labruna et al. (2008)
Antricola guglielmonei	Brazil	Bats	Labruna et al. (2008)
Argas dulus	Dominican Republic	Birds	Keirans et al. (1971)
Argas keiransi	Chile	Birds	Estrada-Peña et al. (2003, 2006)
Argas persicus	Paraguay	Poultry, birds, livestock	Nava et al. (2007)
Argas miniatus	Paraguay, Chile, Brazil	Pultry	González-Acuña & Guglielmone (2005), Nava et al. (2007), Ataliba et al. (2007)
Argas monachus	Argentina, Paraguay	Birds	Keirans et al. (1973), Nava et al. (2007)
Argas neghmei	Argentina, Chile	Poultry, humans	Di Iorio et al. (2010)
Carios mimon	Bolivia, Uruguay, Brazil	Bats, humans	Barros-Battesti et al. (2011)
Nothoaspis amazoniensis	Brazil	Bats	Nava et al. (2010)
Ornithodoros rioplatensis	Uruguay, Argentina, Chile	NR	Venzal et al. (2008)
Ornithodoros amblus	Peru, Chile	Birds	Clifford et al. (1980), Need et al. (1991)
Ornithodoros brasiliensis	Brazil	Humans	Martins et al. (2011)
Ornithodoros coriaceus	Mexico	Humans	Failing et al. (1972)

Species	Localization	Hosts	References
Ornithodoros hasei	Paraguay	NR	Nava et al. (2007)
Ornithodoros hermsi	Mexico	Humans	Dana (2009), Schwan et al. (2007), Parola & Raoult (2001)
Ornithodoros marinkellei	Colombia, Panama, Venezuela, Guyana, Brazil	Bats	Labruna et al. (2011)
Ornithodoros parkeri	Mexico	Humans	Dana (2009), Dworkin et al. (2002)
Ornithodoros puertoricensis	México, Guatemala, Nicaragua, Panama, Colombia, Venezuela, Paraguay , Jamaica, Dominican Republic, Puerto Rico, Haiti	Reptiles	Nava et al. (2007), Venzal et al. (2006, 2008), Bermúdez et al. (2010), Endris et al. (1989)
Ornithodoros rondoniensis	Brazil	Bats	Labruna et al. (2008)
Ornithodoros rostratus	Paraguay, Brazil, Argentina	Reptiles	Venzal et al. (2006), Martins et al. (2011), Guglielmone et al. (2003)
Ornithodoros rudis	Paraguay	Humans	Parola & Raoult (2001)
Ornithodoros spheniscus	Chile	Penguins	González-Acuña & Guglielmone (2005)
Ornithodoros talaje	México, Brazil, Chile[1]	Rodents, domestic animals, humans	Tizu et al. (1995), Parola & Raoult (2001), González-Acuña & Guglielmone (2005)
Ornithodoros turicata	Mexico	Human	Dana (2009)
Ornithodoros yunkeri	Galapagos Islands	Seabirds	Keirans et al. (1984)
Otobius megnini	Argentina, Chile	Humans, cattle	Nava et al. (2006, 2009b)
Oriental region (Indomalayan)			
Argas abdussalami[1]	India	Livestock	Ghosh et al. (2007)
Argas gujaratensis[1,2]	India	Bats	Ghosh et al. (2007)
Argas hermanni	India	Birds	Ghosh et al. (2007)
Argas hoogstraali[1]	India	Bats, wild mammals	Ghosh et al. (2007)
Argas indicus[1,2]	India	Bats, wild mammals	Ghosh et al. (2007)
Argas japonicus	China, Korea	Livestock, poultry	Chen et al. (2010), Yamaguti et al. (1968)
Argas persicus	India, Bangladesh	Poultry, birds, livestock	Keirans et al. (2001), Ntiamoa-Baidu et al. (2004), Ghosh et al. (2007)

Species	Localization	Hosts	References
Argas robertsi	Taiwan, Thailand, India, Indonesia, Sri Lanka	Birds	Hoogstraal et al. (1975), Ghosh et al. (2007)
Argas soneshinei[1,2]	India	Livestock	Ghosh et al. (2007)
Argas vespertilionis	India	Livestock, bats, humans	Gavrilovskaya (2001), Ghosh et al. (2007), de la Fuente et al. (2008a)
Argas wilsoni[1,2]	India	Bats	Ghosh et al. (2007)
Carios batuensis	Indonesia	Bats	Durden et al. (2008)
Carios chiropterphila[1,2]	India	Bats	Ghosh et al. (2007)
Carios faini[1]	India	Bats, wild mammals	Ghosh et al. (2007)
Ornithodoros coniceps	India	Pigeons	Hoogstraal et al. (1979), Ghosh et al. (2007)
Ornithodoros crossi[2]	India	Livestock	Ghosh et al. (2007)
Ornithodoros lahorensis	India	Cattle	Moemenbellah-Fard et al. (2009), Ahmed et al. (2007), Ghosh et al. (2007)
Ornithodoros piriformis[1]	India	Bats	Ghosh et al. (2007)
Ornithodoros savignyi	India	Livestock	Ghosh et al. (2007)
Ornithodoros tholozani	India, Kashmir	Human	Moemenbellah-Fard et al . (2009), Assous & Wilamowski (2009)
Otobius megnini	India	Humans, cattle, dogs	Nava et al. (2006, 2009b), Ghosh et al. (2007)
Australian			
Argas persicus	Southern Australia	Poultry	Petney et al. (2004)
Argas robertsi	Australia	Birds	Hoogstraal et al. (1975)
Carios capensis	Heron island, Australia	Humans	Humphery-Smith et al. (1991)

Table 1. Soft tick distribution ordered by biogeographical regions (historical records). [1]Need confirmation; [2]controversial name. NR, not reported.

2. Pathogens and infectious diseases transmitted by soft ticks

Ticks are among the most competent and versatile arthropod vectors of pathogens. Today, most emerging infectious diseases arise from zoonotic pathogens, and many of them are transmitted by arthropod vectors. Tick-borne infectious diseases are a growing and very serious world health problem and a major obstacle for animal health and production (Rajput et al., 2006). For example, in the United States Lyme disease is transmitted by *Ixodes* ticks and it has become the most common arthropod-borne infectious disease in that country (Díaz, 2009). In Europe, important pathogens transmitted by ticks are *Borrelia* spp.,

Anaplasma spp., *Rickettsia* spp., *Babesia* spp., Tick borne Encephalitis Virus (TBEV), and Crimean-Congo Haemorrhagic Fever Virus (CCHFV) (Heyman et al., 2010). In Africa, tick-borne diseases and tick infestations are among the most commonly documented causes of morbidity (Phiri et al., 2010).

Regarding the pathogens transmitted by argasid ticks, they are mainly viruses together with a number of bacterial species, and they cause severe diseases in humans and animals. The currently recognized viral diseases transmitted by soft ticks are shown in Table 2. Among them, African swine fever (ASF) has received particular attention and will be used as a model in this review. The argasid-borne bacteria are almost exclusively borreliae, which cause relapsing fever in humans (Table 3). Other potential argasid-borne pathogens that have been transmitted experimentally are shown in Table 4. Finally, most vector specimens also contain a range of non-pathogenic microorganisms that can also be transmitted to the host in the tick saliva, some of them also being included in Table 4.

2.1 African swine fever virus

The African swine fever virus (ASFV) belongs to the Asfarviridae family of arboviruses and represents the only known DNA arbovirus to date (Kleiboeker & Scoles, 2001; Labuda & Nuttall, 2008). It affects only porcine species and causes African swine fever (ASF), highly lethal to pigs, which is one of the most important viral diseases of swine included in the A list of the OIE (http://www.oie.int/en/animal-health-in-the-world/oie-listed-diseases-2011/).

In nature ASFV circulates in two types of enzootic cycles -sylvatic and domestic- both of which involve porcine hosts and argasid ticks of the genus *Ornithodoros*, including *O. moubata*, *O. porcinus*, *O. savignyi*, and *O. sonrai* in Africa; members of the *O. erraticus* complex on the Iberian Peninsula, the trans-Caucasus countries and the Russian Federation, and *O. coriaceus*, *O. turicata*, *O. parkeri* and *O. puertoricensis* in North America and the Caribbean (Kleiboeker & Scoles, 2001; Labuda & Nuttall, 2008). The virus replicates in the tissues of these tick species and, depending on the species, can be transmitted transstadially, transovarially and sexually (EFSA panel, 2010c). Among the Old World species, transovarial, transstadial and sexual transmission of ASFV have been described in *O. moubata*; transstadial and sexual transmission have been demonstrated for *O. erraticus* (Endris & Hess, 1994) and only transstadial transmission has been demonstrated for *O. savignyi*. Among the New World species, the transstadial transmission of ASFV has only been demonstrated for *O. coriaceus* and *O. parkeri*, and transovarial transmission has only been demonstrated for *O. puertoricensis* (Kleiboeker & Scoles, 2001). Thus, it can be said that all *Ornithodoros* species investigated so far (i.e., those mentioned above) can become readily infected by ASF, and all of them, except *O. parkeri* (EFSA, 2010c), can also transmit the virus to pigs, thereby playing a potential role not only as reservoirs but also as active biological vectors of ASFV. Interestingly, in spite of evidence suggesting that *O. puertoricensis* could be an efficient vector for ASFV, the presence of this tick in Haiti and the Dominican Republic did not appear to complicate the eradication of ASF from those countries in 1978. This was probably due to a lack of contact between infected pigs and *O. puertoricensis*, since the Dominican Republic II strain of ASFV (one of the strains isolated from that epizootic outbreak) was shown to be capable of infecting and being transmitted by these ticks under experimental conditions (Kleiboeker & Scoles, 2001). Other *Ornithodoros* species remain untested for ASFV infection and transmission and the possibility that they might play some kind of role in the epidemiology of ASF cannot be ruled out.

Soft tick species	Virus	References
Argas robertsi	Kao Shuan virus, Pathum Thani virus, Nyamanini virus, Lake Clarendon virus	Hoogstraal et al. (1975), Hoogstraal (1985), Labuda & Nuttall (2008)
Argas abdussalami	Manawa virus, Bakau virus, Uukuniemi virus	Hoogstraal (1985), Labuda & Nuttall (2008)
Argas africolumbae	Pretoria virus	Labuda & Nuttall (2008)
Argas arboreus	West Nile virus, Quaranfil virus, Nyamanini virus	Hoogstraal (1985), Mumcuoglu et al. (2005)
Argas cooleyi	Mono Lake virus, Sixgun virus, Sapphire II virus, Sunday Canyon virus	Hoogstraal (1985), Calisher et al. (1988), Vermeil et al. (1996), Labuda & Nuttall (2008), de la Fuente et al. (2008a),
Argas hermanni	Chenuda virus, Abu Hammad virus, Royal Farm virus, West Nile virus, Grand Arbaud virus, Nyamanini virus, Quaranfil virus	Hoogstraal (1985), Labuda & Nuttall (2008)
Argas monolakensis	Mono Lake Virus	Schwan et al. (1992), Vermeil et al. (1996), de la Fuente et al. (2008a)
Argas persicus	CCHF virus	Hoogstraal (1985)
Argas pusillus	Issyk-Kul Fever virus	Gavrilovskaya (2001), de la Fuente et al. (2008a)
Argas reflexus	Uukuniemi virus, CCHF virus	Labuda & Nuttall (2008), Tahmasebi et al. (2010)
Argas vespertilionis	Issyk-Kul Fever virus, Sokuluk virus	Hoogstraal (1985), Gavrilovskaya (2001), de la Fuente et al. (2008a)
Carios amblus	Mono lake virus	Labuda & Nuttall (2008)
Carios capensis	Upolu virus, Nyaminini virus, Quaranfil virus, Saumarez Reef vírus, Soldado vírus, Hughes virus	Converse et al. (1975), Hoogstraal (1985), Labuda & Nuttall (2004, 2008)
Carios maritimus	Chenuda virus, West Nile virus	Labuda & Nuttall (2008)
Carios spp.	Chobar Gorge virus	Labuda & Nuttall (2008)
OME/CTVM21 O. moubata cells	Karshi and Langat virus	Bell-Sakyi et al. (2009)
Ornithodoros amblus	Huacho virus, Punta Salinas virus	Hoogstraal (1985)
Ornithodoros coniceps	Baku virus	Hoogstraal et al. (1979)
Ornithodoros coriaceus	ASFV[1], Bluetongue virus	Groocock et al. (1980), Stott et al. (1985), Kleiboeker et al. (1998), Labuda & Nuttall (2004), de la Fuente et al. (2008a)
Ornithodoros denmarki	Soldado virus, Hughes virus, Raza virus, Quaranfil group	Labuda & Nuttall (2004), de la Fuente et al. (2008a)

Soft tick species	Virus	References
Ornithodoros erraticus	Qalyub virus (QYB), ASFV	Miller et al. (1985), Labuda & Nuttall (2004, 2008), Basto et al. (2006), de la Fuente et al. (2008a)
Ornithodoros kohlsi	Matucare virus	Labuda & Nuttall (2008)
Ornithodoros lagophilus	Colorado tick fever virus	Sonenshine et al. (2002)
Ornithodoros lahorensis	CCHF virus	Hoogstraal (1985), Telmadarraiy et al. (2010)
Ornithodoros maritimus	Soldado virus	Labuda & Nuttall (2004), de la Fuente et al. (2008a)
Ornithodoros moubata	ASFV, West Nile virus, HIV[2,3] Hepatitis B virus[1]	Haresnape & Wilkinson (1989), Labuda & Nuttall (2004, 2008), de la Fuente et al. (2008a), Lawrie et al. (2004), Shepherd et al. (1989), Durden et al. (1993), Humphery-Smith et al. (1993), Jupp et al. (1987)
Ornithodoros parkeri	ASFV[1], Karshi and Langat virus	Kleiboeker & Scoles (2001), Turell et al. (1994, 2004)
Ornithodoros porcinus	ASFV	Kleiboeker et al. (1998), Bastos et al. (2009)
Ornithodoros puertoricensis	ASFV[1]	Endris et al. (1991), Kleiboeker et al. (1998), Labuda & Nuttall (2004), de la Fuente et al. (2008a)
Ornithodoros savignyi	AHF virus, Bluetongue virus[1], ASFV[1]	Kleiboeker et al. (1998), Charrel et al. (2007), Bouwknegt et al. (2010)
Ornithodoros sonrai	Karshi and Langat virus, ASFV, Bandia virus	Turell et al. (1994, 2004), Vial et al. (2007), Labuda & Nuttall (2008)
Ornithodoros tadaridae	Estero Real virus	Málková et al. (1985), Labuda & Nuttall (2008)
Ornithodoros tartakovskyi	Karshi and Langat virus	Turell et al. (2004)
Ornithodoros tholozani	Karshi and Langat virus	Labuda & Nuttall (2008)
Ornithodoros turicata	ASFV[1]	Hess et al. (1987), Kleiboeker et al. (1998), Labuda & Nuttall (2004), de la Fuente et al. (2008a)
Otobius lagophilus	Colorado tick fever group	Hoogstraal (1985)

Table 2. Viruses transmitted by or associated to soft ticks. AHF, Alkhurma hemorrhagic fever virus; CCHF, Crimean Congo haemorraghic fever; ASFV, African swine fever virus; QYB, Qalyub virus. [1]Experimental infection; [2]laboratory transmission; [3]mechanical transmission.

The pathogenesis of ASFV in Old World *Ornithodoros* tick species is characterized by a low infectious dose, lifelong infection, and low mortality until after the first oviposition; by contrast, in New World *Ornithodoros* ticks species relatively high nymphal mortality has been reported after infection, and infection does not appear to be lifelong, although it is not known whether the reduction in the number of infected ticks with time is due to differential mortality or to loss of infection (Kleiboeker & Scoles, 2001). In general, *Ornithodoros* ticks have a long life span, and some species can survive up to 15-20 years in their adult stage. Consequently, ASFV-infected soft tick populations can maintain this virus for years, although they do not seem to play an active role in the spreading of the virus over long distances. Recently, *O. erraticus* specimens collected from pig farms in Portugal more than five years after the removal of infectious hosts showed the presence of the virus and the experimental transmissibility of these persistent infections, highlighting the epidemiological role of *O. erraticus* ticks in the persistence of ASFV in the field (Boinas et al., 2011).

The epidemiological role played by soft ticks becomes important when domestic pigs are managed under traditional systems, in which pigs range freely in wild or peridomestic habitats and may enter into contact with ticks. Ticks feed mainly on wild hosts living in burrows and pigs are mostly accidental hosts. The mechanism of ASFV transmission from the sylvatic cycle to domestic pigs is probably through infected ticks feeding on pigs.

ASF affects only porcine species. Wild boars have been shown to be susceptible to ASFV infection in Sardinia (Italy), Spain and Portugal, showing similar clinical signs and case-fatality rates. This was also the case for experimentally infected feral pigs in Florida. The transmission of ASFV between the European wild boar and soft ticks is unlikely to occur since wild boars do not live in burrows; however wild boars and feral pigs can transmit the virus directly to domestic swine as well as between themselves. Whether wild boars have a reservoir role and/or could be infected in areas with outbreaks in domestic pigs remains to be elucidated (McVicar et al., 1981; Sánchez-Vizcaíno, 2006). In Africa, it has been observed that ASFV induces an unapparent infection in three species of wild swine (warthogs, bushpigs and red river hogs); however, current evidence suggests an unlikely role for bushpigs in the maintenance and transmission of ASFV, while the role played by the giant forest hog has not yet been clarified (Jori and Bastos, 2009; Ravaomanana et al., 2011).

The disease is currently endemic in many countries of Africa (mainly located south of the Sahara), Sardinia and the Caucasus. In Africa it is maintained by a cycle of infection between wild suidae and soft ticks. ASFV infection is characterized by low levels of virus in host tissues and low or undetectable levels of viraemia, but this is sufficient to infect soft tick vectors and cause subsequent tick transmission to domestic pigs. In Europe, ASF is still endemic in Sardinia, where wild boars seem to be as susceptible as domestic pigs. Previous studies have failed to find ticks from the *O. erraticus* complex in Sardinia (Encinas-Grandes, pers. com.), but those studies did not rule out the presence of the tick and this aspect deserves further attention. More recently in 2007, ASFV spread to Georgia and later to the Trans-Caucasic countries and the Russian Federation, with devastating effects on pig production (Rowlands et al., 2008). The origin of the outbreak is more probably related to entry through international ports or airports through swine fed with garbage containing ASFV-contaminated wastes. The vector competence of ticks for the ASFV currently circulating in the Caucasus is unknown; however the presence of ticks of the *O. erraticus* group has been reported in the Caucasus (Table 1).

Currently, the eradication of ASF from endemic areas is very difficult to achieve because there is no effective vaccine or treatment and the virus can be transmitted by many other routes besides tick bites. Thus, the prevention of the introduction of the virus into new areas and control of tick populations are of great importance to avoid the risk of ASF spreading from infected areas into new ones, as could be the case of virus spread throughout Europe from the Caucasus. Recommendations based on the development of an integrated strategy involving trans-Caucasus countries, the Russian Federation, and the European Union should facilitate the trans-boundary control of ASF (Wieland et al., 2011). The EFSA Panel on Animal Health and Welfare (EFSA 2010a, b, c) offers more detailed information about ASF, ASFV and its vectors in Europe, also presenting several recommendations regarding the ASFV vectorial ability of soft ticks for effective disease management.

2.2 Other soft tick transmitted viruses

West Nile virus has been isolated from *O. moubata* ticks, suggesting that ticks can become infected after feeding on viremic hosts (Lawrie et al., 2004). The tick maintains the infection through moulting, and can transmit the virus to laboratory rodents during a second blood meal (Lawrie et al., 2004). These findings suggest a potential role for *O. moubata* as a reservoir and vector of West Nile virus.

Ornithodoros ticks can also become infected with the encephalitis-producing Karshi and Langat virus group, and hence they can transmit it vertically and horizontally. These viruses have been passed in *O. moubata* cell lines without changing their biological properties (Bell-Sakyi et al., 2009). Taken together, these observations suggest a potential role for *O. moubata* as a vector of this virus group.

Indirect evidence has shown the presence of RNA from flaviviruses such as Alkhurma virus in *O. savignyi* (Charrel et al., 2007), suggesting the possibility of viral replication in this argasid and, consequently, its potential role as a vector. This possibility should be further investigated.

O. savignyi ticks can also become infected with serotype 8 of the bluetongue virus (BTV8), and this infection has been shown to be transmitted transovarially, suggesting that this soft tick could be a potential vector for bluetongue virus. Although soft ticks do not occur on livestock in Europe, they could play a role in the introduction of bluetongue virus in this region (Bouwknegt et al., 2010).

Several studies have been carried out to determine the presence of Crimean Congo Hemorrhagic Fever (CCHF), hepatitis B and HIV-1 viruses in *O. moubata*, with the conclusion that only the hepatitis B virus could be transmitted mechanically to man by this argasid (Jupp et al., 1987). Later, Shepherd et al. (1989) and Durden et al. (1993) confirmed the absence of laboratory transmission of CCHF virus by *Argas walkerae, O. sonrai, O. porcinus* and *O. savignyi*. Humphery-Smith et al. (1993) confirmed the absence of HIV-1 transmission by *O. moubata,* although these authors commented that this may not be the situation under field conditions.

The absence of CCFH virus in *O. moubata* is in accordance with the notion that the CCFH virus is not associated with argasids. However, two exceptional reports exist of the isolation of

CCHF virus from argasids, although the information should be regarded with caution. The first one reports the isolation of the virus from an *O. lahorensis* larva in Iran (Sureau et al. 1980), although this was not confirmed later; the second report describes the isolation of the virus from *A. persicus* in Uzbeck (Rusia) (Hoogstraal, 1985). Recently, in CCHF endemic areas of Iran *O. lahorensis* and *A. reflexus* ticks collected from infected and non-infected hosts have been found to be infected with the CCHF virus (Telmadarraiy et al., 2010; Tahmasebi et al., 2010). Moreover, in these areas antibodies to the CCHF virus have been found in domestic and wild animals and in birds, in which the virus can replicate and, consequently, be spread over long distances (Chevalier et al., 2004). Although it has not been evaluated whether *O. lahorensis* or *A. reflexus* can transmit the CCHF virus, the above data suggest that these ticks could be real vectors of this virus, reflecting the broad range of animal species that can act as reservoirs for the CCHF virus, and also the varied range of potential animals acting as tick hosts. Should this be confirmed, the real field situation for CCHF could be unexpectedly worrying.

Some arboviruses have been identified in *Argas* spp. ticks such as Kao Shuan, Pathum Thani and Nyamanini viruses (Hoogstraal et al., 1975), the West Nile virus (WNV) (Mumcuoglu et al., 2005), Issyk-Kul Fever virus (Gavrilovskaya, 2001), and Mono Lake virus (Labuda & Nuttall, 2008). Since the main hosts of *Argas* spp. ticks are birds, more research is necessary to know the role of tick-infested migratory birds as distributors of emerging arthropod-borne viral diseases worldwide.

About one fourth of the last pandemics were originated by the spread of vector-borne pathogens (Alcaide et al., 2009). Emerging pathogens are frequently RNA viruses with a broad host range, and tick-borne viruses are found in all the RNA virus families (Labuda and Nuttall, 2004; Reperant, 2010). Since these new pathogens can emerge either through introduction into a new population or when the interaction with the vector changes, it is very important to identify the new vectors and reservoirs of such pathogens.

2.3 Bacteria causing relapsing fevers

The most frequent bacterial disease transmitted by soft ticks is human recurrent (relapsing) fever, causing high fever in patients that abates and then recurs, giving the disease its name. Other argasid-borne bacteria causing disease in animals are less frequent, or simply under-reported.

Human relapsing fever is an arthropod-borne infection caused by *Borrelia* spp. spirochetes, whose reservoir hosts are usually wild rodents (Cutler, 2006, 2009). There are two types of human relapsing fever: the endemic or tick-borne (TBRF) type (Calia & Calia, 2000; Dworkin et al., 2002, 2009), caused by several *Borrelia* species and transmitted mainly -but not only- by ticks of the genus *Ornithodoros* (Table 3), and the epidemic or louse-borne type, caused by *Borrelia recurrentis* and transmitted by the human body louse *Pediculus humanus*; this type is more severe than the tick-borne variety.

Ornithodoros spp. ticks act not only as vectors but also as reservoirs of relapsing fever spirochetes, which seem to be quite vector-specific without crossed infections (Shanbaky & Helmy, 2000). Each *Borrelia* species responsible is identified closely with its tick vector and such species share parallel nomenclature; for example, *Borrelia hermsii* is the agent transmitted by *Ornithodoros hermsii*. Vertebrates and humans become infected during a tick blood meal through contamination of the feeding site by salivary and/or coxal secretions of the tick (Parola & Raoult, 2001). Also, transplacental transmission has been reported (Cutler, 2006).

Soft tick-transmitted *Borrelia* species causing disease in humans			
Soft tick species	**Borrelia species**	**Disease**	**References**
Argas africolumbae	*Borrelia anserina*	TBRF	Gothe et al. (1981)
Argas persicus	*Borrelia anserina*	TBRF	Gothe et al. (1981)
Carios kelleyi	*Borrelia johnsoni*	TBRF	Schwan et al. (2009)
Ornithodoros asperus	*Borrelia caucasica*, *Borrelia microti*, *Borrelia baltazardi*	TBRF	Assous & Wilamowski (2009), Parola & Raoult (2001)
Ornithodoros erraticus	*Borrelia microti*, *Borrelia hispanica*, *Borrelia crocidurae*	TBRF	Gaber et al. (1984), Anda et al. (1996), Masoumi et al. (2009), Cutler (2009)
Ornithodoros graingeri	*Borrellia graingeri*		Parola & Raoult. (2001)
Ornithodoros hermsi	*Borrelia hermsi*	TBRF	Dana (2009), Schwan et al. (2007)
Ornithodoros moubata	*Borrelia duttoni*	TBRF	Cutler (2006), Mans et al. (2008a)
Ornithodoros parkeri	*Borrelia parkeri*	TBRF	Dana (2009), Dworkin et al. (2002)
Ornithodoros porcinus	*Borrelia duttoni*	TBRF	Mitani et al. (2004), Cutler (2006)
Ornithodoros rudis	*Borrelia venezuelensis*	TBRF	Rebaudet & Parola (2006)
Ornithodoros savignyi	*Borrelia crocidurae*	TBRF	Gaber et al. (1984), Helmy (2000), Shanbaky & Helmy (2000)
Ornithodoros sonrai	*Borrelia crocidurae*	TBRF	Vial et al. (2006)
Ornithodoros talaje	*Borrelia mazzottii*	TBRF	Davis (1956), Rebaudet & Parola (2006)
Ornithodoros tartakovskyi	*Borrelia latyschewii*	TBRF	Parola & Raoult (2001), Rebaudet & Parola (2006)
Ornithodoros tholozani	*Borrelia persica*	TBRF	Sidi et al. (2005), Assous & Wilamowski (2009), Moemenbellah-Fard et al. (2009), Masoumi et al. (2009)
Ornithodoros turicata	*Borrelia turicatae*	TBRF	Dana (2009)
Ornithodoros zumpti	*Borrelia tillae*		Rebaudet & Parola (2006)
Soft tick-transmitted *Borrelia* species causing disease in animals			
Species	**Borrelia species**	**Disease**	**References**
Argas spp.	*Borrelia anserina*	Avian spirochetosis	Barbour & Hayes (1986)
Argas miniatus	*Borrelia anserina*[1]	Avian spirochetosis	Lisbôa et al. (2009)
Ornithodoros coriaceus	*Borrelia coraciae*	Bovine epizootic abortion	Hendson & Lane (2000), Barbour & Hayes (1986), Teglas et al. (2006), Chen et al. (2007)

Table 3. Bacteria transmitted by soft ticks. TBRF, tick-borne relapsing fever. [1]Experimental transmission.

At present, TBRF can be considered a zoonotic disease since endemic foci in humans have been detected in zones with high prevalences in animals and high infection rates in ticks (McCall et al., 2007). TBRF is characterized by episodes of recurrent fever and other non-specific symptoms, such as headache and myalgia. If not treated with antibiotics it can be fatal. In Tanzania, TBRF caused by *B. duttoni* is endemic. The infection primarily occurs in children and pregnant women, and is associated with foetal loss and neonatal deaths. Perinatal death ratios of 436/1000 have been reported from disease-endemic regions of the country (Cutler, 2006). The laboratory diagnosis of TBRF is done by detecting the spirochetes in human peripheral blood or, better, by flagelin gene PCR amplification and sequencing (Kawabata et al., 2006; Assous & Wilamowski, 2009). This method can be applied to any infection by *Borrelia* spp. spirochetes and allows the specific identification of the etiologic agent. Currently, any *Borrelia* species could represent a health risk for any country, since an exotic pathogen may be introduced into that country by infected people coming from endemic areas. TBRF is considered an emerging disease and it should be kept in mind by health-care providers, especially when dealing with travellers showing symptoms such as fever and in whom malaria is not detected.

More studies are necessary to determine the geographical distribution of *Borrelia*-infected soft ticks, the prevalences of tick infection, and how these prevalences change, and also to identify any new reservoir.

2.4 Other pathogens transmitted by soft ticks

Soft ticks also transmit other pathogens, most of which are important rickettsiae impacting human and animal health. In addition, some protozoan and filarial species may be also transmitted by argasids (Table 4).

Modern molecular biology techniques have enabled the detection of a large number of rickettsial species in argasids. In many cases, the importance of these rickettsiae as pathogens remains to be determined, as does the epidemiological role played by argasid ticks as their vectors and that of migratory birds as spreaders. As already occurs in ixodids, it is anticipated that increasing numbers of new bacterial species will be detected in argasid ticks.

3. Soft ticks as pathogen vectors in a changing environment

Climate is an important factor in the geographic distribution of arthropod vectors. Environmental and climatic global change is currently exerting a strong impact on the transmission and distribution of tick-borne pathogens (El Kammah et al., 2007). The effect of climate on infectious diseases is largely determined by the unique transmission cycle of each pathogen. Transmission cycles that require a vector are more susceptible to external environmental influences than diseases which include only the pathogen and host (Estrada-Peña, 2009).

Generally, the most significant determinant in the transmission of vector-borne pathogens is the survival rate of the vector involved. Warmer temperatures generally increase the survival and development rates of blood-feeding vectors; however, host availability is more important than climate in determining the abundance and distribution of vector ticks (Patz, et al., 2010). Climatic conditions and the political changes with human biotic, abiotic, and synergistic causal factors mainly affecting agriculture, cover and land properties and their use, have a strong effect on the structure of the vegetation, favouring tick ecology (Randolph, 2008, 2010) and, probably, the expansion of tick populations from heavily infested areas of the planet -such as Africa- to nearby places such Europe (Gray et al., 2009) and to more distant areas such Australia, Latin America, and parts of Asia. The increase in tick populations can enhance the contact rates between hosts and ticks.

Specie	Pathogen	Disease	References
Argas spp.	*Aegyptianella pullorum*	Aegyptianellosis	El Kammah et al. (2007)
Argas arboreus	*Wolbachia persica*[1]		Noda et al. (1997)
Argas persicus	*Rahnella aquatilis, Pseudomonas fluorescens, Enterobacter cloacae, Chryseomonas luteola, Chryseobacterium meningosepticum*		Montasser (2005)
Argas vespertilionis	*Borrelia burgdorferi*	Lyme disease	Hubbard et al. (1998)
Carios capensis	*Rickettsia scc3, Rickettsia hoogstraalii*	Spotted fever	Reeves et al. (2005), Kawabata et al. (2006)
Carios kelleyi	*Rickettsia* spp.[2]		Loftis et al. (2005)
	Borrelia spp.[3] *Borrelia lonestari, Rickettsia felis*		Schwan et al. (2009) Loftis et al. (2005)
	Two undescribed *Rickettsia* spp.		Reeves et al. (2006)
	Bartonella henselae	Cat scratch disease	Loftis et al. (2005)
Carios sawaii	*Rickettsia scc3*	Spotted fever	Kawabata et al. (2006)
Ornithodoros coriaceus	Deltaproteobacteria	Bovine Epizootic Abortion[4]	Teglas et al. (2006), Chen et al. (2007)
Ornithodoros erraticus	*Babesia meri*		Gunders & Hadani (1973)
Ornithodoros lahorensis	*Coxiella burnetii*[5]	Q-fever	Mishchenko et al. (2010)
Ornithodoros moubata	*Rickettsia* spp.[2]	Q-fever	Cutler et al. (2006)
	Proteobacteria simbiont[6], Another specific simbiont[7]		Noda et al. (1997)
	Babesia equi[5]	Babesiosis	Battsetseg et al. (2007)
	Acanthocheilonema viteae[5]	Filariasis	Lucius & Textor (1995)
Ornithodoros sonrai	*Coxiella burnetii*	Q-fever	Mediannikov et al. (2010)
Ornithodoros tartakowskyi	*Dipetalonema viteae*[5]	Filariasis	Londoño (1976)

Table 4. Other bacteria, protozoa and filariae with medical/veterinary interest harboured or transmitted by argasid ticks. [1]Symbiont; [2]novel rickettsial agent; [3]closely related to *Borrelia turicatae*; [4]likely agent; [5]experimental transmission or infection; [6]gamma subgroup of proteobacteria symbiont monophyletic group with *Coxiella burnetii*; [7]symbiont which form a monophyletic group with *Francisella tularensis* and *Wolbachia persica*. NR, not reported.

Currently, a change is being noted in the epidemiology of tick-borne diseases caused by changes in environmental parameters: i.e., small changes in temperature can account for large variations in the spreading area of infectious diseases. Increasing tick populations can boost contact rates between ticks and pathogens and also contact between ticks and domestic and wild animals, modifying the endemicity of tick-borne diseases with a higher risk of clinical cases (Cumming & van Vuuren, 2006). Interestingly, an epidemiological heterogeneity of tick-borne infectious diseases with periodic epidemics is being observed; i.e., those of CCHF, which is now appearing with increasing frequency in new areas of Europe. These changes in disease distribution and the emergence of tick borne diseases in unexpected areas may be associated with pathogen dissemination caused, among others, by the movements of livestock, wild animals, and migratory birds.

To date it has been accepted that many of the etiologic agents of these diseases are transmitted exclusively by hard ticks. This specificity seems to be determined by molecular factors involving ticks (i.e., the intracellular process of blood meal digestion in ticks) and pathogens (infection, replication, aggregation), which condition pathogen infection and development in vectors and vertebrates. However, it is tempting to speculate that there could be some pathogens not exclusively transmitted by either hard or soft ticks, since new conditions favouring ticks and pathogen dissemination could provide the opportunity for the establishment of new tick-pathogen interactions. An example supporting such an idea is the association observed between the CCHF virus and the soft tick species referred to above. Evidently, confirmation of this issue will require evidence that well-known soft-tick pathogens can be transmitted by an ixodid species or, conversely, the transmission by argasids of pathogens normally transmitted by species of ixodid ticks. This highlights the need for a systematic surveillance for as yet unknown associations between pathogens and competent vectors and the occurrence of new emerging diseases.

4. Soft tick location and surveillance

As mentioned above, each tick species requires optimum environmental conditions and biotopes for its development, which determine their geographic distribution and the pathogens they transmit (Parola & Raoult, 2001). Accurate knowledge of the distribution of ticks and the monitoring of changes in their distribution are important to define risk areas for tick-borne diseases and to establish adequate measures for tick control and the prevention of tick-borne disease. In this context, continuous tick surveillance emerges as a permanent need.

Direct methods for tick surveillance are based on the capture and identification of specimens, either from the vegetation (dragging method) or from animal hosts in the area sampled. While these procedures are useful for the surveillance of ixodid ticks owing to their exophilous lifestyle and long feeding times, they will not work with argasid ticks because they are endophilous/nidicolous and fast feeders. This means that vegetation dragging and the removal from animals are inefficient as direct methods for argasid surveillance; instead it is necessary to explore all possible tick refuges in the area sampled before such an area can be considered tick-free (Oleaga-Pérez et al., 1990; Vial et al., 2006). Evidently, this is an impractical procedure for large-scale studies.

These drawbacks have encouraged the development of serological tests (ELISA) as indirect methods for tick surveillance, especially for argasid ticks. Serological methods are based on the detection of specific antibodies against tick salivary proteins in serum samples taken from animal hosts -or humans- living in the area under study. The development of such methods requires the resolution of several issues such as: 1) the host species to be sampled; these are determined first by the host preference of the tick species investigated, and second by factors such as the availability and ease of management of the different animal hosts. Domestic instead of wild animals are preferred. 2) Demonstration that the tick species investigated induces a humoral immune response. 3) Characterization of the response in terms of how many tick bites are necessary to induce detectable antibody levels, and how long antibodies remain at detectable levels after the last tick-host contact. 4) Which antigen should be used and what its sensitivity and specificity are.

Such tests have been developed for *O. erraticus* in southern Europe and for *O. moubata* in Africa. In Spain and Portugal, *O. erraticus* lives in close association with swine on free-range pig farms, where it can transmit TBRF and ASF. Accordingly, elimination of the tick from pig farms would greatly improve the control of such diseases (Oleaga-Pérez et al., 1990; Manzano-Román et al., 2007). As part of an ASF eradication campaign carried out in the 90's in Spain, an ELISA test was developed to detect specific antibodies against *O. erraticus* in pigs. The authors of the test demonstrated first that *O. erraticus* bites induced detectable humoral responses in pigs, and that after secondary contact antibody levels were detectable for at least 3 months (Canals et al., 1990). Then, the authors analysed the specificity of the antigen used in the test, which was a crude salivary gland extract (SGE) obtained from adult *O. erraticus* ticks, with a composition similar to that of tick saliva (Baranda et al., 1997). The SGE demonstrated 100% sensitivity and specificity with sera from experimentally infected pigs (Pérez-Sánchez et al., 1992) and 90% sensitivity and specificity in field conditions (Oleaga-Pérez et al., 1994). Subsequently the SGE-ELISA test was used to analyse anti-*O. erraticus* antibodies in more than 19,000 samples of pig sera from 3,478 farms located in 234 townships in the province of Salamanca (Spain). This allowed the identification of the farms infested with the argasid in the province, the establishment of a significant association between the presence of the tick and the persistence of ASF cases on such farms (Pérez-Sánchez et al., 1994), and consequently the application of specific control measures to avoid tick-pig contact on the tick-infested farms. Recently, a similar serological study has been done in Madagascar to look for the presence of anti-*O. moubata* ticks in domestic pigs and bushpigs, using as antigen an SGE obtained from adult *O. moubata* in a similar way to that of *O. erraticus* (Ravaomanana et al., 2011). The absence of anti-tick antibodies and anti-ASFV in bushpigs suggested that the latter are unlikely to play a significant role in the maintenance and transmission of ASFV in Madagascar. In addition, the presence of antibodies against *O. moubata* in domestic pigs suggests that soft ticks may be able to maintain ASFV within a domestic pig cycle in areas of Madagascar where they remain present.

The above indicates that the *O. erraticus* and *O. moubata* SGEs are suitable antigens for the serological surveillance of these two ticks by ELISA tests, although SGEs have some drawbacks. Their collection is time-consuming and difficult to standardise, their composition is poorly known and they may contain non-specific antigens, giving rise to unexpected cross-reactivity. The alternative to SGE would be the use of an individual salivary antigen of proven specificity. With this aim, Baranda et al. (2000) purified the four main antigens from both the *O. erraticus* and *O. moubata* SGE and studied their diagnostic value. Regarding *O. moubata*, the best candidate for the serodiagnosis of infested animals was its 20A1 antigen. This antigen was later identified as a homologue of the TSGP1 salivary lipocalin of *O. savignyi* (Mans et al., 2008b; Oleaga et al., 2007). Recently, this *O. moubata* TSGP1 has been cloned, obtaining the recombinant form (rOmTSGP1), and shown to have a better diagnostic performance (sensitivity and specificity) than SGE (Díaz-Martín et al., 2011), thereby providing a reliable serologic tool for *O. moubata* surveillance.

Regarding the use of anti-tick ELISA tests for ixodid surveillance, only a few studies have been carried out using similar SGEs as antigens and human sera (Schwartz et al., 1993; Lane et al., 1999; Nebreda et al., 2004). These studies also confirmed the suitability of the method to detect anti-ixodid tick antibodies but found a high degree of cross-reactivity among ixodid species. As in the case of *O. moubata*, the use of a specific recombinant antigen would probably solve these problems.

5. Soft tick control

Tick control is an intrinsically difficult task for a number of reasons: ticks produce abundant progeny (they lay many eggs); they usually have more than one developmental stage in nature, and they often parasitize numerous and diverse hosts. Several methods for tick control have been used but none of them has been efficacious against all ticks and the problems they cause.

Chemical control with acaricides (arsenicals, chlorinated hydrocarbons, organophosphates, carbamates and synthetic pyrethroids) was considered the best method but resistant tick strains to these acaricides have been selected (Foil et al., 2004). Furthermore, acaricides may cause toxicity problems and contamination of the environment and animal products, such as milk and meat (George et al., 2008). In addition, owing to the nidicolous life-style of the argasids, their control through the use of acaricides is very difficult to achieve simply because it is not feasible to ensure that the acaricide will reach all places where the parasites hide (Astigarraga et al., 1995).

The problems associated with acaricides have encouraged the development of alternative methods for tick control, such as anti-tick vaccines or bio-control using entomopathogenic organisms, including bacteria, fungi and nematodes. To date, the only bio-control agents tested against soft ticks have been entomopathogenic fungi (Samish et al., 2008). These have been shown to be effective against many ixodid species in different laboratory and field studies. The most pathogenic species were *Beauveria bassiana* and *Metarhizium anisopliae* (Samish et al., 2004; Ostfeld et al., 2006). These two fungal species have received the greatest attention and have been the object of subsequent studies (Fernandes & Bittencourt, 2008; Polar et al., 2008). However, such studies have been focused almost exclusively on the control of ixodid ticks, and have neglected the control of argasid ticks. One exception is the work by Sewify & Habib (2001), which studied the pathogenic effect of *M. anisopliae* on the argasid tick *A. persicus*. These authors sprayed heavily infested poultry houses with a fungal spore suspension and observed that the argasid population disappeared in 3 weeks. More recently, Zabalgogeazcoa et al. (2008) and Herrero et al. (2011) carried out laboratory trials showing that isolates of *B. bassiana* and *Tolypocladium cylindrosporum* caused up to 70% mortality in *O. erraticus* and up to 40% mortality in *O. moubata*. These results justify further efforts towards the application of entomopathogenic fungal strains as anti-argasid bio-control agents.

Immunological control using anti-tick vaccines offers an attractive alternative to the use of acaricides. In spite of the research efforts invested in this field over the last two decades, only two recombinant anti-hard tick vaccines against *Rhipicephalus (Boophilus)* species have become available commercially (de la Fuente et al., 2007; Willadsen, 2008). The application of these vaccines has shown that it is possible to control tick populations through host vaccination. Nevertheless, the progress in vaccine development against other tick species has been disappointing, and this is especially evident in relation to argasid ticks (de la Fuente & Kocan, 2003; de la Fuente et al., 2008b; Willadsen, 2008). Among other reasons underlying the slow development of new and more effective anti-tick vaccines, the main one is the difficulty involved in identifying tick protective antigens (Willadsen, 2008).

As far as we know, the only attempts to develop anti-argasid vaccines have been those undertaken by our group, which focused on *O. erraticus* and *O. moubata*. We found a concealed antigen from the endothelial gut cells of *O. erraticus*, the so-called Oe45, which induces a protective response in pigs, causing up to 80% mortality in nymphs and a 50% reduction in female fecundity (Manzano-Román et al., 2006, 2007). In *O. moubata*, a salivary anti-haemostatic protein that acts as an antagonist ligand of the host P-selectin molecule has been characterized (García-Varas et al., 2010). This protein, called Om44, does not elicit an immune response in naturally-infected hosts, but when administered as a vaccine in pigs and rabbits it induces a protective immune response that inhibits tick feeding by up to 70%, and the protective response increases with successive infestations. Hence, Om44 is a new example of "silent" salivary antigen according to the new concept introduced for the salivary sialostatin L2 from *I. scapularis* (Kotsyfakis et al., 2008).

Consequently, the search for and identification of new anti-soft tick protective antigens should continue, and tick saliva could be an important antigen source. As demonstrated with Bm86, tick gut proteins may also provide good candidate protective antigens. It would be desirable that the new antigens were shared between soft and hard ticks, since this would allow the development of universal anti-tick vaccines. In the search for protective antigens, new genomic-based experimental approaches, such as Expression Library Immunization (ELI) and RNA interference-based screening of cDNA libraries, have been developed and successfully applied to *Ixodes scapularis* and *Amblyomma americanum* (Almazán et al., 2005, de la Fuente et al., 2010). The results of these studies showed that the use of RNAi gene silencing for the identification of tick protective antigens is a rapid and cost-effective tool for the discovery of candidate vaccine antigens.

6. Conclusions

Soft ticks are distributed worldwide and global climatic changes, along with social factors, influence soft-tick habitats and their hosts. These factors hinder the prediction of the argasid and argasid-borne diseases distribution patterns. Also, several factors could influence the vector competence of soft ticks. A serious swine disease transmitted by argasids is African Swine Fever. This disease jumped between continents in the 60´s and 70´s and recently in the North of Europe, exemplifying the growing possibility that human and animal tick-borne infectious diseases can emerge and colonize previously uninfected areas because the potential distribution of the infection is transcontinental.

Endemic zones for a specific tick-borne pathogen may serve as the origin for its epidemiological dissemination towards new environments, and this dissemination would probably require the adaptation of both the pathogen and the new vector to each other, implying some kind of genetic evolution. The recent characterization of non-specific viruses in argasid vectors and all the argasid-associated pathogens mentioned in this review suggest the great potential of argasids for viral and bacterial disease transmission in any part of the world owing to their extensive geographical distribution and their relatively indiscriminate host feeding.

Here, we show that soft-tick surveillance by serological methods and control thought vaccination could be possible and this opens new avenues for the development and advance of new tests and further research on other argasid species. The possibility that argasids might serve as vectors for many more pathogens that expected requires a greater effort in implementing control measures, such as the search for new protective antigens to be included in a broad spectrum anti-tick vaccine as well as specific coordinated and urgent epidemiological and parasite-surveillance programs. Since there is no single ideal solution for the control of ticks, an integrated control approach is probably the most effective. Vector and reservoir surveillance is an important component of such a strategy.

7. Acknowledgement

We thank the financial support of the Spanish Ministry of Science and Innovation (Project AGL2010-18164) and the Regional Government of Castilla y León (Spain) (Project CSI062A11-2) that allowed part of this research. We also thank Dr. Agustin Estrada-Peña for his helpful comments and suggestions.

8. References

Adeyeye, OA. & Butler, JF. (1989). Population structure and seasonal intra-burrow movement of *Ornithodoros turicata* (Acari: Argasidae) in gopher tortoise burrows. *Journal of Medical Entomology*, Vol. 26, No. 4, (July 1989), pp. 279-283, ISSN 0022-2585.

Ahmed, J., Alp, H., Aksin, M. & Seitzer, U. (2007). Current status of ticks in Asia. *Parasitology Research*, Vol. 101, No. 2, (September 2007), pp. 159-162, ISSN 0932-0113.

Alcaide, M., Rico, C., Ruiz, S., Soriguer, R., Muñoz, J. & Figuerola, J. (2009). Disentangling vector-borne transmission networks: a universal DNA barcoding method to identify vertebrate hosts from arthropod bloodmeals. *Plos One*, Vol. 4, No. 9, (September 2009), pp. 1-6, ISSN 1932-6203.

Almazán, C., Blas-Machado, U., Kocan, KM., Yoshioka, JH., Blouin, EF., Mangold, AJ. & de la Fuente J. (2005). Characterization of three Ixodes scapularis cDNAs protective against tick infestations. *Vaccine*, Vol. 23, No. 35, (August 2005), pp. 4403-16, ISSN 0264-410X.

Anda, P., Sánchez-Yebra, W., Del Mar Vitutia, M., Pérez Pastrana, E., Rodríguez, I., Miller, NS., Backenson, PB. & Benach, JL. (1996). A new *Borrelia* species isolated from patients with relapsing fever in Spain. *Lancet*, Vol. 348, No. 9021, (July 1996), pp. 162-165, ISSN 0140-6736.

Assous, MV. & Wilamowski, A. (2009). Relapsing fever borreliosis in eurasia--forgotten, but certainly not gone!. *Clinical Microbiology and Infection*, Vol. 15, No. 5, (May 2009), pp. 407-414, ISSN 1198-743X.

Astigarraga, A., Oleaga-Pérez, A., Pérez-Sánchez, R. & Encinas-Grandes, A. (1995). A study of the vaccinal value of various extracts of concealed antigens and salivary gland extracts against *Ornithodoros erraticus* and *Ornithodoros moubata*. *Veterinary Parasitolgy*, Vol. 60, No. 1-2, (November 1995), pp. 133-147, ISSN 0304-4017.

Ataliba, AC., Resende, JS., Yoshinari, N. & Labruna, MB. (2007). Isolation and molecular characterization of a Brazilian strain of *Borrelia anserina*, the agent of fowl spirochaetosis. *Research in Veterinary Science*, Vol. 83, No. 2, (October 2007), 145-149, ISSN 0034-5288.

Aydin, L. & Bakirci, S. (2007). Geographical distribution of ticks in Turkey. *Parasitology Research*. Vol. 101, No. 2, (September 2007), pp. 163-166, ISSN 0932-0113.

Baranda, JA., Pérez-Sánchez, R. Oleaga-Pérez, A. & Encinas-Grandes, A. (1997). Antigens of interest for the diagnosis of parasitism in pigs by *Ornithodoros erraticus* and *Ornithodoros moubata*. *The Journal of Parasitology*. Vol. 83, No. 5, (October 1997), pp. 831-838, ISSN 0022-3395.

Baranda, JA., Pérez-Sánchez, R., Oleaga, A., Manzano, R. & Encinas-Grandes, A. (2000). Purification, N-terminal sequencing and diagnostic value of the major antigens of *Ornithodoros erraticus* and *O. moubata*. *Veterinary Parasitology*, Vol. 87, No. 1-2, (January 2000), pp. 193-206, ISSN 0304-4017.

Barbour, AG. & Hayes, SF. (1986). Biology of *Borrelia* species. *Microbiol rev*, Vol. 50, No. 4 (December 1986) pp. 381-400. ISSN 0146-0749

Barros-Battesti, DM., Landulfo, GA., Onofrio, VC., Faccini, JL., Marcili, A., Nieri-Bastos, FA., Venzal, JM., & Labruna, MB. (2011). *Carios mimon* (Acari: Argasidae): description of adults and redescription of larva. *Exp Appl Acarol*. Vol. 54, No. 1, (May 2011), pp. 93-104, ISSN 0168-8162.

Basto, AP., Nix, RJ., Boinas, F., Mendes, S., Silva, MJ., Cartaxeiro, C., Portugal, RS., Leitão, A., Dixon, LK. & Martins, C. (2006). Kinetics of African swine fever virus infection in *Ornithodoros erraticus* ticks. *Journal of General Virology*. Vol. 87, No. 7, (July 2006), pp. 1863-1871, ISSN 0022-1317.

Bastos, AD., Arnot, LF., Jacquier, MD. & Maree, S. (2009). A host species-informative internal control for molecular assessment of African swine fever virus infection rates in the African sylvatic cycle *Ornithodoros* vector. *Medical Veterinary Entomology*. Vol. 23, No. 4, (December 2009), pp. 399-409, ISSN 0269-283X.

Battsetseg, B., Matsuo, T., Xuan, X., Boldbaatar, D., Chee, SH., Umemiya, R., Sakaguchi, T., Hatta, T., Zhou, J., Verdida, AR., Taylor, D. & Fujisaki, K. (2007). Babesia parasites develop and are transmitted by the non-vector soft tick *Ornithodoros moubata* (Acari: Argasidae). *Parasitology*, Vol. 134, No. 1, (January 2007), pp. 1-8, ISSN 0031-1820.

Bell-Sakyi, L., Růzek, D. & Gould, EA. (2009). Cell lines from the soft tick *Ornithodoros moubata*. *Experimental and Applied Acarology*, Vol. 49, No. 3, (November 2009), pp. 209-219, ISSN 0168-8162.

Belozerov, VN., Van Niekerk, DJ. & Butler, HJ. (2003). Population structure of *Argas arboreus* (Acari: Argasidae) ticks associated with seasonally abandoned mixed heronries, dominated by cattle egrets (*Bubulcus ibis*), in South Africa. *Onderstepoort Journal of Veterinary Research*. Vol. 70, No. 4, (December 2003), pp. 325-30, ISSN 0030-2465.

Bermúdez, SE., Miranda, RJ. & Smith, D. (2010). Ticks species (Ixodida) in the summit municipal park and adjacent areas, Panama City, Panama. *Experimaental Applied Acarology*, Vol. 52, No. 4, (December 2010), pp. 439-448, ISSN 0168-8162.

Boinas, FS., Wilson, AJ., Hutchings, GH., Martins, C. & Dixon, LJ. (2011). The persistence of African swine fever virus in field-infected *Ornithodoros erraticus* during the ASF endemic period in Portugal. *PLoS One*. Vol.6, No. 5, ISSN 1932-6203.

Bouwknegt, C., Van Rijn, PA., Schipper, JJ., Hölzel, D., Boonstra, J., Nijhof, AM., Van Rooij, EM. & Jongejan, F. (2010). Potential role of ticks as vectors of bluetongue virus. *Experimental and Applied Acarology*, Vol. 52, No. 2, (April 2010), pp. 183-192, ISSN 0168-8162.

Caeiro, V. (1999). General review of tick species present in Portugal. *Parassitologia*, Vol. 41, No. 1, (September 1999), pp. 11-15, ISSN 0048-2951.

Calia, KE. & Calia, FM. (2000). Tick borne relapsing fever. In: *Tickborne Infectious Diseases: Diagnosis and Management*, Burke A. Cunha (Ed.), pp. 169-183, Informa Healthcare, ISBN: 0-8247-0310-3, New York, USA.

Calisher, CH., Schwan, TG., Lazuick, JS., Eads, RB. & Francy, DB. (1988). Isolation of Mono Lake virus (family Reoviridae, genus Orbivirus, Kemerovo serogroup) from *Argas cooleyi* (Acari: Argasidae) collected in Colorado. *Journal of Medical Entomology* Vol. 25, No. 5, (September 1988), pp. 388-390, ISSN 0022-2585.

Canals, A., Oleaga, A., Pérez, R., Domínguez, J., Encinas, A. & Sánchez-Vizcaíno, JM. (1990) Evaluation of an enzyme-linked immunosorbent assay to detect specific antibodies in pigs infested with the tick *Ornithodoros erraticus* (Argasidae). *Veterinary Parasitology*. Vol. 37, No. 2, (October 1990) pp. 145-153, ISSN 0304-4017.

Charrel, RN., Fagbo, S., Moureau, G., Alqahtani, MH., Temmam, S. & de Lamballerie, X. (2007). Alkhurma hemorrhagic fever virus in *Ornithodoros savignyi* ticks. *Emerging Infectious Diseases*, Vol. 13, No. 1, (January 2007), pp. 153-155, ISSN 1080-6040.

Chen, CI., King, DP., Blanchard, MT., Hall, MR., Aldridge, BM., Bowen, L. & Stott, JL. (2007). Identification of the etiologic agent of epizootic bovine abortion in field-collected *Ornithodoros coriaceus* koch ticks. *Veterinary Microbiology*, Vol. 120, No. 3-4, (March 2007), pp. 320-7, ISSN 0378-1135.

Chen, Z., Yang, X., Bu, F., Yang, X., Yang, X. & Liu, J. (2010). Ticks (Acari: Ixodoidea: Argasidae, Ixodidae) of China. *Experimental and Applied Acarology*, Vol. 51, No. 4, (August 2010), pp. 393-404, ISSN 0168-8162.

Chevalier, V., de la Rocque, S., Baldet, T., Vial, L. & Roger F. (2004). Epidemiological processes involved in the emergence of vector-borne diseases: West Nile fever, Rift Valley fever, Japanese encephalitis and Crimean-Congo haemorrhagic fever. *Revue Scientifique et Technique (International Office of Epizootics)*. Vol. 23, No. 2, (August 2004), pp. 535-55, ISSN 0253-1933.

Cilek, JE. & Knapp, FW. (1992). Occurrence of *Ornithodoros kelleyi* (Acari: Argasidae) in Kentucky. *Journal of Medical Entomology*, Vol. 29, No. 2, (March 1992), pp. 349-51, ISSN 0022-2585.

Clifford, CM., Hoogstraal, H., Radovsky, FJ., Stiller, D. & Keirans, JE. (1980). *Ornithodoros* (alectorobius) *amblus* (Acarina: Ixodoidea: Argasidae): identity, marine bird and human hosts, virus infections, and distribution in Peru. *Journal of Parasitology*, Vol. 66, No.2, (April 1980), pp. 312-323, ISSN 0022-3395.

Converse, JD., Hoogstraal, H., Moussa, MI., Feare, CJ. & Kaiser, MN. (1975). Soldado virus (hughes group) from *Ornithodoros* (alectorobius) *capensis* (Ixodoidea: Argasidae) infesting sooty tern colonies in the Seychelles, Indian Ocean. *American Journal of Tropical Medicine and Hygiene*, Vol. 24, No. 6(pt 1), (November 1975), pp. 1010-1018, ISSN 0002-9637.

Cordero del Campillo, M., Castañón Ordóñez, L. & Reguera Feo, A. (1994). *Indice-catálogo de zooparásitos ibéricos*. Ediciones Universidad de León. ISBN: 9788477194033, León (Spain).

Cornely, M. & Schultz, U. (1992). The tick fauna of eastern Germany. *Angewandte Parasitologie*, Vol. 33, No. 3, (August 1992), pp. 173-183, ISSN 0003-3162.

Cumming, GS. & Van Vuuren, DP. (2006). Will climate change affect ectoparasite species ranges?. *Global Ecology and Biogeography*, Vol. 15, No. 5, (September 2006), pp. 486–497, ISSN 1466-822X.

Cutler, SJ., Browning, P., & Scott, JC. (2006). *Ornithodoros moubata*, a soft tick vector for Rickettsia in east Africa?. *Annals of the New York Academy of Sciences*. Vol. 1078, (October 2006), pp. 373-377, ISSN 0077-8923.

Cutler, SJ. (2006). Possibilities for relapsing fever re-emergence. *Emerging Infectious Diseases*. Vol. 12, pp. 369–374, ISSN 1080-6040

Cutler, SJ. (2009). Relapsing fever - a forgotten disease revealed. *Journal of Applied Microbiology*, Vol. 108, No. 4, (April 2009), pp. 1115-22, ISSN 1364-5072.

Dana, AN. (2009). Diagnosis and treatment of tick infestation and tick-borne diseases with cutaneous manifestations. *Dermatologic Therapy*, Vol. 22, No.4, (July 2009), pp. 293-326, ISSN 1396-0296.

Davis, GE. (1956). A relapsing fever spirochete, *Borrelia mazzottii* (sp. nov.) from *Ornithodoros talaje* from Mexico. *American Journal of Hygiene*, Vol. 63, No. 1, (January 1956), pp. 13-7, ISSN 0096-5294.

De la Fuente, J. & Kocan, KM. (2003). Advances in the identification and characterization of protective antigens for development of recombinant vaccines against tick infestations. *Expert Review of Vaccines*. Vol. 2, No. 4, (August 2003), pp. 583-593, ISSN 1476-0584.

De la Fuente, J., Almazán, C., Canales, M., Pérez de la Lastra, JM., Kocan, KM. & Willadsen, P. (2007). A ten-year review of commercial vaccine performance for control of tick infestations on cattle. *Animal Health Research Reviews*. Vol. 8, No. 1, (June 2007), pp. 23-28, ISSN 1466-2523.

De la Fuente, J., Estrada-Peña, A., Venzal, JM., Kocan, KM., & Sonenshine, DE. (2008a). Overview: ticks as vectors of pathogens that cause disease in humans and animals. *Frontiers in Bioscience*, Vol.1, No. 13, (May 2008), pp. 6938-6946, ISSN 1093-9946

De la Fuente, J., Kocan, KM., Almazán, C. & Blouin, EF. (2008b). Targeting the tick-pathogen interface for novel control strategies. *Frontiers in Bioscience*, Vol. 1, No. 13, (May 2008), pp. 6947-6956, ISSN 1093-9946

De la Fuente, J., Manzano-Román, R., Naranjo, V., Kocan, KM., Zivkovic, Z., Blouin, EF., Canales, M., Almazán, C., Galindo, RC., Step, DL. & Villar, M. (2010). Identification of protective antigens by RNA interference for control of the lone star tick,

Amblyomma americanum. *Vaccine*, Vol. 28, No. 7, (February 2010), pp. 1786-1795, ISSN 0264-410X.

Di Iorio, O., Turienzo, P., Nava, S., Mastropaolo, M., Mangold, AJ., Acuña, DG. & Guglielmone, AA. (2010). *Asthenes dorbignyi* (Passeriformes: Furnariidae) host of *Argas neghmei* (Acari: Argasidae). *Experimental and Applied Acarology*, Vol. 51, No. 4, (August 2010), pp. 419-422, ISSN 0168-8162.

Diaz, JH. (2009). Endemic tickborne infectious diseases in Louisiana and the Gulf South. *Journal of the Louisiana State Medical Society*, Vol. 161, No. 6, pp. 325-326, ISSN 0024-6921.

Díaz-Martín, V., Manzano-Román, R., Siles-Lucas, M., Oleaga, A. & Pérez-Sánchez, R. (2011). Cloning, characterization and diagnostic performance of the salivary lipocalin protein TSGP1 from *Ornithodoros moubata*. *Veterinary Parasitology*. Vol. 178, No. 1-2, (May 2011), pp. 163-172, ISSN 0304-4017.

Dikaev, B. (1981). Argasid tick fauna (Argasidae) of the Chechen-Ingush ASSR. *Parazitologiia*. Vol. 15, No. 1, (January 1981), pp. 76-78, ISSN 0031-1847.

Durden, LA., Logan, TM., Wilson, ML. & Linthicum, KJ. (1993). Experimental vector incompetence of a soft tick, *Ornithodoros sonrai* (Acari: Argasidae), for Crimean-Congo hemorrhagic fever virus. *Journal of Medical Entomology*, Vol. 30, No. 2, (March 1993), pp. 493-496, ISSN 0022-2585

Durden, LA., Merker, S. & Beati, L. (2008). The tick fauna of Sulawesi, Indonesia (Acari: Ixodoidea: Argasidae and Ixodidae). *Experimental and Applied Acarology* Vol. 45, No. 1-2, (June 2008), pp. 85-110, ISSN 0168-8162.

Dworkin, MS., Schwan, TG. & Anderson DE Jr. (2002). Tick-borne relapsing fever in North America. *The Medical Clinics of North America*, Vol. 86, No. 2, (March 2002), pp. 417-33, ISSN 0025-7125

Dworkin, MS., Schwan, TG., Anderson, DE Jr. & Borchardt, SM. (2008). Tick-borne relapsing fever. *Infectious Disease Clinics of North America*, Vol. 22, No. 3, (September 2008), pp. 449-68, ISSN 0891-5520.

El Kammah, KM., Oyoun, LM. & Abdel-Ahafy, S. (2007). Detection of microorganisms in the saliva and midgut smears of different tick species (Acari: Ixodoidea) in Egypt. *Journal of the Egyptian Society of Parasitology*, Vol. 37, No. 2, (August 2007), pp. 533-539, ISSN 0253-5890.

EFSA (2010a). Scientific Opinion on Geographic Distribution of Tick-borne Infections and their Vectors in Europe and the other Regions of the Mediterranean Basin. *EFSA Journal*, Vol. 8, No. 9, pp. 1723, ISSN 1831-4732.

EFSA (2010b). Scientific Opinion on the Role of Tick Vectors in the Epidemiology of Crimean-Congo Hemorrhagic Fever and African Swine Fever in Eurasia. *EFSA Journal*, Vol. 8, No. 8, pp. 1703, ISSN 1831-4732.

EFSA (2010c). Scientific Opinion on African Swine Fever. *EFSA Journal*, Vol. 8, No. 3, pp. 1556, ISSN 1831-4732.

Endris, RG., Keirans, JE., Robbins, RG. & Hess, WR. (1989). *Ornithodoros* (Alectorobius) *puertoricensis* (Acari: Argasidae): redescription by scanning electron microscopy. *Journal of Medical Entomology* Vol. 26, No. 3, (May 1989), pp. 146-154, ISSN 0022-2585.

Endris, RG., Haslett, TM. & Hess, WR. (1991). Experimental transmission of African swine fever virus by the tick *Ornithodoros* (Alectorobius) *puertoricensis* (Acari: Argasidae).

Journal of Medical Entomology, Vol. 28, No. 6, (November 1991), pp. 854-858, ISSN 0022-2585.

Endris, RG., & Hess, WR. (1994). Attempted transovarial and venereal transmission of African swine fever virus by the Iberian soft tick *Ornithodoros (Pavlovskyella) marocanus* (Acari: Ixodoidea: Argasidae). *Journal of Medical Entomology*, Vol. 31, No. 3, pp. 373-81, ISSN 0022-2585.

Estrada-Peña, A., Venzal, JM., González-Acuña, D. & Guglielmone, AA. (2003). *Argas* (Persicargas) *keiransi* n. sp. (Acari: Argasidae), a parasite of the Chimango, *Milvago c. chimango* (Aves: Falconiformes) in Chile. *Journal of Medical Entomol*ogy Vol. 40, No. 6, (November 2003), pp. 766-769, ISSN 0022-2585.

Estrada-Peña, A., Venzal, JM., González-Acuña, D., Mangold, AJ. & Guglielmone, AA. (2006). Notes on new world *Persicargas* ticks (Acari: Argasidae) with description of female *Argas* (p.) *keiransi*. *Journal of Medical Entomology* Vol. 43, No. 5, (September 2006), pp. 801-9, ISSN 0022-2585.

Estrada-Peña, A. (2009). Tick-borne pathogens, transmission rates and climate change. *Frontiers in Bioscience*, Vol. 1, No. 14, (January 2009), pp. 2674-2687, ISSN 1093-9946.

Estrada-Peña, A., Mangold, AJ., Nava, S., Venzal, JM., Labruna, MB. & Guglielmone, AA. (2010). A review of the systematics of the tick family argasidae (Ixodida). *Acarologia*, Vol. 50, No. 3, (September 2010), pp. 317–333, ISSN 0044-586-X.

Failing, RM., Lyon, CB. & Mckittrick, JE. (1972). The pajaroello tick bite. The frightening folklore and the mild disease. *California Medicine*, Vol. 116, No. 5, (May 1972), pp. 16-19, ISSN 0008-1264.

Fernandes, EK. & Bittencourt, VR. (2008). Entomopathogenic fungi against South American tick species. *Experimental and Applied Acarology*, Vol. 46, No. 1-4, (December 2008), pp. 71-93, ISSN 0168-8162.

Filippova, NA. (1966). Argasid ticks (Argasidae). *Fauna SSSR*. Paukoobraznye, Vol. 4, No. 3, pp. 255

Foil, LD., Coleman, P., Eisler, M., Fragoso-Sanchez, H., Garcia-Vazquez, Z., Guerrero, FD., Jonsson, NN., Langstaff, IG., Li, AY., Machila, N., Miller, RJ., Morton, J., Pruett, JH. & Torr, S. (2004). Factors that influence the prevalence of acaricide resistance and tick-borne diseases. *Veterinary Parasitology*, Vol. 125, No.1-2, (October 2004), pp. 163-181, ISSN 0304-4017.

Gaber, MS., Khalil, GM., Hoogstraal, H. & Aboul-Nasr, AE. (1984). *Borrelia crocidurae* localization and transmission in *Ornithodoros erraticus* and *O. savignyi*. *Parasitology*, Vol. 88, No.3, (June 1984), pp. 403-413, ISSN 0031-1820.

García-Varas, S, Manzano-Román, R., Fernández-Soto, P., Encinas-Grandes, A., Oleaga, A. & Pérez-Sánchez, R. (2010). Purification and characterisation of a p-selectin-binding molecule from the salivary glands of *Ornithodoros moubata* that induces protective anti-tick immune responses in pigs. *International Journal of Parasitology*, Vol. 40, No. 3, (March 2010), pp. 313-26, ISSN 0020-7519.

Gavrilovskaya, IN. (2001). *Issyk-Kul* virus disease, In: *The encyclopedia of arthropod-transmitted infections of man and domesticated animals*. Cabi Publishing, pp. 231-234, ISBN-13: 978-0851994734, NY.

George, JE., Pound, JM. & Davey, RB. (2008). Acaricides for controlling ticks on cattle and the problem of acaricides resistance. In: *Ticks: biology, disease and control*. Alan S.

Bowman & Pat Nuttall (Eds.), pp. 408-423, Cambridge University Press, ISBN 978-0-521-86761-0, Cambridge, UK.

Ghosh, S., Bansal, GC., Gupta, SC., Ray, D., Khan, MQ., Irshad, H., Shahiduzzaman, M., Seitzer, U. & Ahmed, JS. (2007). Status of tick distribution in Bangladesh, India and Pakistan. *Parasitology Research* Vol. 101, No. 2, (September 2007), pp. 207-216, ISSN 0932-0113

Gilot, B. & Pautou, G. (1982). Evolution of populations of ticks (Ixodidae and Argasidae) in relation to artificialization of the environment in the French Alps. Epidemiologic effects. *Acta Tropica,* Vol. 39, No. 4, (December 1982), pp. 337-354, ISSN 0001-706X.

González-Acuña, D. & Guglielmone, AA. (2005). Ticks (Acari: Ixodoidea: Argasidae, Ixodidae) of Chile. *Experimental and Applied Acarology* Vol. 35, No. 1-2, pp. 147-63, ISSN 0168-8162.

Gothe, R., Buchheim, C. & Schrecke, W. (1981). *Argas* (*Persicargas*) *persicus* and *Argas* (*Argas*) *africolumbae* as natural vectors of *Borrelia anserina* and *Aegyptianella pullorum* in upper Volta. *Berliner und Munchener Tierarztliche Wochenschrift*, Vol. 94, No. 14, (July 1981), pp. 280-285, ISSN 0005-9366.

Gray, JS., Dautel, H., Estrada-Peña, A., Kahl, O. & Lindgren, E. (2009). Effects of climate change on ticks and tick-borne diseases in Europe. *Interdisciplinary Perspectives on Infectious Diseases,* Volume 2009 (2009), Article ID 593232, 12 pages, doi:10.1155/2009/593232.

Groocock, CM., Hess, WR. & Gladney, WJ. (1980). Experimental transmission of African swine fever virus by *Ornithodoros coriaceus*, an argasid tick indigenous to the United States. *American Journal of Veterinary Research*, Vol.41, No. 4, (April 1980), pp. 591-594, ISSN 0002-9645.

Guglielmone, AA., Estrada-Peña, A., Keirans, JE. & Robbins, RG. (2003). *Ticks (Acari: Ixodida) of the Neotropical zoogeographic region*. Houten Editors, ISBN 9874368284, Atalanta, 2003.

Guglielmone, AA., Robbins, RG., Apanaskevich, DA., Petney, TN., Estrada-Peña, A., Horak, IG., Shao, R. & Barker, SC. (2010). The Argasidae, Ixodidae and Nuttalliellidae (Acari: Ixodida) of the world: a list of valid species names. *Zootaxa,* Vol. 2528, pp. 1–28, ISSN 1175-5326.

Gugushvili, GK. (1972). Hosts of *Ornithodoros verrucosus* and *O. alactagalis* ticks in the Georgian SSR. I. Results of the precipitation test. *Meditsinskaia parazitologiia i parazitarnye bolezni,* Vol. 41, No. 3, (May 1972), pp. 259-264, ISSN 0025-8326.

Gunders, AE. & Hadani, A. (1973). An argasid tick, *Ornithodoros erraticus* (Lucas) a natural vector of *Nuttalia meri Gunders.* Preliminary communication. *Zeitschrift für Tropenmedizin und Parasitologie,* Vol. 24, No. 4, (December 1973), pp. 536-538, ISSN 0044-359X.

Haresnape, JM. & Wilkinson, PJ. (1989). A study of African swine fever virus infected ticks (*Ornithodoros moubata*) collected from three villages in the asf enzootic area of Malawi following an outbreak of the disease in domestic pigs. *Epidemiology and Infection,* Vol. 102, No. 3, (June 1989), pp. 507-522, ISSN 0950-2688.

Helmy, N. (2000). Seasonal abundance of *Ornithodoros (O.) savignyi* and prevalence of infection with Borrelia spirochetes in Egypt. *Journal of the Egyptian Society of Parasitology,* Vol. 30, No. 2, (August 2000), pp. 607-619, ISSN 0253-5890.

Hendson, M. & Lane, RS. (2000). Genetic characteristics of *Borrelia coriaceae* isolates from the soft tick *Ornithodoros coriaceus* (Acari: Argasidae). *Journal of Clinical Microbiology*, Vol. 38, No. 7, (July 2000), pp. 2678-2682, ISSN 0095-1137.

Herrero, N., Pérez-Sánchez, R., Oleaga, A., Zabalgogeazcoa, I. (2011). Tick pathogenicity, thermal tolerance and virus infection in *Tolypocladium cylindrosporum*. *Annals of Applied Biology*. Doi:10.1111/J.1744-7348.2011.00485.X, ISSN 0003-4746

Hess, WR., Endris, RG., Haslett, TM., Monahan, MJ. & Mccoy, JP. (1987). Potential arthropod vectors of African swine fever virus in North America and the Caribbean basin. *Veterinary Parasitology*, Vol. 26, No. 1-2, (December 1987), pp. 145-155, ISSN 0304-4017.

Heyman, P., Cochez, C., Hofhuis, A., Van der Giessen, J., Sprong, H., Porter, SR., Losson, B., Saegerman, C., Donoso-Mantke, O., Niedrig, M. & Papa, A. (2010). A clear and present danger: tick-borne diseases in Europe. *Expert Review of Anti-infective Therapy*, Vol. 8, No. 1, (January 2010), pp. 33-50, ISSN 1478-7210.

Hoogstraal, H., Guirgis, SS., Khalil, GM. & Kaiser, MN. (1975). The subgenus *Persicargas* (Ixodoidea: Argasidae: Argas). 27. The life cycle of *A.* (*P.*) *robertsi* population samples from Taiwan, Thailand, Indonesia, Australia, and Sri Lanka. *The Southeast Asian Journal of Tropical Medicine and Public Health*, Vol. 6, No. 4, (December 1975), pp. 532-539, ISSN 0125-1562.

Hoogstraal, H., Wassef, HY., Easton, ER. & Dixon, JE. (1977). Observations on the subgenus *Argas* (Ixodoidea: Argasidae: Argas). 12. *Argas* (A.) *africolumbae*: variation, bird hosts, and distribution in Kenya, Tanzania, and South and South-West Africa. *Journal of Medical Entomology*, Vol. 13, No. 4-5, (January 1977), pp. 441-445, ISSN 0022-2585.

Hoogstraal, H., Clifford, CM. & Keirans, JE. (1979). The *Ornithodoros* (*alectorobius*) *capensis* group (Acarina: Ixodoidea: Argasidae) of the palearctic and oriental regions. *O. (A.) coniceps* identity, bird and mammal hosts, virus infections, and distribution in Europe, Africa, and Asia. *Journal of Parasitology*, Vol. 65, No. 3, (June 1979), pp. 395-407, ISSN 0022-3395.

Hoogstraal, H. (1985). Argasid and Nuttalliellid ticks as parasites and vectors. *Advances in Parasitology*, Vol. 24, pp. 135-238, ISSN 0065-308X.

Horak, IG., Mckay, IJ., Henen, BT., Heyne, H., Hofmeyr, MD. & De Villiers, AL. (2006). Parasites of domestic and wild animals in South Africa. xlvii. Ticks of tortoises and other reptiles. *The Onderstepoort Journal of Veterinary Research*, Vol. 73, No. 3, (September 2006), pp. 215-227, ISSN 0030-2465.

Howell, CJ. (1966). Studies on karyotypes of South African argasidae. I. *Ornithodoros savignyi*. (Audouin) (1827). *The Onderstepoort Journal of Veterinary Research*, Vol. 33, No. 1, (June 1966), pp. 93-98, ISSN 0030-2465.

Hubbard, MJ., Baker, AS. & Cann, KJ. (1998). Distribution of *Borrelia burgdorferi* s.l. spirochaete DNA in British ticks (Argasidae and Ixodidae) since the 19th century, assessed by PCR. *Medical and Veterinary Entomology*, Vol. 12, No. 1, (January 1998), pp. 89-97, ISSN 0269-283X

Humphery-Smith, I., Thong, YH., Moorhouse, D., Creevey, C., Gauci, M. & Stone, B. (1991). Reactions to argasid tick bites by island residents on the Great Barrier Reef. *Medical Journal of Australia*, Vol. 155, No. 3, (August 1991), pp. 181-186, ISSN 0025-729X.

Humphery-Smith, I., Donker, G., Turzo, A., Chastel, C. & Schmidt-Mayerova, H. (1993). Evaluation of mechanical transmission of HIV by the African soft tick, *Ornithodoros moubata*. *AIDS*. Vol. 7, No. 3, (March 1993), pp. 341-347, ISSN 0269-9370.

Jaenson, TG., Tälleklint, L., Lundqvist, L., Olsen, B., Chirico, J. & Mejlon, H. (1994). Geographical distribution, host associations, and vector roles of ticks (Acari: Ixodidae, Argasidae) in Sweden. *Journal of Medical Entomology*, Vol. 31, No.2, (March 1994), pp. 240-256, ISSN 0022-2585.

Jongejan, F. & Uilenberg, G. (2004). The global importance of ticks. *Parasitology*, Vol. 129, No. suppl, pp. s3-s14, ISSN 0031-1820

Jori, F. & Bastos, AD. (2009). Role of wild suids in the epidemiology of African swine fever. *Ecohealth*, Vol. 6, No. 2, (June 2009), pp. 296-310, ISSN 1612-9202.

Jupp, PG., Joubert, JJ., Cornel, AJ., Swanevelder, C. & Prozesky, OW. (1987). An experimental assessment of the tampan tick *Ornithodoros moubata* as vector of hepatitis B virus. *Medical Veterinary Entomology*, Vol. 1, No. 4, (October 1987), pp. 361-368, ISSN 0269-283X.

Karbowiak, G. & Supergan, M. (2007). The new locality of *Argas reflexus fabricius*, 1794 in Warsaw, Poland. *Wiadomosci Parazytologiczne*,Vol. 53, No. 2, pp. 143-144, ISSN 0043-5163.

Kawabata, H., Ando, S., Kishimoto, T., Kurane, I., Takano, A., Nogami, S., Fujita, H., Tsurumi, M., Nakamura, N., Sato, F., Takahashi, M., Ushijima, Y., Fukunaga, M. & Watanabe, H. (2006). First detection of Rickettsia in soft-bodied ticks associated with seabirds, Japan. *Microbiology and Immunology*, Vol. 50, No. 5, pp. 403-406, ISSN 0385-5600.

Keirans, JE., Clifford, CM. & Capriles, JM. (1971). *Argas* (argas) *dulus*, new species (Ixodoidea: Argasidae), from nests of the palm chat *Dulus dominicus* in the Dominican Republic. *Journal of Economic Entomology*. Vol. 64, No. 6, (November 1971), pp. 1410-1413, ISSN 0022-0493.

Keirans, JE., Radovsky, FJ. & Clifford, CM. (1973). *Argas* (*argas*) *monachus*, new species (Ixodoidea: Argasidae), from nests of the monk parakeet, *Myiopsitta monachus*, in Argentina. *Journal of Medical Entomology*, Vol. 10, No. 5, (November 1973), pp. 511-516, ISSN 0022-2585.

Keirans, JE., Clifford, CM. & Hoogstraal, H. (1984). *Ornithodoros* (*alectorobius*) *yunkeri*, new species (Acari: Ixodoidea: Argasidae), from seabirds and nesting sites in the Galapagos Islands. *Journal of Medical Entomology*, Vol. 21, No. 3, (May 1984), pp. 344-350, ISSN 0022-2585.

Keirans, JE. & Durden, LA. (2001). Invasion: exotic ticks (Acari: Argasidae, Ixodidae) imported into the United States. A review and new records. *Journal of Medical Entomology*, Vol. 38, No. 6, (November 2001), pp. 850-861, ISSN 0022-2585.

Khoury, C., Bianchi, R., Massa, AA., Severini, F. Di Luca, M. & Toma, L. (2011). A noteworthy record of *Ornithodoros* (*Alectorobius*) *coniceps* (Ixodida: Argasidae) from Central Italy. *Experimental and Applied Acarology*, Vol 54, No. 2, (June 2011), pp. 205-209, ISSN 0168-8162.

Kleiboeker, SB., Burrage, TG., Scoles, GA., Fish, D. & Rock, DL. (1998). African swine fever virus infection in the argasid host, *Ornithodoros porcinus porcinus*. *Journal of Virology*, Vol. 72, No. 3, (March 1998), pp. 1711-1724, ISSN 0022-538X.

Kleiboeker, SB. & Scoles, GA. (2001). Pathogenesis of African swine fever virus in *Ornithodoros* ticks. *Animal Health Research Reviews*, Vol. 2, No.2, (December 2001), pp. 121-128, ISSN 1466-2523.

Kotsyfakis, M., Anderson, JM., Andersen, JF., Calvo, E., Francischetti, IM., Mather, TN., Valenzuela, JG. & Ribeiro, JM. (2008). Cutting edge: immunity against a "silent" salivary antigen of the lyme vector *Ixodes scapularis* impairs its ability to feed. *Journal of Immunology*, Vol. 81, No. 8, (October 2008), pp. 5209-5212, ISSN 0022-1767.

Labruna, MB., Terassini, FA., Camargo, LM., Brandão, PE., Ribeiro, AF. & Estrada-Peña, A. (2008). New reports of *Antricola guglielmonei* and *Antricola delacruzi* in Brazil, and a description of a new argasid species (Acari). *Journal of Parasitology*, Vol. 94, No. 4, (August 2008), pp. 788-792, ISSN 0022-3395.

Labruna, MB., Nava, S., Terassini, FA., Onofrio, VC., Barros-Battesti, DM., Camargo, LM. & Venzal, JM. (2011). Description of adults and nymph, and redescription of the larva, of *Ornithodoros marinkellei* (Acari: Argasidae), with data on its phylogenetic position. *Journal of Parasitology*, Vol. 97, No. 2, (April 2011), pp. 207-217, ISSN 0022-3395.

Labuda, M. & Nuttall, PA. (2004). Tick-borne viruses. *Parasitology*. Vol. 129, pp. 221-245, ISSN 0031-1820.

Labuda, M. & Nuttall, PA. (2008). Viruses transmitted by ticks. In: *Ticks: biology, disease and control*. Alan S. Bowman & Pat Nuttall (Eds.), pp. 253-280, Cambridge University Press, ISBN 978-0-521-86761-0,Cambridge. UK.

Lane, RS., Moss, RB., Hsu, YP., Wei, T., Mesirow, ML. & Kuo, MM. (1999). Anti-arthropod saliva antibodies among residents of a community at high risk for Lyme disease in California. *The American Journal of Tropical Medicine and Hygiene*, Vol. 61, No. 5, (November 1999), pp. 850-859, ISSN 0002-9637.

Lawrie, CH., Uzcátegui, NY., Gould, EA. & Nuttall, PA. (2004). Ixodid and Argasid tick species and West Nile Virus. *Emerging Infectious Diseases*, Vol. 10, No. 4, (April 2004), pp. 653-657, ISSN 1080-6040.

Lisbôa, RS., Teixeira, RC., Rangel, CP., Santos, HA., Massard, CL. & Fonseca, AH. (2009). Avian spirochetosis in chickens following experimental transmission of *Borrelia anserina* by *Argas* (*Persicargas*) *miniatus*. *Avian Diseases*, Vol. 53, No. 2, (June 2009), pp. 166-168, ISSN 0005-2086.

Loftis, AD., Gill, JS., Schriefer, ME., Levin, ML., Eremeeva, ME., Gilchrist, MJ. & Dasch, GA. (2005). Detection of *Rickettsia*, *Borrelia*, and *Bartonella* in *Carios kelleyi* (Acari: Argasidae). *Journal of Medical Entomology*, Vol. 42, No. 2, (May 2005), pp. 473-480, ISSSN 0022-2585.

Londoño, I. (1976). Transmission of microfilariae and infective larvae of *Dipetalonema viteae* (Filarioidea) among vector ticks, *Ornithodoros tartakowskyi* (Argasidae), and loss of microfilariae in coxal fluid. *Journal of Parasitology*, Vol. 62, No. 5, (October 1976), pp. 786-788, ISSN 0022-3395.

Lucius, R. & Textor, G. (1995). *Acanthocheilonema viteae*: rational design of the life cycle to increase production of parasite material using less experimental animals. *Applied Parasitology*, Vol. 36, No. 1, (February 1995), pp. 22-33, ISSN 0943-0938.

Málková, D., Holubová, J., Cerný, V., Daniel, M., Fernández, A., de la Cruz, J., Herrera, M. & Calisher, CH. (1985). Estero real virus: a new virus isolated from argasid ticks *Ornithodoros tadaridae* in Cuba. *Acta Virologica*, Vol. 29, No. 3, (May 1985), pp. 247-250, ISSN 001-723X.

Manilla, G. (1990). *Ornithodoros* (Alectorobius) *maritimus* (Ixodoidea, Argasidae) a new species in Italy and observations on the coniceps-capensis group. *Parassitologia*. Vol. 32, No. 2, (August 1990), pp. 265-74, ISSN 0048-2951.

Mans, JB., Gothe, R. & Neitz, AWH. (2008a). Tick toxins: perspectives on paralysis and other forms of toxicoses caused by ticks. In: *Ticks: biology, disease and control*. Alan S. Bowman & Pat Nuttall (Eds.), pp. 92-107, Cambridge University Press, ISBN 978-0-521-86761-0, Cambridge, UK.

Mans, B.J., Ribeiro, J.W. & Andersen, J.A. (2008b). Structure, function and evolution of biogenic amine-binding proteins in soft ticks. *Journal of Biological Chemistry*, Vol. 283, pp. 18721–18733, ISSN 0021-9258.

Manzano-Román, R., Encinas-Grandes, A & Pérez-Sánchez, R. (2006). Antigens from the midgut membranes of *Ornithodoros erraticus* induce lethal anti-tick immune responses in pigs and mice. *Veterinary Parasitology*, Vol. 135, No. 1, (January 2006), pp. 65-79, ISSN 0304-4017.

Manzano-Román, R., García-Varas, S., Encinas-Grandes, A. & Pérez-Sánchez, R. (2007). Purification and characterization of a 45-kda concealed antigen from the midgut membranes of *Ornithodoros erraticus* that induces lethal anti-tick immune responses in pigs. *Veterinary Parasitology*. Vol. 145, No. 3-4, (April 2007), pp. 314-325, ISSN 0304-4017.

Martins, JR., Doyle, RL., Barros-Battesti, DM., Onofrio, VC. & Guglielmone, AA. (2011). Occurrence of *Ornithodoros brasiliensis* Aragão (Acari: Argasidae) in São Francisco de Paula, RS, Southern Brazil. *Neotropical Entomology*, Vol. 40, No. 1 (February 2011), pp. 143-144, ISSN 1519-566X.

Maruashvili, GM. (1965). Studies on natural foci of some diseases in Georgia, USSR. In: *Studies on natural foci of some diseases in Georgia, USSR*, pp. 469-475, ISBN 19651000816.

Masoumi, Asl H., Goya, MM., Vatandoost, H., Zahraei, SM., Mafi, M., Asmar, M., Piazak, N. & Aghighi, Z. (2009). The epidemiology of tick-borne relapsing fever in Iran during 1997-2006. *Travel Medicine and Infectious Disease*, Vol. 7, No. 3, (May 2009), pp. 160-164, ISSN 1477-8939

McCall, PJ., Hume, JC., Motshegwa, K., Pignatelli, P., Talbert, A. & Kisinza, W. (2007). Does tick-borne relapsing fever have an animal reservoir in East Africa?. *Vector Borne and Zoonotic Diseases*, Vol. 7, No. 4, (September 2007), pp. 659-666, ISSN 1530-3667.

McVicar, JW., Mebus, CA., Becker, HN., Belden, RC. & Gibbs, EP. (1981). Induced African swine fever in feral pigs. *Journal of the American Veterinary Medical Association*, Vol. 179, No. 5, (September 1981), pp. 441-446, ISSN 0003-1488.

Mediannikov, O., Fenollar, F., Socolovschi, C., Diatta, G., Bassene, H., Molez, JF., Sokhna, C., Trape, JF. & Raoult, D. (2010). *Coxiella burnetii* in humans and ticks in rural Senegal. *PloS Neglected Tropical Diseases*, Vol. 4, No. 4, (April 2010), pp. 654, ISSN 1935-2727.

Miller, BR., Loomis, R., Dejean, A. & Hoogstraal, H. (1985). Experimental studies on the replication and dissemination of qalyub virus (Bunyaviridae: Nairovirus) in the putative tick vector, *Ornithodoros* (*Pavlovskyella*) *erraticus*. *The American Journal of Tropical Medicine and Hygiene* Vol. 34, No.1, (January 1985), pp. 180-187, ISSN 0002-9637.

Mishchenko, OA., Tsvetkova, SM., Borisevich, SV. & Grabarev, PA. (2010). Experimental study of relations of the argasid ticks *Alveonasus lahorensis* with *Coxiella burneti*. *Meditsinskaia parazitologiia i parazitarnye bolezni*, Vol. 2, pp. 40-42, ISSN 0025-8326.

Mitani, H., Talbert, A. & Fukunaga, M. (2004). New world relapsing fever Borrelia found in *Ornithodoros porcinus* ticks in central Tanzania. *Microbiology and Immunology*, Vol. 48, No. 7, pp. 501-505, ISSN 0385-5600.

Moemenbellah-Fard, MD., Benafshi, O., Rafinejad, J. & Ashraf, H. (2009). Tick-borne relapsing fever in a new highland endemic focus of western Iran. *Annals of Tropical Medicine and Parasitology* Vol. 103, No. 6, (September 2009), pp. 529-537, ISSN 0003-4983.

Montasser, AA. (2005). Gram-negative bacteria from the camel tick *Hyalomma dromedarii* (Ixodidae) and the chicken tick *Argas persicus* (Argasidae) and their antibiotic sensitivities. *Journal of the Egyptian Society of Parasitology*, Vol. 35, No. 1, (April 2005), pp. 95-106, ISSN 0253-5890.

Mumcuoglu, KY., Banet-Noach, C., Malkinson, M., Shalom, U. & Galun, R. (2005). Argasid ticks as possible vectors of west Nile virus in Israel. *Vector Borne Zoonotic Diseases*. Vol. 5, No. 1, pp. 65-71, ISSN 1530-3667.

Nava, S., Caparrós, JA., Mangold, AJ. & Guglielmone, AA. (2006). Ticks (Acari: Ixodida: Argasidae, Ixodidae) infesting humans in northwestern Cordoba province, Argentina. *Medicina (B aires)*. Vol. 66, No. 3, pp. 225-228, ISSN 0025-7680.

Nava, S., Lareschi, M., Rebollo, C., Benítez Usher, C., Beati, L., Robbins, RG., Durden, LA., Mangold, AJ. & Guglielmone, AA. (2007). The ticks (Acari: Ixodida: Argasidae, Ixodidae) of Paraguay. *Annals of Tropical Medicine and Parasitology* Vol. 101, No. 3, (April 2007), pp. 255-70, ISSN 0003-4983.

Nava, S., Guglielmone, AA. & Mangold, AJ. (2009a). An overview of systematics and evolution of ticks. *Frontiers in Bioscience*, Vol. 14, (January 2009), pp. 2857-2877, ISSN 1093-9946.

Nava, S., Mangold, AJ. & Guglielmone, AA. (2009b). Field and laboratory studies in a neotropical population of the spinose ear tick, *Otobius megnini*. *Medical and Veterinary Entomology*, Vol. 23, No. 1, (March 2009), pp. 1-5, ISSN 0269-283X.

Nava, S., Venzal, JM., Terassini, FA., Mangold, AJ., Camargo, LM. & Labruna, MB. (2010). Description of a new Argasid tick (Acari: Ixodida) from bat caves in Brazilian Amazon. *Journal of Parasitology*, Vol. 96, No. 6, (December 2010), pp. 1089-1101, ISSN 0022-3395.

Nebreda Mayoral, T., Merino, FJ., Serrano, JL., Fernández-Soto, P., Encinas, A. & Pérez-Sánchez, R. (2004). Detection of antibodies to tick salivary antigens among patients from a region of Spain. *European Journal of Epidemiolgy*. Vol. 19,No. 1, pp. 79-83, ISSN 0393-2990.

Need, JT., Dale, WE., Keirans, JE. & Dasch, GA. (1991). Annotated list of ticks (Acari: Ixodidae, Argasidae) reported in Peru: distribution, hosts, and bibliography. *Journal of Medical Entomology*, Vol. 28, No. 5, (September 1991), pp. 590-597, ISSN 0022-2585.

Noda, H., Munderloh, UG. & Kurtti, TJ. (1997). Endosymbionts of ticks and their relationship to *Wolbachia* spp. and tick-borne pathogens of humans and animals. *Applied and Environmental Microbiology*,Vol. 63, No. 10, (October 1997), pp. 3926-3932, ISSN 0099-2240.

Ntiamoa-Baidu, Y., Carr-Saunders, C., Matthews, BE., Preston, PM. & Walker, AR. (2004). An updated list of the ticks of Ghana and an assessment of the distribution of the ticks of Ghanaian wild mammals in different vegetation zones. *Bulletin of Entomological Research*, Vol. 94, No.3, (June 2004), pp. 245-60, ISSN 0007-4853.

Nyangiwe, N., Gummow, B. & Horak, IG. (2008). The prevalence and distribution of *Argas walkerae* (Acari: Argasidae) in the eastern region of the eastern cape province, South Africa. *Onderstepoort Journal of Veterinary Research*, Vol. 75, No. 1, (March 2008), pp. 83-86, ISSN 0030-2465.

Oleaga-Pérez, A., Pérez-Sánchez, R. & Encinas-Grandes, A. (1990). Distribution and biology of *Ornithodoros erraticus* in parts of Spain affected by African swine fever. *Veterinary Record*, Vol. 126, No. 2, (January 1990), pp.32-37, ISSN 0042-4900.

Oleaga-Pérez, A., Pérez-Sánchez, R., Astigarraga, A. & Encinas-Grandes, A. (1994) Detection of pig farms with *Ornithodoros erraticus* by pig serology. Elimination of non-specific reactions by carbohydrate epitopes of salivary antigens. *Veterinary Parasitology*, Vol. 52, No. 1-2, (March 1994), pp. 97-111, ISSN 0304-4017.

Oleaga, A., Escudero-Población, A., Camafeita, E. & Pérez-Sánchez R. (2007). A proteomic approach to the identification of salivary proteins from the argasid ticks *Ornithodoros moubata* and *Ornithodoros erraticus*. *Insect Biochemistry and Molecular Biology*. Vol. 37, No. 11, (November 2007), pp. 1149-59, ISSN 0965-1748.

Ostfeld, RS., Price, A., Hornbostel, VL. & Benjamin, AB. (2006). Controlling ticks and tick-borne zoonoses with biological and chemical agents. *Bioscience*. Vol. 5, pp. 383–394, ISSN 0006-3568.

Pantaleoni, RA., Baratti, M., Barraco, L., Contini, C., Cossu, CS., Filippelli, MT., Loru, L. & Romano, M. (2010). *Argas* (*Persicargas*) *persicus* (Oken, 1818) (Ixodida: Argasidae) in Sicily with considerations about its Italian and West-Mediterranean distribution. *Parasite*. Vol. 17, No. 4, (December 2010), pp. 349-355, ISSN 1252-607X.

Parola, P. & Raoult, D. (2001). Ticks and tickborne bacterial disease in humans: an emerging infection threat. *Clinical Infectious Disases*,Vol. 32, pp. 897-928, ISSN 1058-4838.

Patz, JA., Githeko, AK., Mccarty, JP., Hussein, S., Confalonieri, U. & de Wet, UN. (2010). Climate change and infectious diseases. Chapter 6. In: *Climate change and health*. Fact sheet No. 266.
http://www.who.int/globalchange/publications/climatechangechap6.pdf

Pérez-Sánchez, R., Oleaga-Pérez, A. & Encinas-Grandes, A. (1992). Analysis of the specificity of the salivary antigens of *Ornithodoros erraticus* for the purpose of serological detection of swine farms harbouring the parasite. *Parasite Immunology*, Vol. 14, No. 2, (March 1992), pp.201-216, ISSN 0141-9838.

Pérez-Sánchez, R., Astigarraga, A., Oleaga-Pérez, A. & Encinas-Grandes, A. (1994). Relationship between the persistence of African swine fever and the distribution of *Ornithodoros erraticus* in the province of Salamanca, Spain. *Veterinary Record*, Vol. 135, No. 9, (August 1994), pp. 207-209, ISSN 0042-4900.

Petney, TN., Andrews, RH., Mcdiarmid, LA. & Dixon, BR. (2004). *Argas persicus* sensu stricto does occur in Australia. *Parasitology Research*, Vol. 93, No.4, (July 2004), pp. 296-299, ISSN 0932-0113.

Peter, RJ., Van den Bossche, P., Penzhorn, BL. & Sharp, B. (2005). Tick, fly, and mosquito control-lessons from the past, solutions for the future. *Veterinary Parasitology*, Vol. 132, No. 3, (September 2005), pp. 205-15, ISSN 0304-4017.

Phiri, BJ., Benschop, J. & French, NP. (2010). Systematic review of causes and factors associated with morbidity and mortality on smallholder dairy farms in eastern and southern Africa. *Preventive Veterinary Medicine*, Vol. 94, No. 1-2, (April 2010), p. 1-8, ISSN 0167-5877.

Poggiato, M. (2008). *Argas reflexus*, the pigeon tick. A case report. *Recenti Progressi in Medicina*. Vol. 99, No. 4, (April 2008), pp. 204-206, ISSN 2038-1840.

Polar, P., Moore, D., Kairo, MTK. & Ramsubhag, A. (2008). Topically applied myco-acaricides for the control of cattle ticks: overcoming the challenges. *Experimental and Applied Acarology*, Vol. 46, pp. 119–148, ISSN 0168-8162.

Rajput, ZI., Hu, SH., Chen, WJ., Arijo, AG. & Xiao, CW. (2006). Importance of ticks and their chemical and immunological control in livestock. *Journal of Zhejiang University Science-B*. Vol. 7, No. 11, (November 2006), pp. 912-921, ISSN 1673-1581.

Randolph, SE. (2008). Dynamics of tick-borne disease systems: minor role of recent climate change. *Revue Scientifique et Technique (International Office of Epizootics)*,Vol. 27, No. 2, (August 2008), pp. 367-381, ISSN 0253-1933.

Randolph, SE. (2010). To what extent has climate change contributed to the recent epidemiology of tick-borne diseases?. *Veterinary Parasitology*, Vol. 167, pp. 92–94, ISSN 0304-4017.

Ravaomanana, J., Jori, F., Vial, L., Pérez-Sánchez, R., Blanco, E., Michaud, V. & Roger, F. (2011). Assessment of interactions between African swine fever virus, bushpigs (*Potamochoerus larvatus*), *Ornithodoros* ticks and domestic pigs in north-western Madagascar. *Transboundary and Emerging Diseases*, Vol. 58, No. 3, (June 2011), pp. 247-254, ISSN 1865-1674.

Rawlings, JA. (1995). An overview of tick-borne relapsing fever with emphasis on outbreaks in Texas. *Texas Medicine* Vol. 91, No. 5, (May 1995), pp. 56-59, ISSN 0040-4470

Rebaudet, S. & Parola, P. (2006). Epidemiology of relapsing fever borreliosis in Europe. *FEMS Immunology and Medical Microbiology*, Vol. 48, No.1, (October 2006), pp. 11-15, ISSN 0928-8244.

Reeves, WK., Loftis, AD., Priestley, RA., Wills, W., Sanders, F. & Dasch, GA. (2005). Molecular and biological characterization of a novel coxiella-like agent from *Carios capensis*. *Annals of the New York Academy of Sciences*, Vol. 1063, (December 2005), pp. 343-345, ISSN 0077-8923.

Reeves, WK., Loftis, AD., Sanders, F., Spinks, MD., Wills, W., Denison, AM. & Dasch, GA. (2006). Borrelia, Coxiella, and Rickettsia in *Carios capensis* (Acari: Argasidae) from a brown pelican (*Pelecanus occidentalis*) rookery in South Carolina, USA. *Experimantal Applied Acarology*, Vol. 39, No. 3-4, pp. 321-329, ISSN 0168-8162.

Reperant, LA. (2010). Applying the theory of island biogeography to emerging pathogens: toward predicting the sources of future emerging zoonotic and vector-borne diseases. *Vector Borne Zoonotic Diseases*. Vol. 10, No. 2, (March 2010), pp. 105-10, ISSN 1530-3667.

Rowlands, RJ., Michaud, V., Heath, L., Hutchings, G., Oura, C., Vosloo, W., Dwarka, R., Onashvili, T. & Albina, E., Dixon, LK. (2008). African swine fever virus isolate, Georgia. *Emerging Infectious Diseases*, Vol. 14, No. 12, (December 2008), ISSN 1080-6040.

Samish, M., Ginsberg, H. & Glazer, I. (2004). Biological control of ticks. *Parasitology*. Vol. 129, pp. 389-403, ISSN 0031-1820.

Samish, M., Ginsberg, H. & Glazer, I. (2008). Anti.ticj biological control agents: assessment and future perspectives. In: *Ticks: biology, disease and control*. Alan S. Bowman & Pat Nuttall (Eds.), pp. 447-469, Cambridge University Press, ISBN 978-0-521-86761-0, Cambridge, UK.

Sánchez-Vizcaíno, JM. (2006). African Swine Fever. In: *Diseases of Swine*. 9th edition. Straw, B., Zimmerman, J., D'Allaire, S., Taylor, D. (Eds.), pp. 291-298, Blackwell Publishing Ltd., ISBN: 9780813817033, Oxford, UK.

Schwan, TG., Corwin, MD. & Brown, SJ. (1992). *Argas (argas) monolakensis*, new species (Acari: Ixodoidea: Argasidae), a parasite of California gulls on islands in mono lake, California: description, biology, and life cycle. *Journal of Medical Entomology*, Vol. 29, pp. 78-97, ISSN 0022-2585.

Schwan, TG., Raffel, SJ., Schrumpf, ME. & Porcella, SF. (2007). Diversity and distribution of *Borrelia hermsii*. *Emerging Infectious Diseases*, Vol. 13, No. 3, (March 2007), pp. 436-42, ISSN 1080-6040.

Schwan, TG., Raffel, SJ., Schrumpf, ME., Gill, JS. & Piesman, J. (2009). Characterization of a novel relapsing fever spirochete in the midgut, coxal fluid, and salivary glands of the bat tick *Carios kelleyi*. *Vector Borne and Zoonotic Diseases*, Vol. 9, No. 6, (December 2009), pp. 643-647, ISSN 1530-3667.

Schwartz, BS., Nadelman, RB., Fish, D., Childs, JE., Forseter, G. & Wormser, GP. (1993). Entomologic and demographic correlates of anti-tick saliva antibody in a prospective study of tick bite subjects in Westchester County, New York. *The American Journal of Tropical Medicine and Hygiene*, Vol. 48, No. 1, (January 1993), pp. 50-7, ISSN 0002-9637.

Sewify, GH. & Habib, SM. (2001). Biological control of the tick fowl *Argas persicus* by the entomopathogenic fungi *Beauveria bassiana* and *Metarhizium anisopliae*. *Journal of Pest Science*. Vol. 74, pp. 121–123, ISSN 1612-4758.

Shanbaky, NM. & Helmy, N. (2000). First record of natural infection with *Borrelia* in *Ornithodoros* (*Ornithodoros*) *savignyi*. Reservoir potential and specificity of the tick to *Borrelia*. *Juornal of the Egyptian Society of Parasitology*, Vol. 30, No. 3, (December 2000), pp. 765-780, ISSN 0253-5890.

Shepherd, AJ., Swanepoel, R., Cornel, AJ. & Mathee, O. (1989). Experimental studies on the replication and transmission of crimean-congo hemorrhagic fever virus in some African tick species. *American Journal of Tropical Medicine and Hygiene* Vol. 40, No. 3, (March 1989), pp. 326-331, ISSN 0002-9637.

Sidi, G., Davidovitch, N., Balicer, RD., Anis, E., Grotto, I. & Schwartz, E. (2005). Tick-borne relapsing fever in Israel. *Emerging Infectious Diseases*, Vol. 11, No. 11, (November 2005), pp. 1784-1786, ISSN 1080-6040.

Siuda, K. (1996). Bionomical and ecological characteristic of ticks (Acari: Ixodida) of significant medical importance on the territory of Poland. *Roczniki Akademii Medycznej w Bialymstoku*. Vol. 41, No. 1, pp. 11-19, ISSN 1427-941X.

Sonenshine, DE. (1992). *Biology of ticks Vol. 1.* Oxford University Press, ISBN-13: 978-0195059106, New York, USA.

Sonenshine, DE., Lane, RS. & Nicholson, WL. (2002). Ticks (Ixodida). In: *Medical and Veterinary Entomology*, G. Mullen and L. Durden (Eds). pp. 517-558. Academic Press, ISBN: 978-0-12-372500-4, Boston, USA.

Steinlein, DB., Durden, LA. & Cannon, WL. (2001). Tick (Acari) infestations of bats in New Mexico. *Journal of Medical Entomology*, Vol. 38, No. 4, (July 2001), pp. 609-11, ISSN 0022-2585.

Stott, JL., Osburn, BI. & Alexander, L. (1985). *Ornithodoros coriaceus* (Pajaroello tick) as a vector of bluetongue virus. *American Journal of Veterinary Research* Vol. 46, No. 5, (May 1985), pp. 1197-1199, ISSN 0002-9645.

Sureau, P., klein, JM., Casals, J., Digoutte, JP., Salaun, JJ., Piazak, N. & Calvo, MA. (1980). Isolement des virus thogoto, wad medani, wanowrie et de la fievre hemorragique de crimée-congo en Iran a partir de tiques dánimaux domestiques. *Annales de L'Institut Pasteur, Série Virologie*. Vol. 131e, pp. 185-200, ISSN 0924-4204

Tahmasebi, F., Ghiasi, SM., Mostafavi, E., Moradi, M., Piazak, N., Mozafari, A., Haeri, A., Fooks, AR. & Chinikar, S. (2010). Molecular epidemiology of Crimean- Congo hemorrhagic fever virus genome isolated from ticks of Hamadan province of Iran. *Journal of Vector Borne Diseases*, Vol. 47, No. 4, (September 2010), pp. 211-216, ISSN 0972-9062.

Teglas, MB., Drazenovich, NL., Stott, J & Foley, JE. (2006). The geographic distribution of the putative agent of epizootic bovine abortion in the tick vector, *Ornithodoros coriaceus*. *Veterinary Parasitology*, Vol. 140, No. 3-4, (September 2006), pp. 327-33, ISSN 0304-4017.

Telmadarraiy, Z., Ghiasi, SM, Moradi, M., Vatandoost, H., Eshraghian, MR., Faghihi, F., Zarei, Z., Haeri, A. & Chinikar, S. (2010). A survey of crimean-congo haemorrhagic fever in livestock and ticks in Ardabil province, Iran during 2004-2005. *Scandinavian Journal of Infectious Diseases*, Vol. 42, No. 2, pp. 137-141, ISSN 0036-5548.

Tizu, T., Schumaker, S. & Barros, DM. (1995). Life cycle of *Ornithodoros* (*Alectorobius*) *talaje* (Acari: Argasidae) in laboratory. *Journal of Medical Entomology*, Vol. 32, No. 3, (May 1995), pp. 249-254, ISSN 0022-2585.

Turell, MJ. & Durden, LA. (1994). Experimental transmission of langat (tick-borne encephalitis virus complex) virus by the soft tick *Ornithodoros sonrai* (Acari: Argasidae). *Journal of Medical Entomology*, Vol. 31, No. 1, (January 1994), pp. 148-151, ISSN 0022-2585.

Turell, MJ., Mores, CN., Lee, JS., Paragas, JJ., Shermuhemedova, D., Endy, TP. & Khodjaev, S. (2004). Experimental transmission of karshi and langat (tick-borne encephalitis virus complex) viruses by *Ornithodoros* ticks (Acari: Argasidae). *Journal of Medical Entomology*, Vol. 41, No. 5, (September 2004), pp. 973-977, ISSN 0022-2585.

Ushijima, Y., Oliver, JH. Jr, Keirans, JE., Tsurumi, M., Kawabata, H., Watanabe, H. & Fukunaga, M. (2003). Mitochondrial sequence variation in *Carlos capensis* (*Neumann*), a parasite of seabirds, collected on Torishima Island in Japan. *Journal of Parasitology*, Vol. 89, No. 1, (February 2003), pp. 196-198, ISSN 0022-3395.

Udvardy, MDF. (1975). A classification of the biogeographical provinces of the world. IUCN Occasional Paper no. 18. Morges, Switzerland: IUCN

Venzal, JM. & Estrada-Peña, A. (2006). Larval feeding performance of two neotropical *Ornithodoros* ticks (Acari: Argasidae) on reptiles. *Experimantal Appleid Acarology*, Vol. 39, No. 3-4, pp. 315-20, ISSN 0168-8162.

Venzal, JM., Estrada-Peña, A., Mangold, AJ., González-Acuña, D. & Guglielmone, AA. (2008). The *Ornithodoros* (*Alectorobius*) *talaje* species group (Acari: Ixodida: Argasidae): description of *ornithodoros* (*Alectorobius*) *rioplatensis* n. sp. from southern

South America. *Journal of Medical Entomology*, Vol. 45, No. 5, (September 2008), pp. 832-40, ISSN 0022-2585.

Vermeil, C., Marjolet, M. & Chastel, C. (1996). Argas et arbovirus. Actualités. *Bulletin de la Societé de Pathologie Exotique*, Vol. 89, pp. 363-365, ISSN 0037-9085.

Vial, L., Durand, P., Arnathau, C., Halos, L., Diatta, G., Trape, JF. & Renaud, F. (2006). Molecular divergences of the *Ornithodoros sonrai* soft tick species, a vector of human relapsing fever in West Africa. *Microbes and Infection*, Vol. 8, No. 11, (September 2006), pp. 2605-2611, ISSN 1286-4579.

Vial, L., Wieland, B., Jori, F., Etter, E., Dixon, L. & Roger, F. (2007). African swine fever virus DNA in soft ticks, Senegal. *Emerging Infectious Diseases*, Vol. 13, No. 12, (December 2007), pp. 1928-1931, ISSN 1080-6040.

Vial, L. (2009). Biological and ecological characteristics of soft ticks (Ixodida: Argasidae) and their impact for predicting tick and associated disease distribution. *Parasite*, Vol. 16, No. 3, (September 2009), pp. 191-202, ISSN 1252-607X.

Walton, GA. (1951). *Ornithodoros savignyi* (Audouin) 1826, Argasidae, in the Embu District of Kenya Colony. *East African Medical Journal*, Vol. 28, No. 4, (April 1951), pp. 189, ISSN 0012 835X.

Whitney, MS., Schwan, TG., Sultemeier, KB., McDonald, PS. & Brillhart, MN. (2007). Spirochetemia caused by *Borrelia turicatae* infection in 3 dogs in Texas. *Veterinary Clinical Pathology*,Vol. 36, No. 2, (June 2007), pp. 212-216, ISSN 0275-6382.

Wieland, B., Dhollander, S., Salman, M. & Koenen, F. (2011). Qualitative risk assessment in a data-scarce environment: A model to assess the impact of control measures on spread of African Swine Fever. *Preventive Veterinary Medicine*, Vol. 99, No. 1, (April 2011), pp. 4-14, ISSN 0167-5877.

Willadsen, P. (2008). Antigen cocktails: valid hypothesis or unsubstantiated hope? *Trends in Parasitology*. Vol. 24 No., 4 (April 2008) pp. 164-167, ISSN 1471-4922.

Yamaguti, N., Clifford, CM. & Tipton, VJ. (1968). *Argas* (Argas) *japonicus*, new species, associated with swallows in Japan and Korea. (Ixodoidea Argasidae). *Journal of Medical Entomology*, Vol. 5, No. 4, (October 1968), pp. 453-459, ISSN 0022-2585.

Zabalgogeazcoa, I., Oleaga, A & Pérez-Sánchez, R. (2008). Pathogenicity of endophytic entomopathogenic fungi to *Ornithodoros erraticus* and *Ornithodoros moubata* (Acari: Argasidae). *Veterinary Parasitology*, Vol. 158, No. 4, (December 2008), pp. 336-343, ISSN 0304-4017.

8

Parasitic Nematodes of some Insects from Manipur, India

M. Manjur Shah, N. Mohilal, M. Pramodini and L.Bina
Section of Parasitology,
Department of Life Sciences,
Manipur University,
Imphal, Manipur
India

1. Introduction

Manipur is situated in the north east of India. The state covers an area of 22,356 sq.kms of which the hilly region is about 91.75%, while the remaining 8.25% of the geographical area constitutes the central valley region. It lies between $23^{0}51$`N and $25^{0}41$`N latitudes and $93^{0}2$`E to $94^{0}47$`E longitudes. Generally, two types of climatic conditions are found in this state according to latitude, topography and direction of the prevailing wind system. Tropical monsoon type of climate prevails in the valley area whereas the cool temperate climate prevails in the hilly areas. The average maximum temperature of this state is 31^{0}C, the minimum temperature is 5^{0}C and the rainfall is about 2077mm per annum. Manipur being part of The North East India represents an important part of the Indo-Myanmar biodiversity hot spot recognized recently in the year 2005 among 34 Biodiversity hotspot of the world.

The present work mainly concerns with the nematodes of insects of Manipur. Nematodes are regarded as the most numerous multicellular animals on earth. There are over 20,000 described species classified in the phylum Nematoda. Most of the free-living nematodes are microscopic; many of the parasitic species invade the body fluids such as blood or lymph channels of their hosts. They exhibit a wide range of feeding habits. Many feed entirely on the microorganisms present in decaying vegetable matter (saprophytic), others live on plants and wander destructively through the tissues and suck their sap. In vertebrates they may parasitize every organ often causing destructive and painful diseases and producing immeasurable hardships. Their life cycle ranges from very simple to extremely complicated. The majority of the nematodes are oviparous, but some are ovoviviparous. All nematode juveniles whether they hatch in water or soil or within the animal host must undergo a series of 4 moults before reaching maturity. Entomophilic or insect nematodes are distributed in 27 families among nine major groups of nematodes viz., Rhabditoid, Tylenchoid, Aphelenchoid, Strongyloid, Oxyuroid, Ascaridoid, Spiruroid, Filaroid and Mermithoid. The first eight groups belong to the Rhabditea (plant and animal parasitic form) and the 9th belong to the Enoplea (mostly free living, microbotrophic aquatic nematodes). The Order Oxyurida contains parasites that parasitize both invertebrate and vertebrate hosts. The nematodes parasitizing the vertebrate hosts belong to the superfamily

Oxyuroidea and those nematodes parasitizing the invertebrate hosts belong to the superfamily Thelastomatoidea. The families listed under the latter superfamily are Thelastomatidae, Travassosinematidae, Protrelloididae, Hystrignathidae and Pseudonymidae [Adamson & Waerebeke, 1992a,b,c]. With the discovery of haplodiploid reproduction [Adamson, 1984] in this group of nematodes in which males develop from unfertilized eggs (haploid) and females from fertilized eggs (diploid) more attention is being paid to the above group of nematodes in the recent time. The present information will provide an impetus on understanding the biodiversity of the region. We all know that biodiversity ensures the essential ecological functions on which life depends. The well being and survival of human populations are dependent on millions of species of plants, animals and microbes. India is one of the twelve mega biodiversity regions of the world with 7.7% genetic resources of the microorganisms, plants and animals as well as the ecosystem, which they inhabit.

Entomophilic nematodes vary greatly in size and shape, have insects as intermediate or as definitive hosts, may be facultative or obligatory in their host relations and often involve other microorganisms in their relationships with their hosts. Though there are no report on important pathogens of man or domestic animals in these groups, entomophilic nematodes cause debilitation, sterility (partial/complete) or death of a large number of insects belonging to various Orders and families. They have evolved to parasitize every kind of insects , so it is not too surprising to find them killing, sterilizing or otherwise debilitating millions of different kinds of insects such as mosquitoes, blackflies, chironomid flies, grasshoppers, moths, ants, bees and many other insects and invertebrates. The nematodes recovered were found to represent four families viz., Thelastomatidae, Travassosinematidae, Pseudonymidae and Protrelloididae. Parasitism by the members of the superfamily Thelastomatoidea revealed 16 species of nematodes spread over 11 known genera. The article encompasses diagnosis on four families and 11 genera, key to genera of four families and key to species of 10 genera.

2. Materials and methods

Insects were anaesthesised with chloroform and dissected immediately in normal saline. Gut was teased out with fine needle and the contents were mixed with saline. The nematodes were picked up using horse hair under low power stereoscopic binocular microscope. The parasitic nematodes collected from insect hosts namely *Periplaneta americana* Linn, *Gryllotalpa africana* Beauvois, *Hydrophilus triangularis* Say were killed and fixed in TAF (Triethanolamine formaline) fixative [Courtney *et al.,* 1955]. They were dehydrated by slow method (anhydrous $CaCl_2$) and mounted on glass slides in anhydrous glycerine. Glass wool or wire of suitable thickness was used to avoid the flattening of the nematode specimens. Measurements were taken using ocular micrometer and illustrations were drawn using drawing tube attached to Nikon (Alphaphot2-YS2 and Optiphot2) microscopes. Photomicrography was done using Olympus BX50 DIC Microscope with C5050 digital camera. De Man's ratios/formula [De Man,1884] was used to denote the dimensions of the nematodes *i.e.,* a=total body length/maximum body width, b=total body length/distance from anterior end to the base of oesophagus, c=total body length/tail length, V=distance of vulva from anterior end x 100/total body length.

3. Key to families of Thelastomatoidea

1. Vulva posterior to base of oesophagus..2
- Vulva anterior to base of oesophagus.........................Protrelloididae Chitwood, 1932
2(1). Cervical cuticle with transverse rows of spines.......Hystrignathidae Travassos, 1920
- Cervical cuticle without spines...3
3(2). Eggs with filaments...4
- Eggs without filaments...................................Thelastomatidae Travassos, 1929
4(3). Egg filaments twisted around shell, polar egg filaments absent...............................
....Pseudonymidae (Kloss, 1958) Adamson, 1989
- Egg filaments not twisted around shell, polar egg filaments present...................
....Travassosinematidae Rao, 1958

4. Family: Thelastomatidae Travassos, 1929

4.1 Key to genera of Thelastomatidae Travassos, 1929

1. Egg bearing spine-like outgrowths......................................*Gryllophila* Basir,1942a
- Egg without spine-like outgrowths..2
2(1). Buccal cavity provided with cuticular modifications..3
Buccal cavity without cuticular modifications...4
3(2). Buccal cavity with 3 tooth-like projections, eggs elongate and has longitudinal lines..*Severianoia* (Schwenk, 1926) Travassos, 1929
- Buccal cavity with intermediate thickenings of the cuticle which form small teeth, eggs oval without longitudinal lines..............................*Fontonema* Chitwood,1930
4(2). Isthmus surrounded by nerve ring...5
- Isthmus not surrounded by nerve ring...9
5(4). Egg with operculum..*Suifunema* Chitwood,1932
- Egg without operculum...6
6(5). Corpus clavate...7
- Corpus pyriform..*Aoruroides* Travassos & Kloss,1958
7(6). Egg elongate, flattened on one side..8
- Egg oval to ellipsoidal...*Johnstonia* Basir,1956
8(7). 4 pairs of caudal papillae in male..............................*Galinanema* Spiridonov,1984
- 5 pairs of caudal papillae in male.........................*Golovatchnema* Spiridonov,1984
9(4). End bulb with valve...10
- End bulb without valve....................................*Robertia* Travassos & Kloss,1960
10(9). Spicule present..11
- Spicule absent...21
11(10). Caudal papillae 3 pairs..12
- Caudal papillae 4-5pairs...14
12(11). Female tail filiform...*Euryconema* Chitwood,1932
- Female tail not filiform...13
13(12). Cephalic extremity with expanded 2nd annule..
....*Leidynemella* Chitwood & Chitwood, 1934
- Cephalic extremity with simple 2nd annule..........................*Cameronia* Basir,1948a
14(11). Female tail not filiform; 4 pairs of caudal papillae in male...............................15
- Female tail filiform;4-5 pairs of caudal papillae in male......................................16
15(14). Ovary monodelphic...*Galebia* Chitwood,1932

-	Ovary didelphic	*Wetanema* Dale, 1967
16(14).	Female tail filiform ; caudal papillae 4 pairs in male	17
-	Female tail filiform ; caudal papillae 5pairs in male	*Leidynema* Schwenk in Travassos, 1929
17(16).	Ovary didelphic, uteri amphidelphic	18
-	Ovary didelphic, uterus prodelphic	*Hammerschmidtiella* Chitwood,1932
18(17).	Vulva near midbody	19
-	Vulva at posterior third of body	20
19(18).	Egg oval to ellipsoidal	*Thelastoma* Leidy,1849
-	Egg elongate	*Tetleyus* Dale, 1964
20(18).	Excretory pore posterior to base of oesophagus	*Cephalobellus* Cobb,1920
	Excretory pore anterior to base of oesophagus	*Desmicola* Basir,1956
21(10).	Oral opening surrounded by membranous flaps	*Coronostoma* Rao,1958
-	Oral opening not surrounded by membranous flaps	22
22(21).	Egg ellipsoidal to elongate	23
	Egg broadly oval	25
23(22).	Egg ellipsoidal	24
-	Egg elongate	*Cranifera* Kloss,1960
24(23).	3 pairs of caudal papillae in male	*Blattophila* Cobb,1920
	4 pairs of caudal papillae in male	*Aorurus* Leidy,1849
25(22).	2 pairs of caudal papillae in male	*Buzionema* Kloss,1966
-	4 pairs of caudal papillae in male	26
26(25).	Gonads didelphic	27
-	Gonads monodelphic	*Blatticola* Schwenk, 1926
27(26).	Vulva at posterior-third of body, anterior vulval lip not swollen	*Cordonicola* Ali & Farooqui, 1969
-	Vulva at midbody, anterior vulval lip swollen	*Corydiella* Rao & Rao, 1965

4.2 Genus: *Cameronia* Basir, 1948a

4.2.1 Generic diagnosis

Female: Cephalic extremity formed by single annulus and simple second annulus. Oesophagus consisting of a cylindrical corpus, an isthmus which may be distinct or indistinct and a valvular bulb. Cardia lobed or simple. Vulva in the posterior third of body, vagina directed anteriorly. Gonads amphidelphic. Eggs elongate, elliptical, flattened on one side, fused in pairs or more along their flattened surfaces with ridges and furrows or simply attached to one another forming a chain. Polar egg filaments present or absent. Tail conical or with a terminal spike.

Male: Cephalic extremity formed by single annulus. Oesophagus consisting of a cylindrical corpus, distinct or indistinct isthmus with a bulb. Spicule single or absent. Caudal papillae comprising 3-5 pairs. Tail very short, rounded, with or without a spine like process on its ventral side.

4.2.2 Species

Cameronia triovata Shah, 2007a (Figs. 1 & 2); **Host:** *Gryllotalpa africana* Beauvois ; **Habitat:** Gut ; **Locality:** Imphal, Manipur, India.

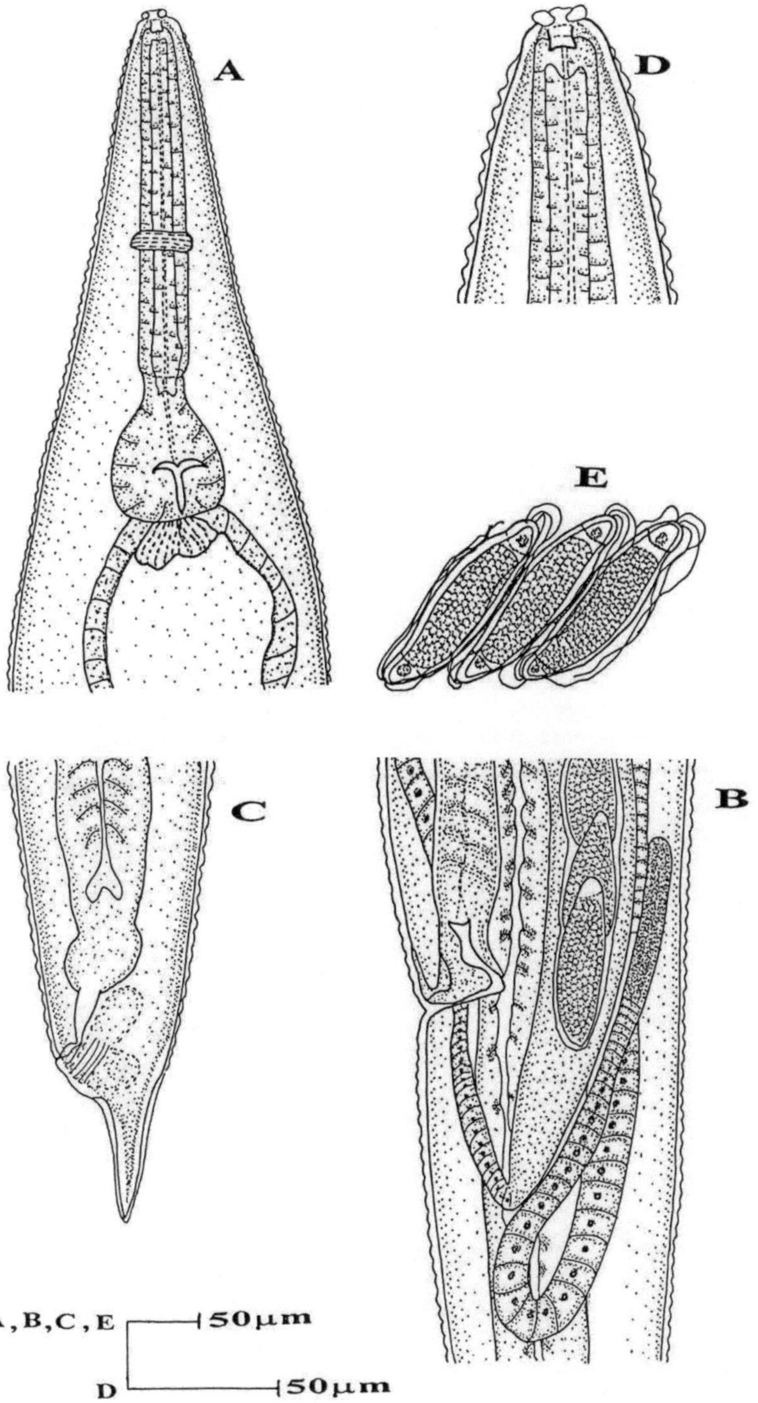

Fig. 1. *Cameronia triovata* Shah, 2007a: A-Female anterior end, B-Female vulval region, C-Female posterior end (lateral view), D-Female cephalic end, E-Eggs.

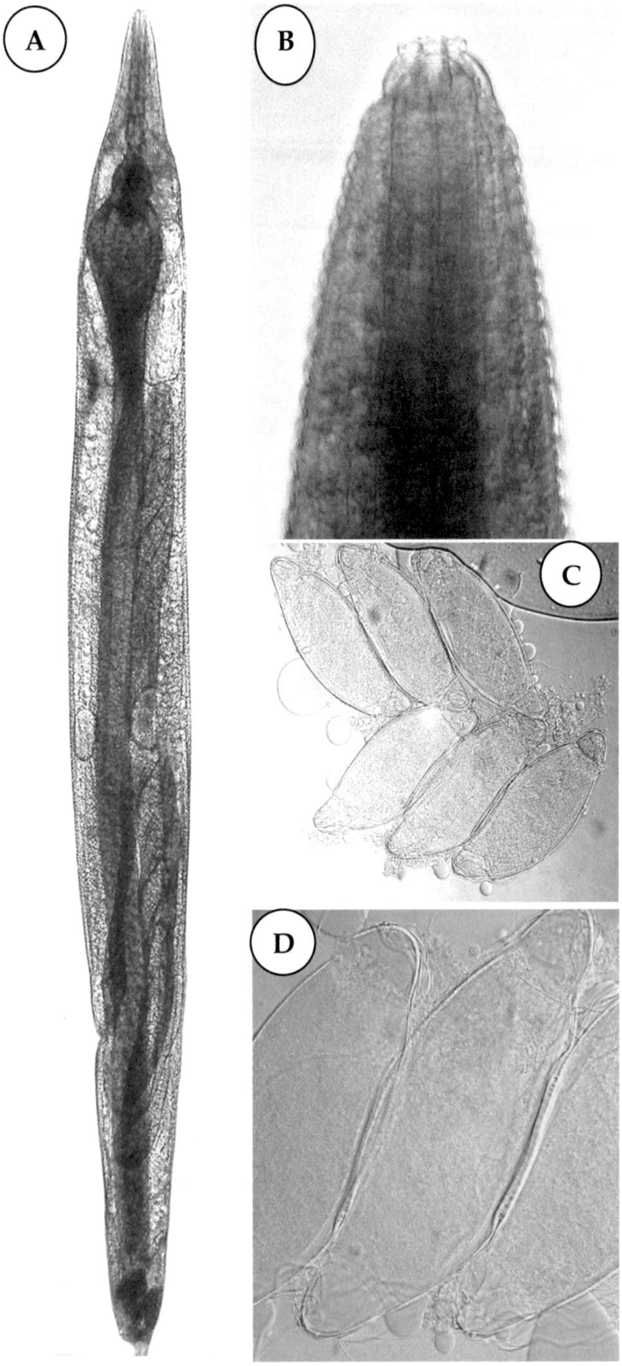

Fig. 2. Photomicrographs of *Cameronia triovata* Shah, 2007a: A-Female entire showing vulval opening, excretory pore and eggs within uterus (lateral view), B-Female cephalic end showing cephalic annule and buccal cavity, C-Eggs joining on lateral sides in three numbers, D-Eggs magnified showing polar filaments, ridges and furrows on lateral sides of attachment.

4.2.3 Species

Cameronia manipurensis Shah, 2007a (Figs.3 & 4); **Host**: *Gryllotalpa africana* Beauvois ; **Habitat:** Gut ; **Locality:** Imphal, Manipur, India

4.2.4 Key to species of *Cameronia* Basir, 1948a

1.	Eggs laid fused...2
-	Eggs laid not fused...5
2(1).	2 eggs fused..3
-	eggs fused...*C. triovata* Shah,2007a
3(2).	2 eggs fused and not ridged.. *C. biovata* Basir,1948a
-	2 eggs fused and ridged..4
4(3).	Spicule 32µm long.................................. *C. klossi* Parveen & Jairajpuri,1984
-	Spicule 38-43µm long................................ *C. travassosi* Farooqui 1968a
5(1).	Male=less than 2.160mm long; oesophagus=less than 564µm long in female..6
-	Male=2.160-2.270mm long; oesophagus=564-644µm long in female...................... ....*C. laplatae* Reboredo & Camino, 2001
6(5).	Spicule present..7
-	Spicule absent.............. *C. aspiculata*(Farooqui,1970)Adamson & Waerebeke,1992a
7(6).	Female tail conical..8
	Female tail with a terminal spike.. ....*C. psilocephala* (Rao,1958) Adamson & Waerebeke,1992a
8(7).	Lobed cardia present.. *C. basiri* Rizvi & Jairajpuri,2002
-	Lobed cardia absent..9
9(8).	Male tail with a thorn-like process on its ventral side.................................... ....*C. multiovata* Leibersperger,1960
-	Male tail without a thorn like process on its ventral side.................................. 10
10(9).	Egg=111-126 x 39-43µm; spicule=19-22µm... ....*C. nisari* (Parveen & Jairajpuri,1985a) Adamson & Waerebeke, 1992a
-	Egg = 102.06-109.35 x 32.80-38.88µm; spicule=10.36-13.18µm.............................. ....*C. manipurensis* Shah,2007a

4.3 Genus: *Thelastoma* Leidy, 1849

4.3.1 Generic diagnosis

Female: Cephalic extremity formed by circumoral annule and enlarged second annule. Mouth surrounded by eight labial papillae. Amphids present. Lateral alae present or absent. Buccal cavity simple. Oesophagus consisting of an anterior cylindrical corpus, an isthmus and a posterior valvular bulb. Excretory pore pre- or post-oesophageal bulb or at the level of the base of the bulb. Tail long filiform about one-third to one-fourth of the total body-length. Vagina short, muscular and anteriorly directed with well developed vulval lip. Vulva at or posterior to mid-body. Eggs broadly oval.

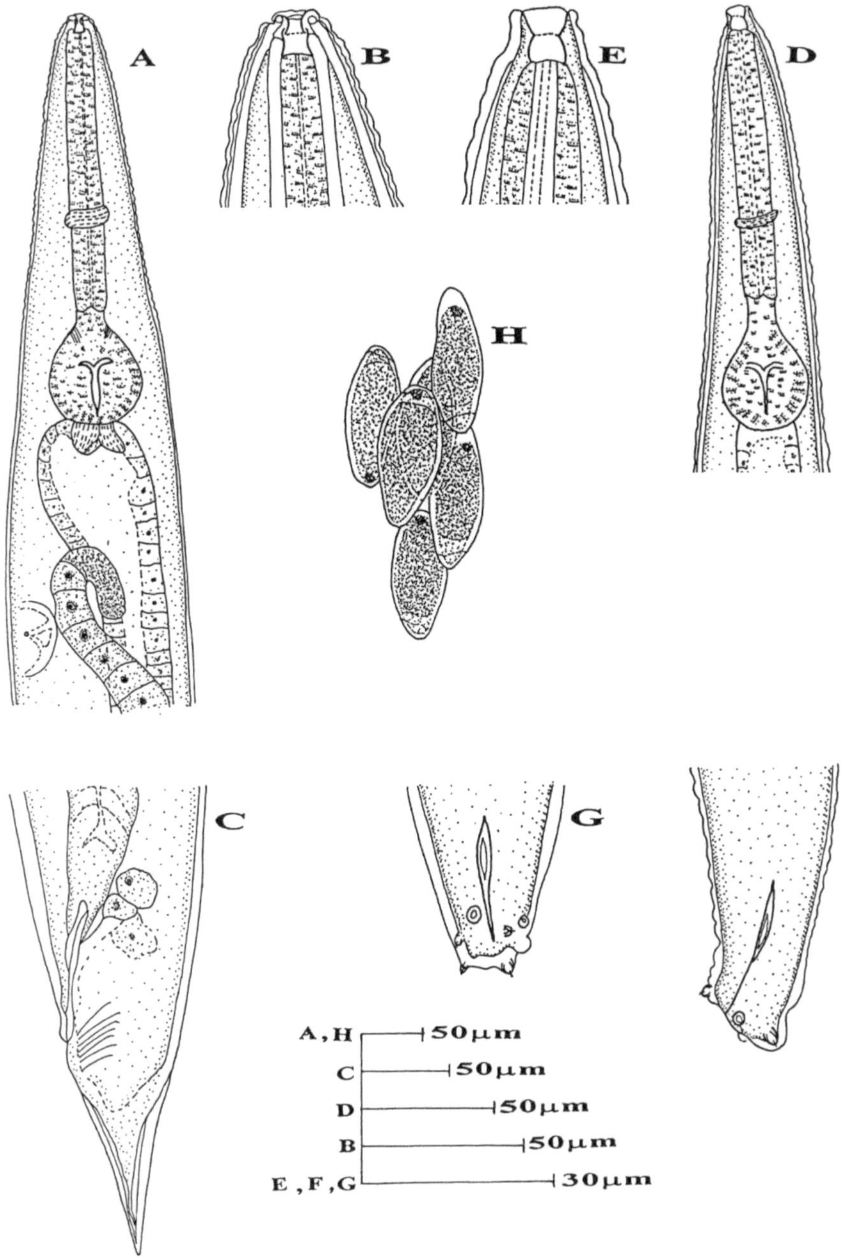

Fig. 3. *Cameronia manipurensis* Shah, 2007a: A-Female anterior end, B-Female cephalic end, C-Female posterior end (lateral view), D-Male anterior end, E-Male cephalic end, F-Male posterior end (lateral view), G-Male posterior end (ventral view), H-Eggs.

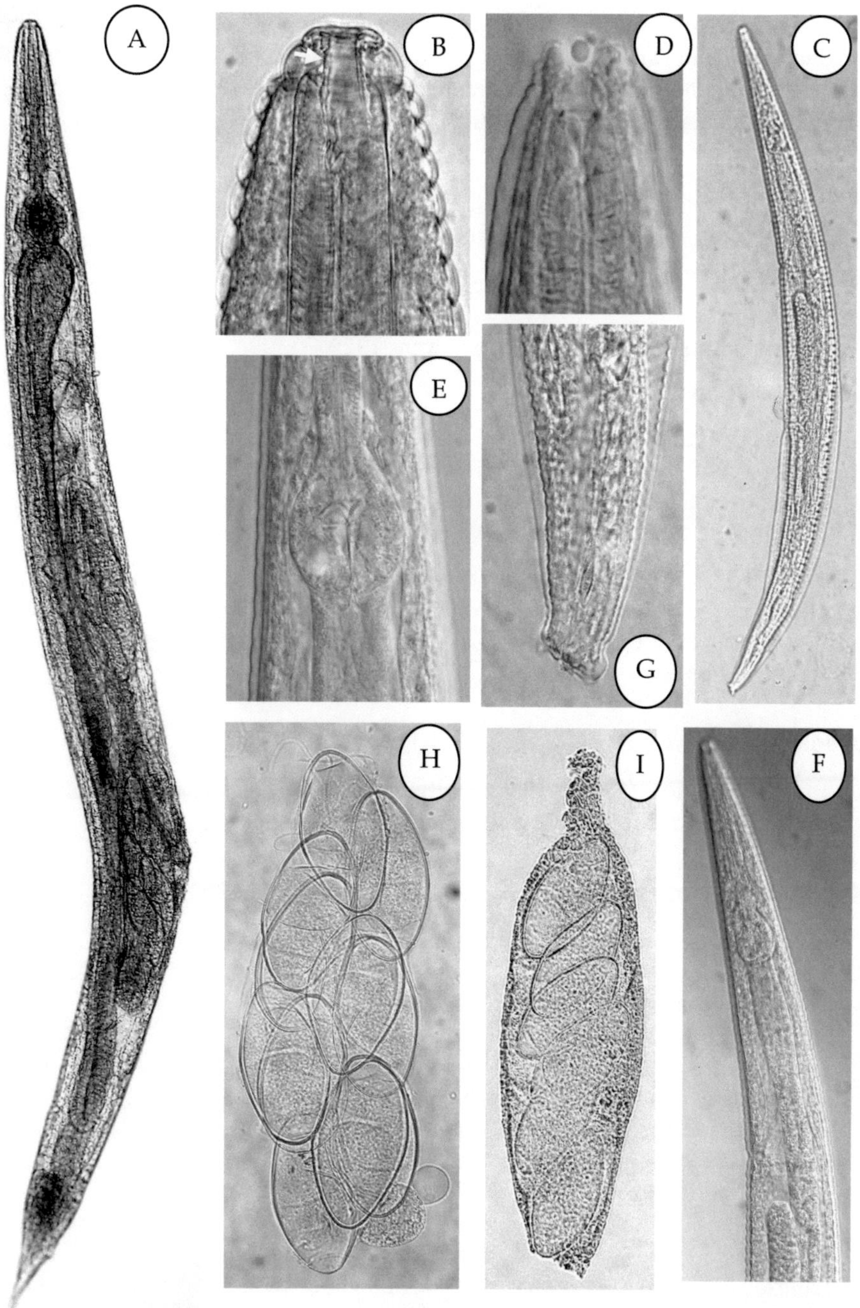

Fig. 4. Photomicrographs of *Cameronia manipurensis* Shah, 2007a: A-Female entire showing eggs (lateral view), B-Female anterior end showing buccal cavity (lateral view), C-Male entire (lateral view), D-Male anterior end showing buccal cavity (lateral view), E-Male cardia (lateral view), F-Portion of male anterior showing excretory pore (lateral view), G-Male posterior end showing spicule (lateral view), H-Eggs showing mode of attachment with one another, I-Eggs within uterus.

Male: Cephalic extremity formed by single expanded annule. Lateral alae present or absent. Tail elongated and filiform. Four pairs of caudal papillae, consisting one pair pre- anal, one pair ad-anal and one median duplex post anal papillae on genital cone. One pair of papillae on caudal appendage some distance away from the anus. Testis single. Spicule present or absent.

4.3.2 Species

Thelastoma periplaneticola Leibersperger, 1960 (Figs.5 & 6); **Host:** *Periplaneta americana* Linn.; **Habitat:** Gut; **Locality:** Imphal, Manipur, India

4.4 Genus: *Leidynema* Schwenk in Travassos, 1929

4.4.1 Generic diagnosis

Female: Cephalic extremity formed by two annules. Lateral alae present. Eggs large, elongate and crescent-shaped. Female tail long, filiform or attenuated. Oesophageal corpus divided into narrow anterior and broad posterior portions of roughly equal length, isthmus short, and bulb spherical. Intestine with blind diverticulum. Vulva near midbody.

Male: Cephalic extremity formed by single expanded annule. Lateral alae present or absent. Spicule present or absent. Caudal extremity in males abruptly truncate with or without short terminal spine (spine-like process on its ventral side) or with several protuberances. Caudal papillae 3-5 pairs.

4.4.2 Species

Leidynema appendiculatum (Leidy, 1850) Chitwood, 1932 (Figs. 7 & 8); Host : *Periplaneta americana* Linn.;Habitat: Gut ; Locality: Imphal, Manipur, India

4.4.3 Key to species of *Leidynema* Schwenk in Travassos, 1929

1.	Males with several protuberances in posterior region..*L. portentosae* Van Waerebeke, 1978
-	Males without protuberances in the posterior region.......................................2
2(1).	Spicule=63µm long in male..*L. socialis* (Leidy,1850)Adamson & Waerebeke,1992a
-	Spicule less than 63µm long in male...3
3(2).	Lateral alae present in females only...4
-	Lateral alae present in both sexes...6
4(3).	Lateral alae in female ends in backwardly pointed projection...*L. schwencki* Farooqui,1967
-	Lateral alae in female do not end in backwardly pointed projection.......................5
5(4).	Lateral alae in female extending along whole length of body without spinous process; cuticular bosses present...................................*L. delatorrei* Chitwood,1932
-	Lateral alae in female start from mid-body and continuous upto tip of tail with spinous process; cuticular bosses absent........*L. stylopygi* Biswas&Chakravarty,1963
6(3).	Female oesophagus 1/5th –1/6th of body length; males with five pairs of caudal papillae..*L. periplaneti* Farooqui,1967
-	Female oesophagus 1/8th of body length; males with 3-5 pairs of caudal papillae.......................................*L. appendiculatum* (Leidy,1850) Chitwood,1932

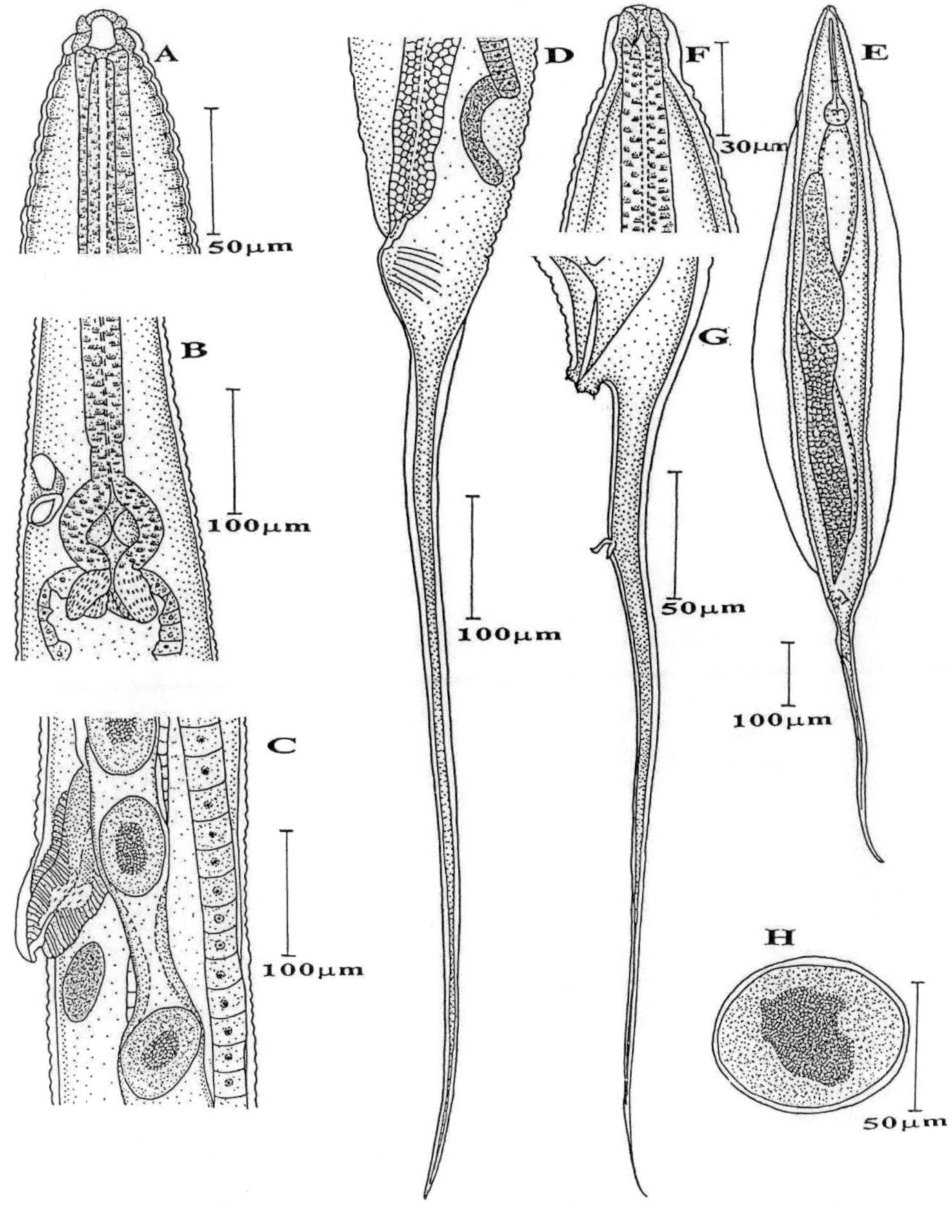

Fig. 5. *Thelastoma periplaneticola* Leibersperger, 1960: A-Female anterior end, B-Female oesophageal region, C-Female vulval region showing lip, D-Female posterior end (lateral view), E-Male entire, F-Male anterior end, G-Male posterior end (lateral view), H-Egg (Shah, 2007b)

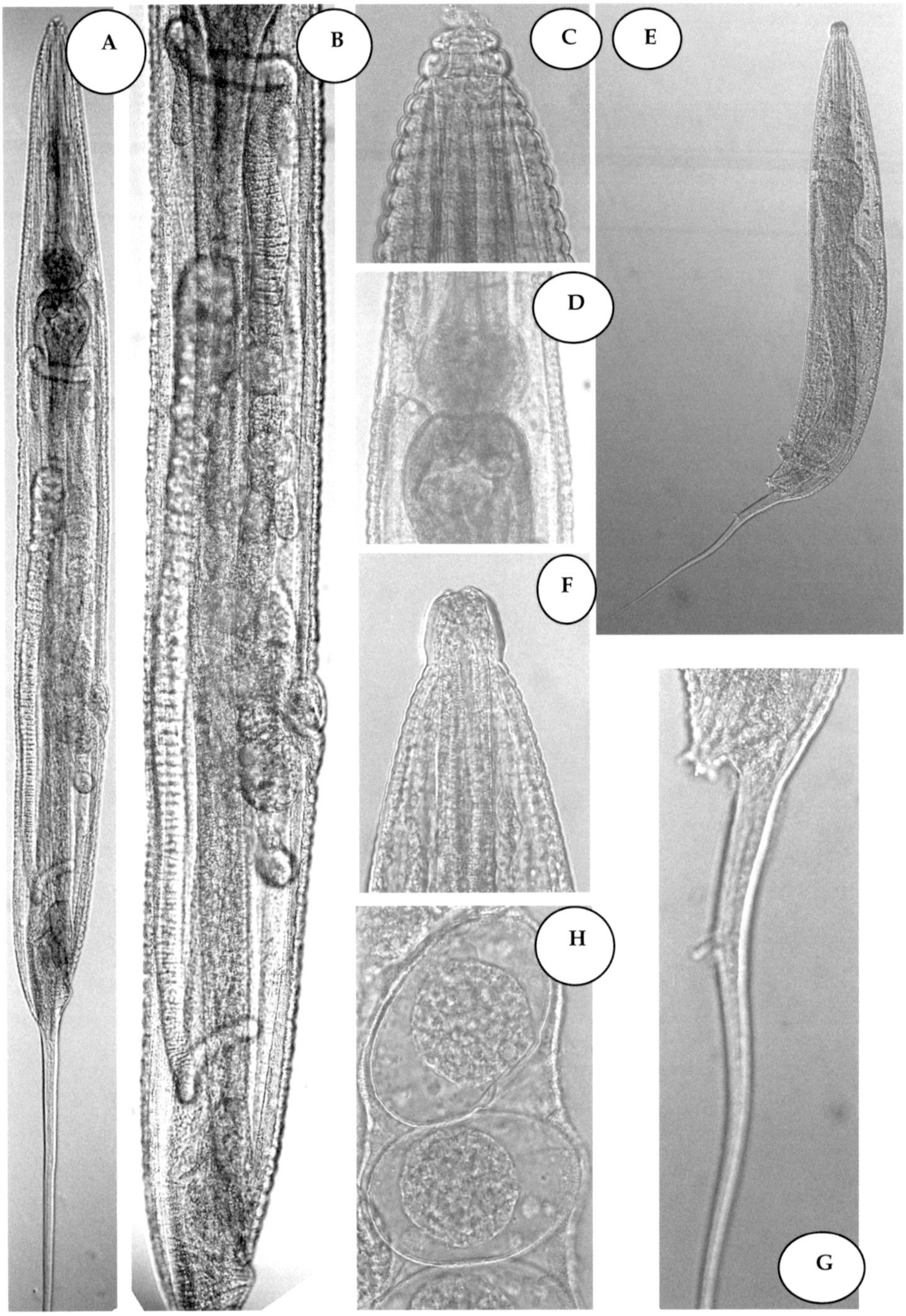

Fig. 6. Photomicrographs of *Thelastoma periplaneticola* Leibersperger, 1960: A-Female entire (lateral view), B-Female gonads, vulval lips and cloacal opening, C-Female cephalic end showing buccal cavity, D-Female excretory pore, E-Male entire (lateral view), F-Male cephalic end showing buccal cavity, G-Male posterior end showing papillae at genital cone and tail (lateral view), H-Eggs (Shah, 2007b).

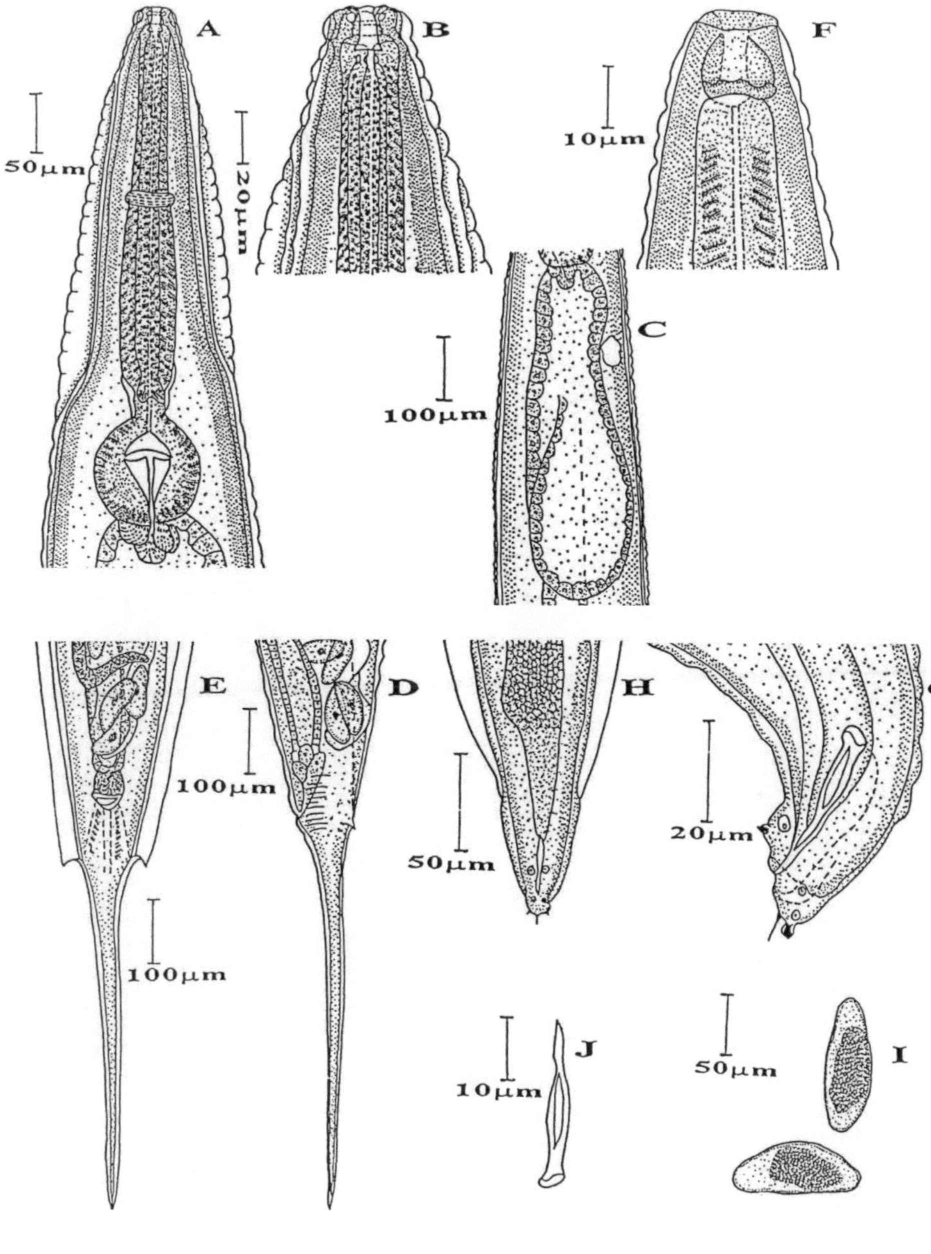

Fig. 7. *Leidynema appendiculatum* (Leidy, 1850) Chitwood, 1932: A-Female anterior end, B-Female cephalic end, C-Female showing intestinal diverticulum, D-Female posterior end (lateral view), E-Female posterior end (ventral view), F-Male cephalic end, G-Male posterior end (lateral view), H-Male posterior end (ventral view), I-Eggs, J-Spicule (Shah, 2007b).

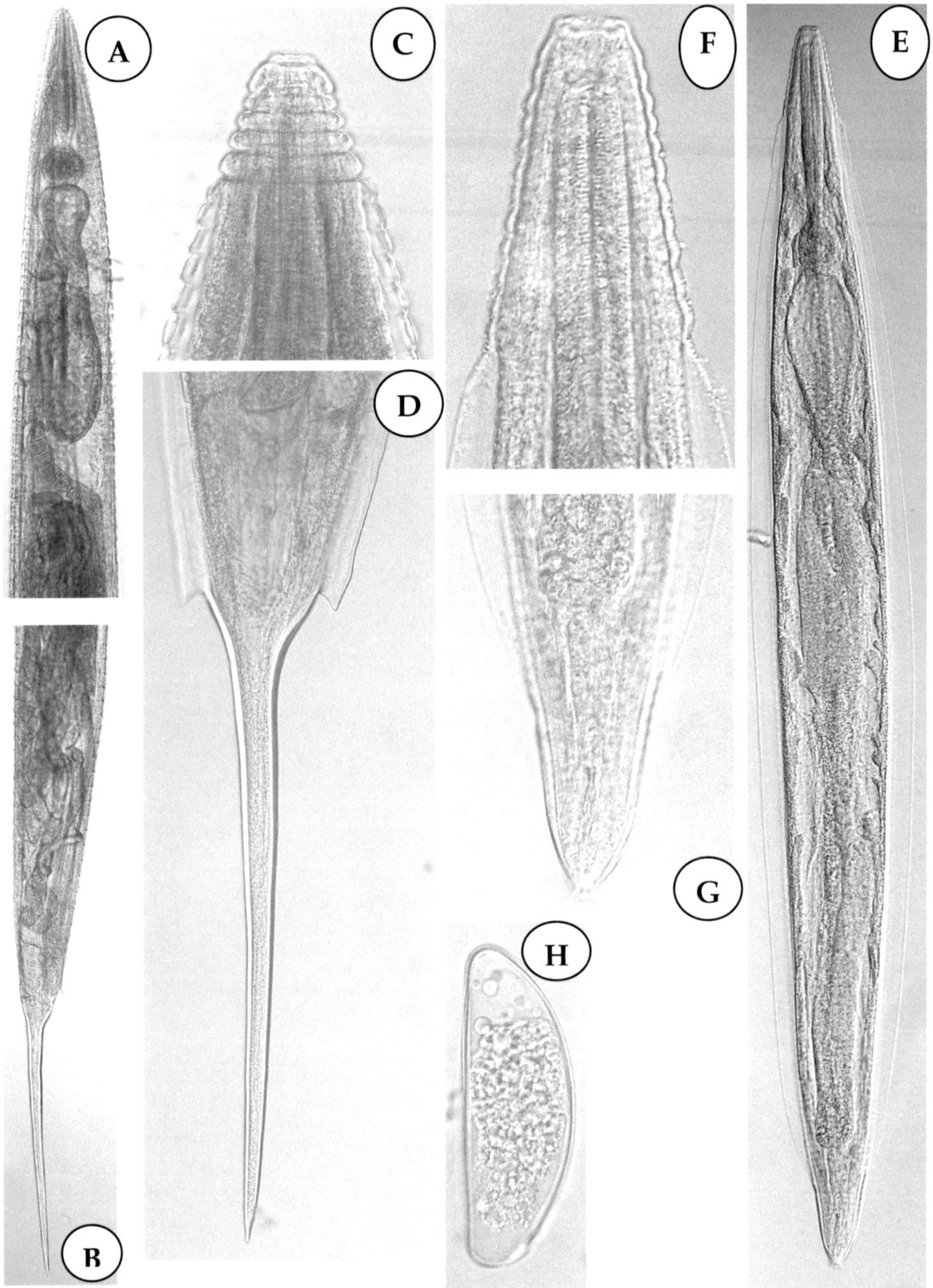

Fig. 8. Photomicrographs of *Leidynema appendiculatum* (Leidy, 1850) Chitwood, 1932: A-Female anterior half showing excretory pore and intestinal diverticulum (lateral view), B-Female posterior half (lateral view) showing coiled uterus, C-Female cephalic end showing buccal cavity and prominent cephalic annules, D-Female posterior end (ventral view) showing lateral alae, F-Male entire (ventral view) showing lateral alae, G-Male posterior end showing spicule (ventral view), H-egg (Shah, 2007b).

4.5 Genus: *Gryllophila* Basir, 1942a

4.5.1 Generic diagnosis

Female: Cephalic extremity formed by circumoral annule and posterior expanded annule. Mouth opening surrounded by eight labiopapillae and a pair of amphids. Oesophageal corpus cylindrical, isthmus cylindrical. Vulva in posterior quarter of the body. Vagina long and anteriorly directed. Uterus extending anteriorly and flexing posteriorly before dividing into two branches. Gonad amphidelphic. Eggs very large, with or without spine-like outgrowths, elongate, deposited in string held together by uterine secretions. Tail conical to attenuate.

Male: Cephalic extremity formed by single expanded annule. Caudal extremity with prominent genital cone. Caudal papillae 3-6 pairs, single median papilla present or absent. Spicule single. Caudal appendage, narrowing abruptly posterior to last pair of caudal papillae, rest of the papillae borne on genital cone.

4.5.2 Species

Gryllophila skrjabini (Sergiev, 1923) Basir, 1956 (Figs. 9 & 10); Host: *Gryllotalpa africana* Beauvois; Locality: Imphal, Manipur, India

4.5.3 Key to species of *Gryllophila* Basir, 1942a

1. Egg-shell with spine-like outgrowths..............*G. skrjabini* (Sergiev, 1923) Basir,1956
- Egg-shell without spine-like outgrowths..2
2(1). Caudal papillae three pairs with a single median papilla.................................
....*G. nihali* Rizvi, Jairaipuri & Shah, 2002
- Caudal papillae 5-6 pairs without a single median papilla...........................3
3(2). Caudal papillae in male five pairs...4
- Caudal papillae in male six pairs...........................*G. basiri* Parveen & Jairajpuri, 1981
4(3). Presence of four lobules in the first ring and 14 lobules in the second in the cephalic region..................................*G. cephalobulata* Camino & Maiztegui, 2002
- Absence of lobules in the cephalic region...................*G. gryllotalpae* Farooqui, 1970

4.6 Genus: *Hammerschmidtiella* Chitwood, 1932

4.6.1 Generic diagnosis

Female: Body spindle shaped. Cephalic extremity formed by two annules and cervical region with variable number and arrangement of enlarged annules. Oesophageal corpus with a pseudobulb, cylindrical isthmus. Vulva in anteriorthird of the body, vagina and uterus posteriorly directed. Didelphic, prodelphic. Eggs elongate, pear-shaped, oval/ovoid that are flattened on one side, tail attenuate to filiform.

Male: Cephalic extremity formed by single expanded annule. Oesophageal corpus clavate. Caudal extremity abruptly truncate, posterior to anus with spine-like appendage. Caudal papillae absent or if present consisting of one pair subv-entral preanal, one pair lateral adanal, one pair sub-ventral just posterior to anus and one duplex papilla at the base of the caudal appendage. Spicule present or absent.

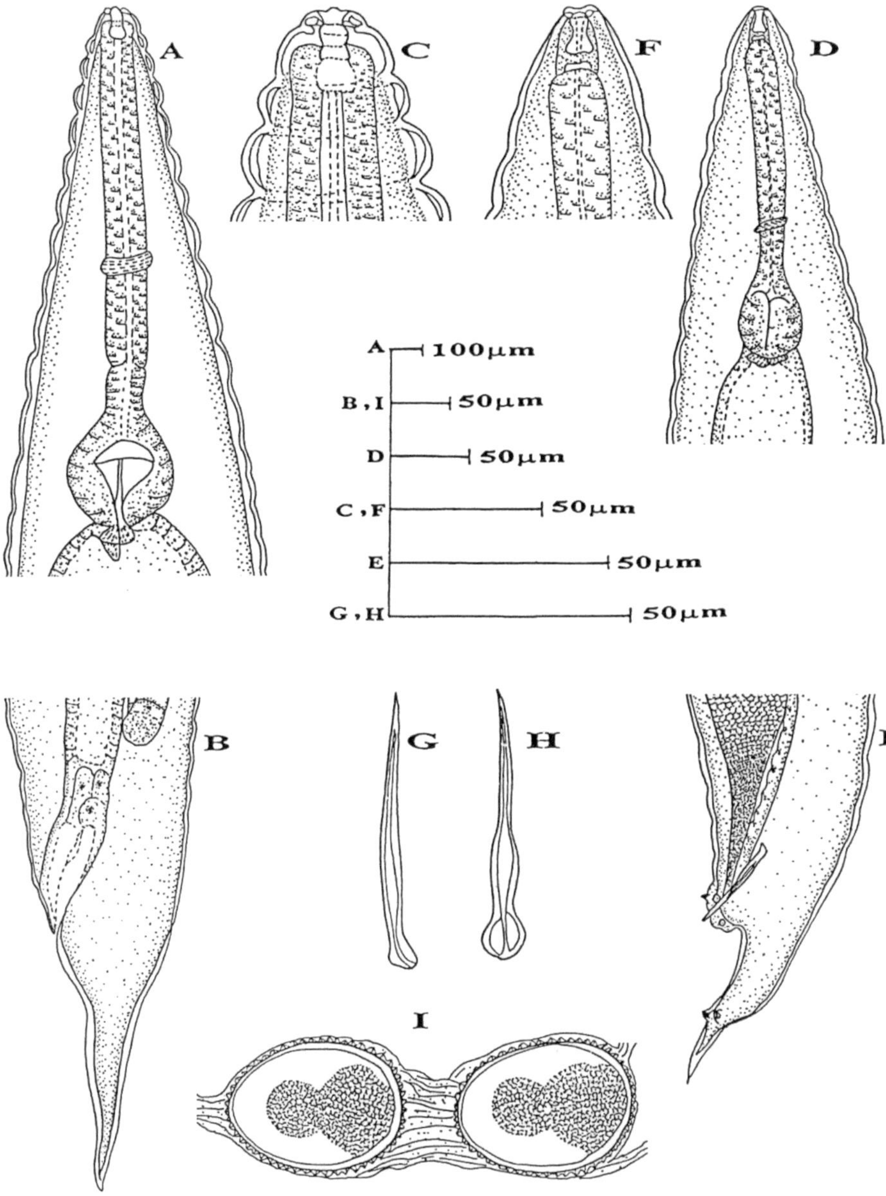

Fig. 9. *Gryllophila skrjabini* (Sergiev, 1923) Basir, 1956: A-Female anterior end, B-Female posterior end (lateral view), C-Female cephalic end, D-Male anterior end, E-Male posterior end (lateral view), F-Male cephalic end, G-Spicule (lateral view), H-Spicule (ventral view), I-Eggs (Shah, 2007b).

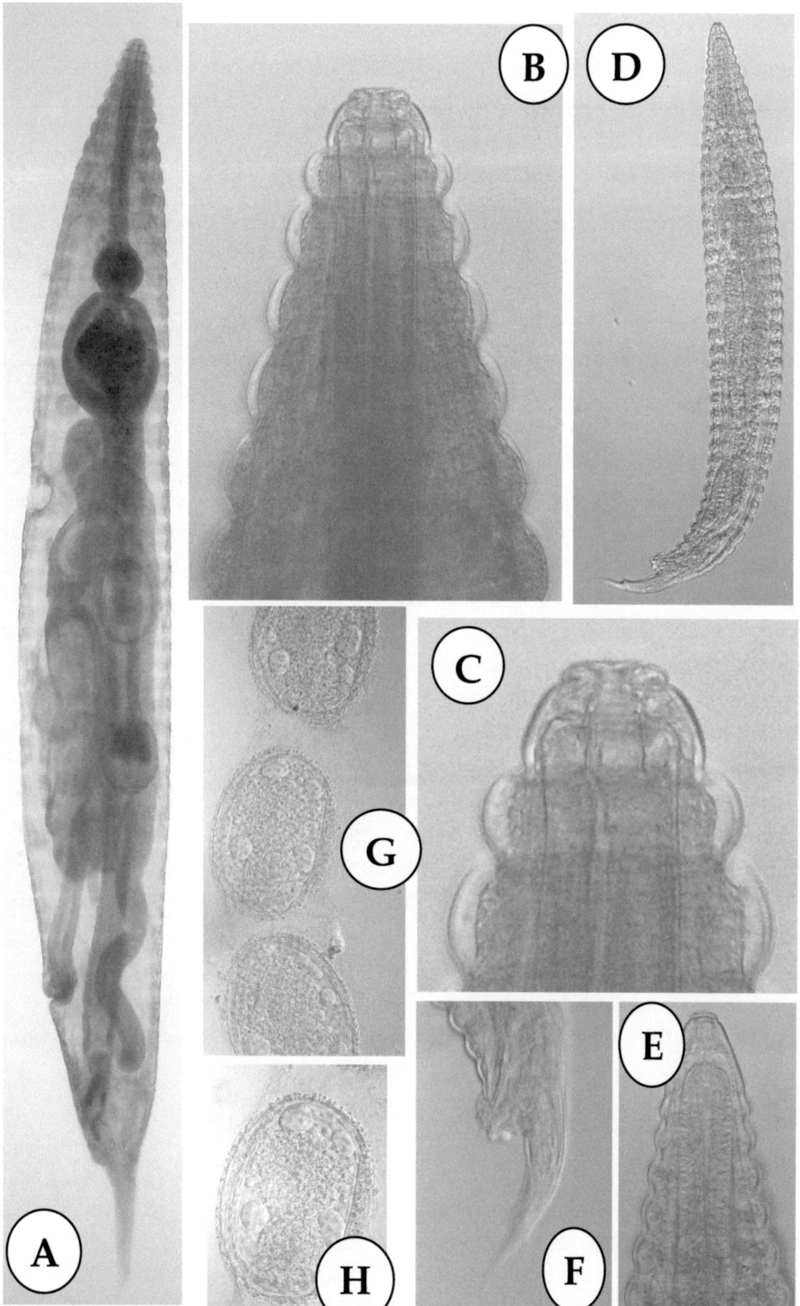

Fig. 10. Photomicrographs of *Gryllophila skrjabini* (Sergiev, 1923) Basir, 1956: A-Female entire (lateral view) showing uterus, excretory pore, vulva and anal opening, B-Female cephalic end with circumoral annule, C-Female cephalic end showing buccal cavity and annules, D-Male entire (lateral view), E-Male anterior end showing buccal cavity (lateral view), F-Male posterior end showing spicule (lateral view), G-Eggs, H-Egg showing spine-like outgrowths on the shell surface (Shah, 2007b).

4.6.2 Species

Hammerschmidtiella diesingi (Hammerschmidt, 1838) Chitwood, 1932 (Figs. 11 & 12); Host: *Periplaneta americana* Linn. ; Habitat: Gut; Locality: Imphal, Manipur, India

4.6.3 Key to species of *Hammerschmidtiella* Chitwood, 1932

1. Presence of pear-shaped eggs..............*H. hochi* Jex, Schneider, Rose & Cribb, 2005
- Oval eggs or ovoid eggs that are flattened on one side....................................2
2(1). Male with multiple crest or ridges behind anus............*H. cristata* Spiridonov,1984
- Multiple crest or ridges behind anus absent in male..3
3(2). Presence of highly curved corpus over end bulb in female oesophagus.................
....*H. poinari* Gupta & Kaur, 1978
- Corpus not curved in female oesophagus 4
4(3). Vulva provided with three cuticularised plates ....*H. basiri* Singh & Kaur, 1988
- Vulva without plates...5
5(4). Caudal papillae and spicule present in male...6
- Caudal papillae and spicule absent in male...*H. aspiculus* Biswas & Chakravarty, 1963
6(5). Spicule=18µm long...7
- Spicule more than 18µm long...9
7(6). Female=1.926-2.022mm long..*H. acreana* Kloss, 1966
- Female more than 2.022mm long 8
8(7). Female=2.20-3.77mm and tail=0.250-0.290mm; male=0.520-0.560mm........................
..........................*H. mackenziei* (Zervos, 1987a) Adamson & Waerebeke, 1992a
- Female=3.0-3.33mm and tail 0.78mm; male= 0.81-0.96 mm......*H. manohari* Rao, 1958
9(6). Female=1.81mm long; spicule=20µm long....................*H. singhi* Rao & Rao, 1965
- Female=more than 1.81mm long; spicule=more than 20µm long.......................10
10(9). Male=0.487-0.853mm long.........*H. diesingi* (Hammerschmidt, 1838) Chitwood, 1932
- Male = more than 0.853mm long...11
11(10). Caudal papillae in male=5pairs, gubernaculums present ....
....*H. andersoni* Adamson & Nasher, 1987
- Caudal papillae = 3 pairs, gubernaculum absent....*H. nayrai* Serrano Sanchez, 1945

5. Family Protrelloididae Chitwood, 1932

5.1 Diagnosis

Mouth with or without trilobed circumoral elevation. Cuticle without spines. Anterior region may or may not possess transverse striations. Oesophagus consisting of corpus which may be clavate or cylindrical, isthmus distinct or indistinct and a posterior valvular bulb. Vulva anterior to base of the oesophagus. Gonads amphidelphic. Eggs with or without cuticular crest or grooves. Tail of female attenuate to conical terminating in narrow spine or short and subconical or short and rounded with two cuticular wing like projections. Male caudal extremity tapering posterior to anus and ending in digitiform appendage or short and subconical or narrowing, with long appendage or short and bluntly rounded or subconical. Caudal papillae 3-8 pairs or completely absent. Spicule single or absent.

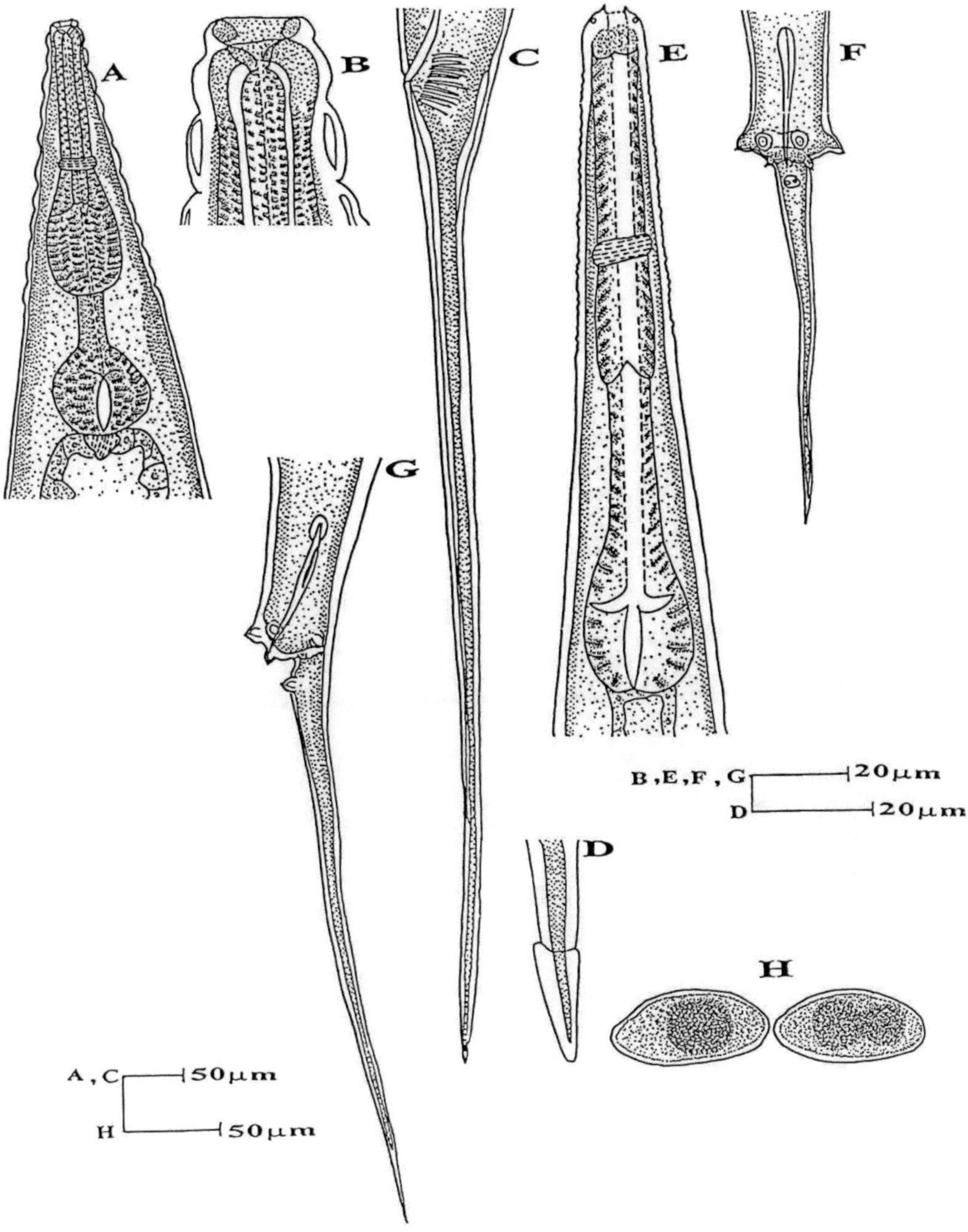

Fig. 11. *Hammerschmidtiella diesingi* (Hammerschmidt, 1838) Chitwood, 1932: A-Female anterior end, B-Female cephalic end, C-Female posterior end (lateral view), D-Female tail tip showing cap-like structure, E-Male anterior end, F-Male posterior end (ventral view), G-Male posterior end (lateral view), H-Eggs (Shah, 2007b).

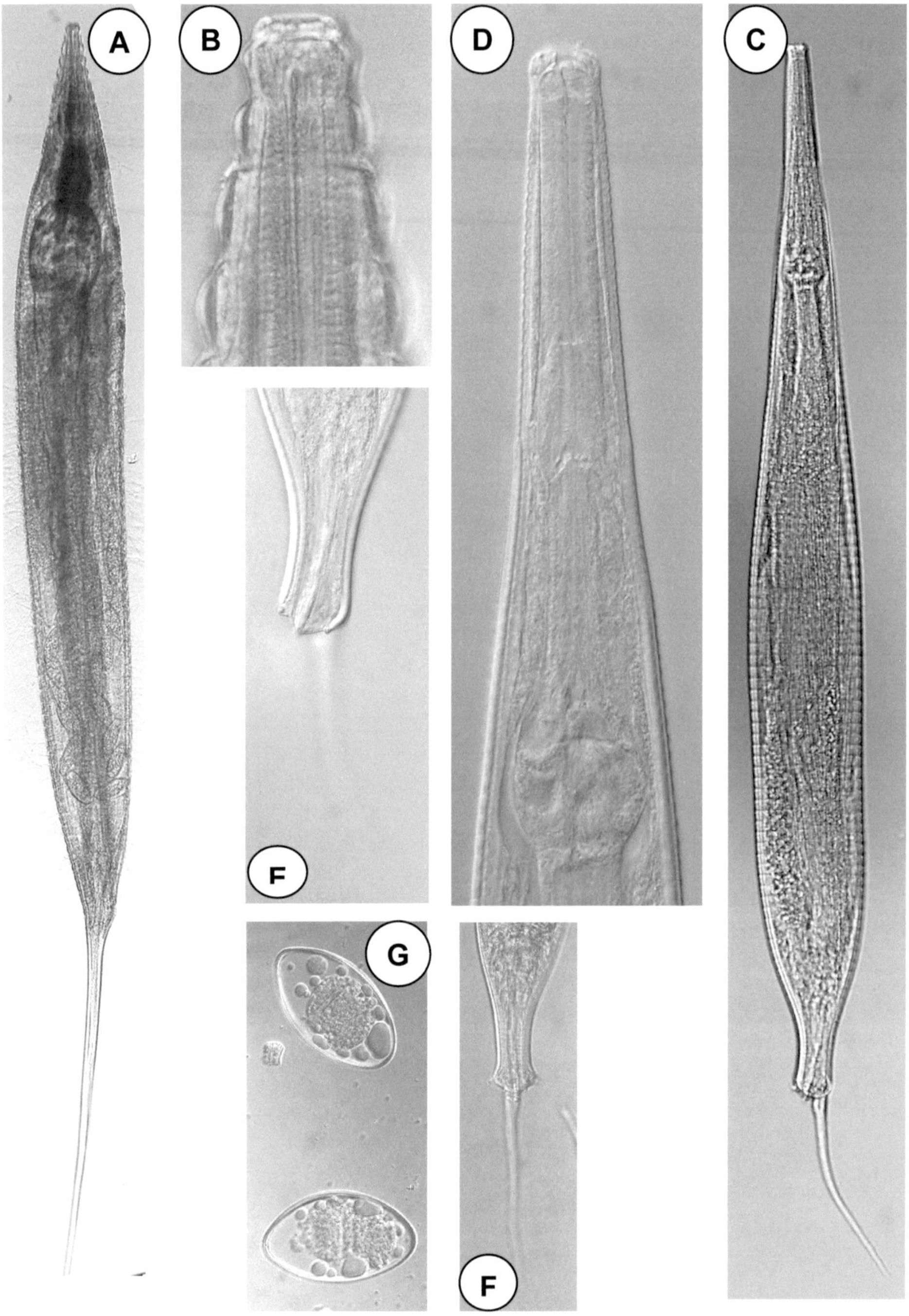

Fig. 12. Photomicrographs of *Hammerschmidtiella diesingi* (Hammerschmidt, 1838) Chitwood, 1932:A-Female entire (lateral view) showing excretory pore, vulva and anal opening, B-Female cephalic end showing buccal cavity, C-Male entire (ventral view), D-Male anterior end showing buccal cavity, E-Male posterior end showing spicule (ventral view), F-Male posterior end showing spicule and papillae (ventral view), G-Eggs. (Shah, 2007b).

5.2 Key to genera of Protrelloididae Chitwood, 1932

1. Cephalic extremity in female formed by lip cone and second annule large...........2
- Cephalic extremity in female simple, second annule normal..*Protrellatus* Farooqui, 1970

2(1). 4 pairs of caudal papillae in male...3
- 3 pairs of caudal papillae in male.......................................*Protrellus* Cobb,1920

3(2). Egg with cuticular modifications...4
- Egg without cuticular modification..............................*Protrellata* Chitwood, 1932

4(3). Female tail conically attenuated; male tail digitiform......*Protrelloides* Chitwood,1932
- Female tail short, male tail not digitiform...........................*Napolitana* Kloss,1959a

5.3 Genus: *Protrellus* Cobb, 1920

5.3.1 Generic diagnosis

Female: Cephalic extremity formed by lip cone and expanded second annule. Oesophageal corpus clavate. Isthmus short. Vulva anterior to base of oesophagus. Vagina and common uterus posteriorly directed, paired uteri opposed. Eggs elongate, oval or ellipsoidal, shell usually bearing longitudinal ridges or excrescences or a circular crest either laterally or towards one of the poles. Tail short, conical to attenuate.

Male: Corpus cylindrical. Caudal extremity subconical. Spicule present. Testis single. Caudal papillae 3-5 pairs.

5.3.2 Species

Protrellus shamimi Shah *et al.*, 2005 (Fig.13);**Host :** *Periplaneta americana* Linn.

Habitat : Gut; **Locality:** Imphal, Manipur, India

5.3.3 Key to species of *Protrellus* Cobb, 1920

1. Female = less than 8.58 mm long..2
- Female = 8.58 - 10.37 mm long..*P. eurycotesi* Kloss, 1961

2(1). Female tail conical,with filiform projection..3
- Female tail short, no filiform projection...4

3(2). Female=2.964-4.758mm; four pairs of caudal papillae in male.. *P. dixoni* Zervos,1987b
- Female=5.6-7.66 mm; three pairs of caudal papillae in male.. *P. rasolefi* Van Waerebeke, 1969

4(2). Egg with crest or bosses...5
- Egg without crest or bosses 9

5(4). Female oesophagus = 0.633 mm long..*P. kunckeli* (Galeb, 1877) Schwenk, 1926
- Female oesophagus less than 0.633 mm long...6

6(5). Excretory pore conspicuous...7
- Excretory pore inconspicuous..................*P. ischnopterae*(Kloss,1966) Zervos,1987a

7(6). Length of egg=90-95µm ....*P. manni* (Chitwood, 1932)Chitwood, 1933
- Length of egg less than 90µm 8

8(7). Spicule = 17μm long, two pairs of caudal papillae in male.................................
....*P. aurifluus* (Chitwood, 1932) Basir, 1956
- Spicule = 36.45 - 38.88μm long, five pairs of caudal papillae in male.........................
.... *P. shamimi* Shah, Rizvi & Jairajpuri, 2005
9(4). Eggs with lateral grooves...
..........*P. phyllodromi* (Basir, 1942b) Skrjabin, Schikhobalova & Lagodovskaya, 1966
- Eggs without lateral grooves...10
10(9). Excretory pore with lip..11
- Excretory pore without lip...12
11(10). Eggs larger than 77μm, oesophagus 180 mm and excretory pore to 0.290 mm from anterior end.. *P. dalei* Zervos, 1987a
- Eggs less than 77μm, oesophagus 0.39-0.43 mm and excretory pore to 0.180mm from anterior end .... *P. behorefi* Van Waerebeke, 1969
12(10). Female = 6 mm long, tail acutely pointed.................................. *P. aureus* Cobb, 1920
- Female = 5.029-5.147mm long, tail subulate......*P. ituana* (Kloss, 1966) Zervos, 1987a

6. Family Pseudonymidae Kloss, 1958

6.1 Diagnosis

The family Pseudonymidae is diagnosed by the presence of filaments coiled around egg shell and in the absence of polar egg filaments.

6.2 Key to the genera of Pseudonymidae Kloss, 1958

1. Cephalic extremity formed by circumoral annule and expanded second annule in female..2
- Cephalic extremity formed by circumoral annule and simple second annule in female..3
2(1). Anterior cuticle in female with transverse rows of scales....*Stegonema* Travassos,1954
- Anterior cuticle in female without transverse rows of scales..............................
....*Pseudonymus* Diesing,1857
3(1). Eggs broadly oval with filaments coiled around shell......................................4
- Eggs elongate with filaments..*Itaguaiana* Kloss,1959a
4(3). Vulva with protruding anterior lip near posterior third of body; male tail conical, 7 pairs of caudal papillae ....*Zonothrix* Todd,1942
- Vulva slightly posterior to midbody; male tail subconical, 5 pairs of caudal papillae ....*Jarryella* Van Waerebeke & Remillet,1973

6.3 Genus: *Pseudonymus* Diesing, 1857

6.3.1 Generic diagnosis

Female: Cephalic extremity formed by circumoral annule and expanded second annule. Oesophageal corpus clavate. Isthmus a constriction between corpus and bulb. Vulva near posterior-third of the body. Vagina short, anteriorly directed. Gonads amphidelphic. Eggs broadly oval with filaments twisted around shell, polar egg filaments absent. Tail filiform or bluntly attenuated or conically attenuated or conical.

Male: Cephalic extremity formed by single annule. Corpus cylindrical. Caudal papillae 3-6 pairs. Spicule present or absent. Caudal appendage consists of one or two parts.

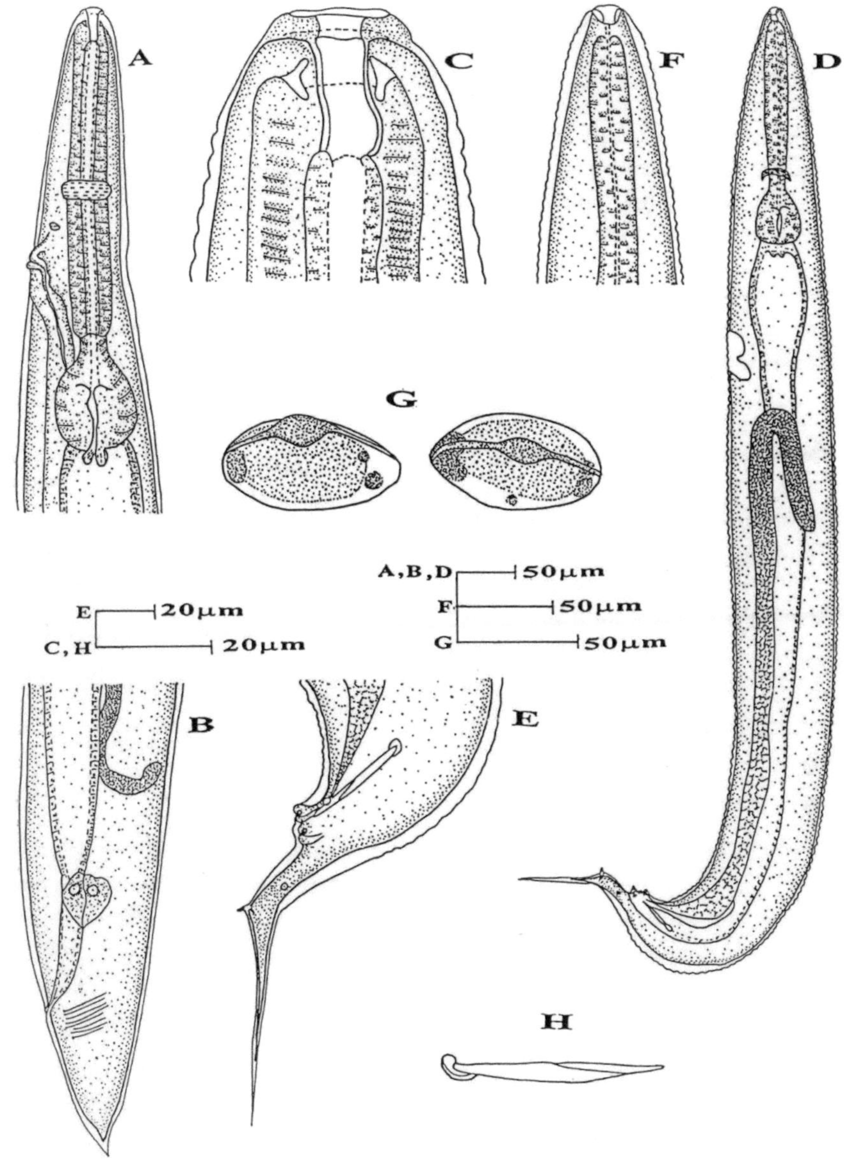

Fig. 13. *Protrellus shamimi* Shah, Rizvi & Jairajpuri,2005: A-Female anterior end, B-Female posterior end (lateral view), C-Female cephalic end, D-Male entire (lateral view), E-Male posterior end (lateral view), F-Male cephalic end, G- Eggs, H-spicule.

6.3.2 Species

Pseudonymus basiri Shah and Rizvi, 2004b (Fig.14)

Host: *Hydrophilus triangularis* Say; Habitat: **Gut ; Locality:** Imphal, Manipur, India

6.3.3 Key to species of *Pseudonymus* Diesing, 1857

1.	Cephalic cuticular annule two	2
-	Cephalic cuticular annule more than two	5
2(1).	Female tail conical	3
-	Female tail filiform	*P. leptocercus* Todd,1944
3(2).	Eggs 78-88 µm in length	*P. brachycercus* Todd, 1944
-	Eggs less than 78 µm in length	4
4(3).	Caudal papillae three pairs	*P. hydrophili* (Galeb,1878) Basir, 1956
-	Caudal papillae six pairs	*P. basiri* Shah & Rizvi,2004b
5(1).	Cephalic cuticular annule =6	*P. klossi* Farooqui, 1967
-	Cephalic cuticular annule more than six	6
6 (5).	Female tail filiform	7
-	Female tail conical	8
7(6).	Cephalic cuticular annules nine	*P. spirotheca* (Gyory,1856) Diesing,1857
-	Cephalic cuticular annules 30	*P. multiannulata* Fotedar,1964
8(6).	Cephalic cuticular annules less than 60	9
-	Cephalic cuticular annules more than 60	*P. reuhmi* Gupta & Kaur, 1978
9(8).	Oesophagus 0.45 mm in length	*P. islamabadi* (Basir, 1941) Basir,1956
-	Oesophagus less than 0.45 mm in length	10
10(9).	Caudal papillae three pairs	*P. vazi* Travassos, 1954
-	Caudal papillae five pairs	*P. toddi* (Travassos, 1954) Kloss, 1959c

6.4 Genus: *Zonothrix* Todd, 1942

6.4.1 Generic diagnosis

Female: Cephalic extremity formed by circumoral annule and simple second annule. Oesophageal end bulb gently clavate with or without pseudobulb. Isthmus a constriction between corpus and bulb. Cardia may or may not be modified into a branch-like structure posteriorly. Vulva with protruding anterior lip near posterior-third of the body. Vagina short, anteriorly directed. Gonads amphidelphic. Eggs broadly oval with filaments coiled around shell. Tail conical

Male: Cephalic extremity formed by single annule. Corpus cylindrical. Caudal extremity conical. Spicule present. Caudal papillae consisting of one pair pre-anal sub-ventral, one pair adanal sub-lateral, three pairs circumanal of which one pair pre-anal, one pair adanal and one pair post-anal and two pairs on tail, of which one is sub-lateral and one sub-ventral.

6.4.2 Species

Zonothrix alata Shah & Rizvi, 2004b (Fig.15); **Host:** *Hydrophilus triangularis* Say

Habitat: Gut; **Locality:** Imphal, Manipur, India

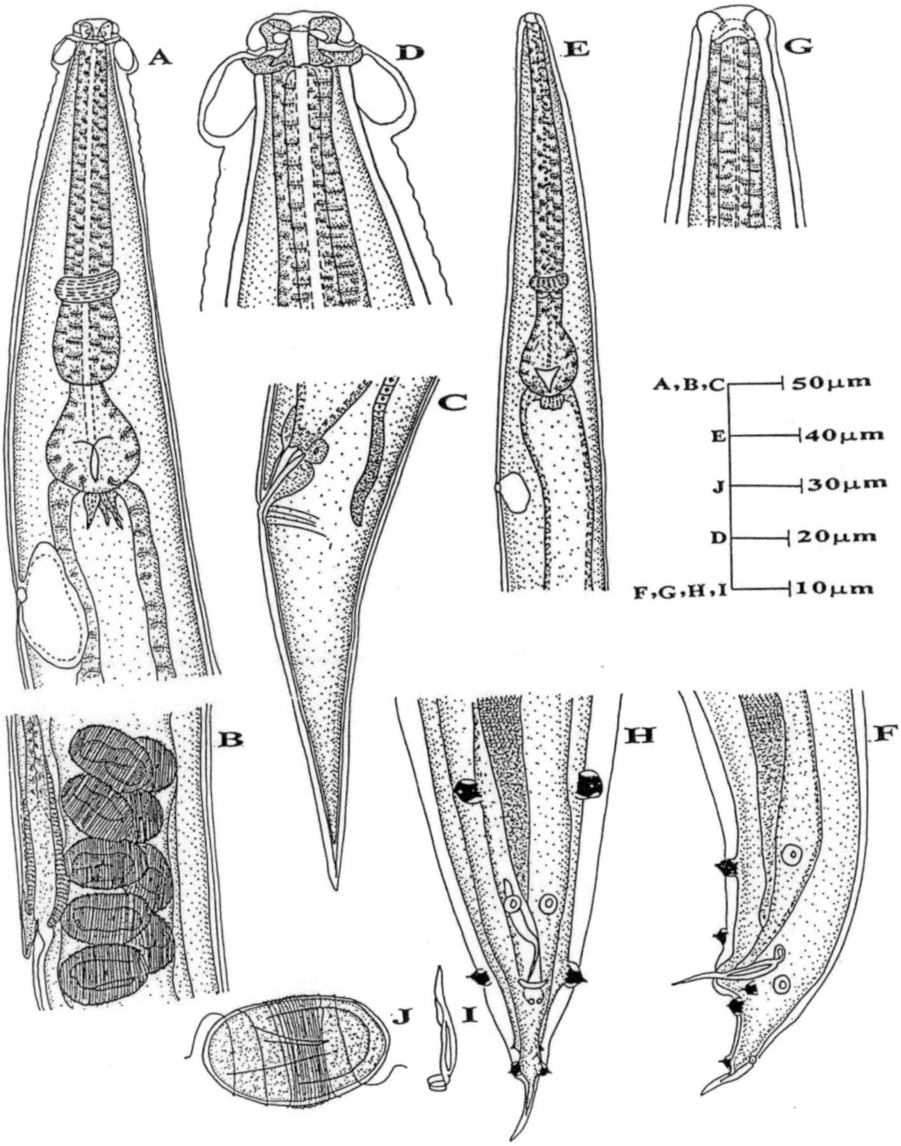

Fig. 14. *Pseudonymus basiri* Shah & Rizvi, 2004b: A-Oesophagus of female, B-Vulva region and eggs in uterus, C-Tail end of female, D-Head cephalic of female, E-Oesophagus of male, F-Tail end of male, lateral, G-Head cephalic end of male, H-Tail end of male (ventral), I-Spicule, J-An embryonated egg.

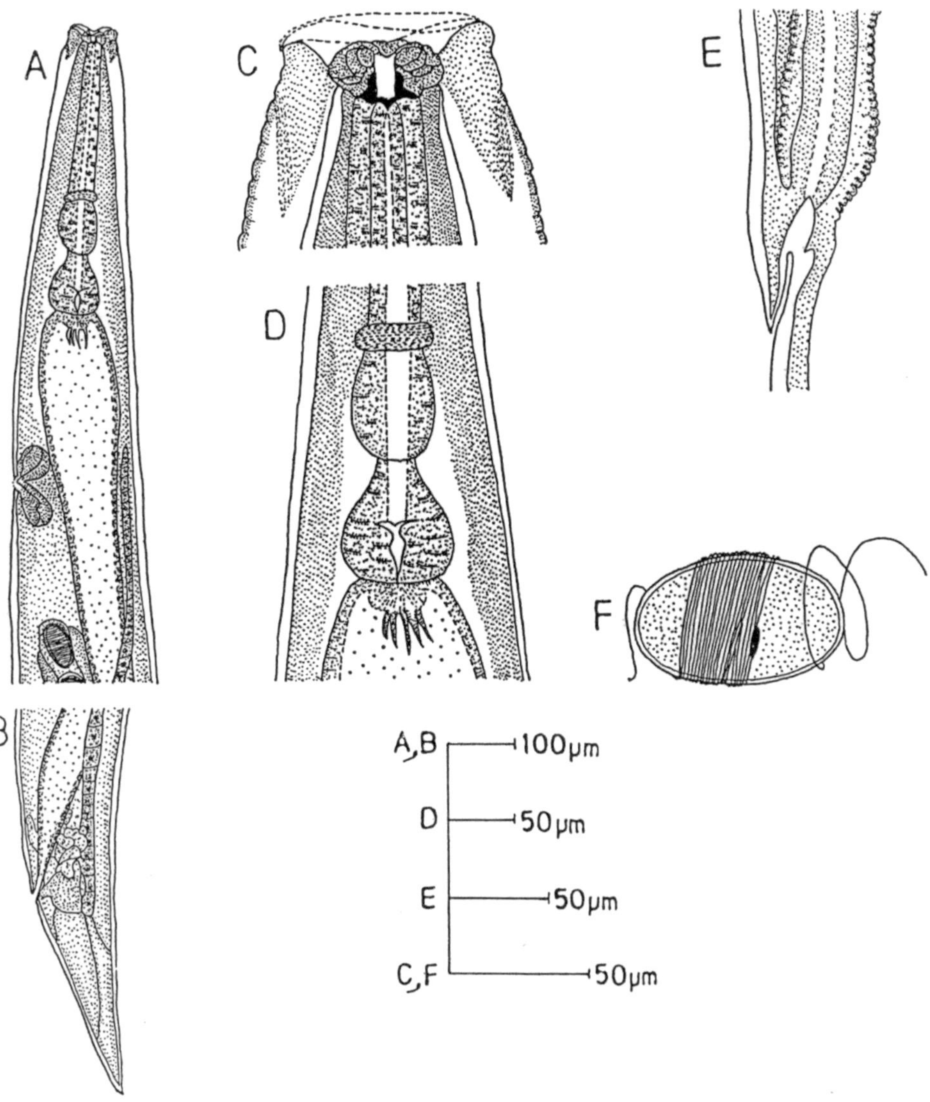

Fig. 15. *Zonothrix alata* Shah & Rizvi, 2004b: A-Anterior region of female, B-Tail end of female, C-Cephalic end of female, D-Basal region of oesophagus, E-Vulva region, F-An egg.

6.4.3 Key to species of *Zonothrix* Todd, 1942

1. Body of female C-shaped after fixation..2
- Body of female coiled after fixation...............................*Z. izecksohni* Kloss, 1959b

2(1). Posterior end of corpus in female narrower than oesophageal bulb..................... 3
- Posterior end of corpus in female almost as broad as oesophageal bulb................ .... *Z. hydroi* (Galeb, 1878) Todd, 1942

3(2). Mature female more than 2 mm and less than 5mm long 4
- Mature female less than 2 mm long .... *Z. helocharesae* Kloss, 1959c

4(3). Swollen annulation present in cephalic extremity of female 5
- Swollenannulation absent in cephalic extremity of female................................. .... *Z. tropisterna* Todd, 1942

5(4). Cephalic annule in female not inflated..6
Cephalic annule in female inflated .... *Z. alata* Shah & Rizvi,2004b

6(5). Female tail narrowing behind anus and not continuing as a spine-like caudal extension...7
- Female tail not as above 8

7(6). Female tail conical ; Ex.=*Coleostoma luederwaldi*..................... *Z. gladius* Kloss, 1959c
- Female tail conically attenuated; Ex.= *Dytiscus marginicollis*............................ ....*Z. mehdii* (Farooqui, 1967) Adamson & Waerebeke,1992b

8(6). Caudal extremity of female terminating in a short spine-like structure 9
- Caudal extremity of female without spine-like appendage................................. 10

9(8). Caudal spine of female=26-35 µm long..................................*Z. galebi* Kloss, 1959c
- Caudal spine of female less than 10 µm long........................ *Z. paraense* Kloss, 1959

10(8). Distance between vulva and anus 20-28% total body length, tail of female 5-8% of body length; seven pairs of caudal papillae in male.. ....*Z. columbianus* Adamson & Buck, 1990
- Distance between vulva and anus less than 15% of total body length, tail of female 10% of body length; six pairs of caudal papillae in male........ *Z. adversa* Kloss, 1958

7. Family Travasosinematidae Rao, 1958

7.1 Diagnosis

Cephalic extremity simple or formed by 6-12 hood-like expansion. Mouth surrounded by 3-8 labial papillae. Lateral alae present or absent. Oesophagus consisting of cylindrical or clavate corpus, isthmus distinct or just a constriction between corpus and a posterior endbulb. Vulva posterior to midbody. Gonads amphidelphic. Eggs with polar filaments and not twisted around shell. Males with single testes. Spicule single or absent. Caudal papillae 2-9 pairs or completely absent.

7.2 Key to genera of Travassosinematidae Rao, 1958

1. Spicule present..*Isobinema* Rao,1958
- Spicule absent...2

2(1). Buccal cavity annulated...*Chitwoodiella* Basir,1948b
- Buccal cavity not annulated..3

3(2). 2-5 pairs of caudal papillae in male..4
- 9-10 pairs of caudal papillae in male.................................*Pteronemella* Rao,1958

4(3). Vulva posterior to midbody..5
- Vulva at 2/3 of body length...*Mirzaiella* Basir, 1942
5(4). Female tail with a spike-like caudal appendage...6
- Female tail without a spike-like caudal appendage.............. *Binema* Travassos,1925
6(5). Spines present on the body of female...................................*Indiana* Chakravarty, 1943
- Spines absent on body of female 7
7(6). Cephalic extremity provided with 6-12 hood-like projections 8
- Cephalic extremity simple, without hood-like projections...*Mohibiella* Farooqui,1970
8(7). Eggs with polar filaments...9
- Eggs without polar filaments..*Travassosinema* Rao,1958
9(8). Mouth with 6 lips, buccal cavity divided into 2 parts, a narrow and a broad posterior chamber occupied by leaf-like plates.........................*Singhiella* Rao,1958
- Mouth with 12 hood-like formations arranged in 2 circles of 6, in tandem, buccal cavity not divided into two parts............................*Pulchrocephala* Travassos,1925

7.3 Genus: *Binema* Travassos, 1925

7.3.1 Generic diagnosis

Cephalic extremity formed by a circumoral ring and short second annule. Lateral alae present or absent in both sexes. Isthmus distinct or it is a constriction between corpus and bulb with or without a ring-like sub-ganglion at its middle of isthmus. Buccal cavity absent or present in females. Vulva posterior to midbody. Gonads amphidelphic. Eggs broadly oval with polar filaments deposited in capsules containing 2-3 eggs or non-encapsulated and laid in pairs. Tail conical or rounded with short or long caudal appendage or flagella-like, with or without fine striations near its tips. Caudal extremity in male conical to subulate or filiform or spike-like. Caudal papillae 5-10 pairs. Single median papilla present or absent. Spicule single or absent.

7.3.2 Species

Binema ornata Travassos, 1925 (Figs. 16 & 18); Host : *Gryllotalpa africana* Beauvois ;**Habitat :** Gut ; **Locality :** Imphal, Manipur, India

7.3.3 Species

Binema korsakowi (Sergiev, 1923) Basir, 1956 (Figs. 17 & 18); **Host :** *Gryllotalpa africana* Beauvois ; **Habitat:** Gut; **Locality:** Imphal, Manipur, India

7.3.4 Species

Binema mirzaia (Basir, 1942a) Basir, 1956 (Figs. 19 & 21) ; **Host:** *Gryllotalpa africana* Beauvois ; **Habitat:** Gut ;**Locality:** Imphal, Manipur, India

7.3.5 Species

Binema anulinervus Shah & Rizvi, 2004a (Figs. 20 & 21); **Host :** *Gryllotalpa africana* Beauvois ; **Habitat :** Gut ; **Locality:** Imphal, Manipur, India

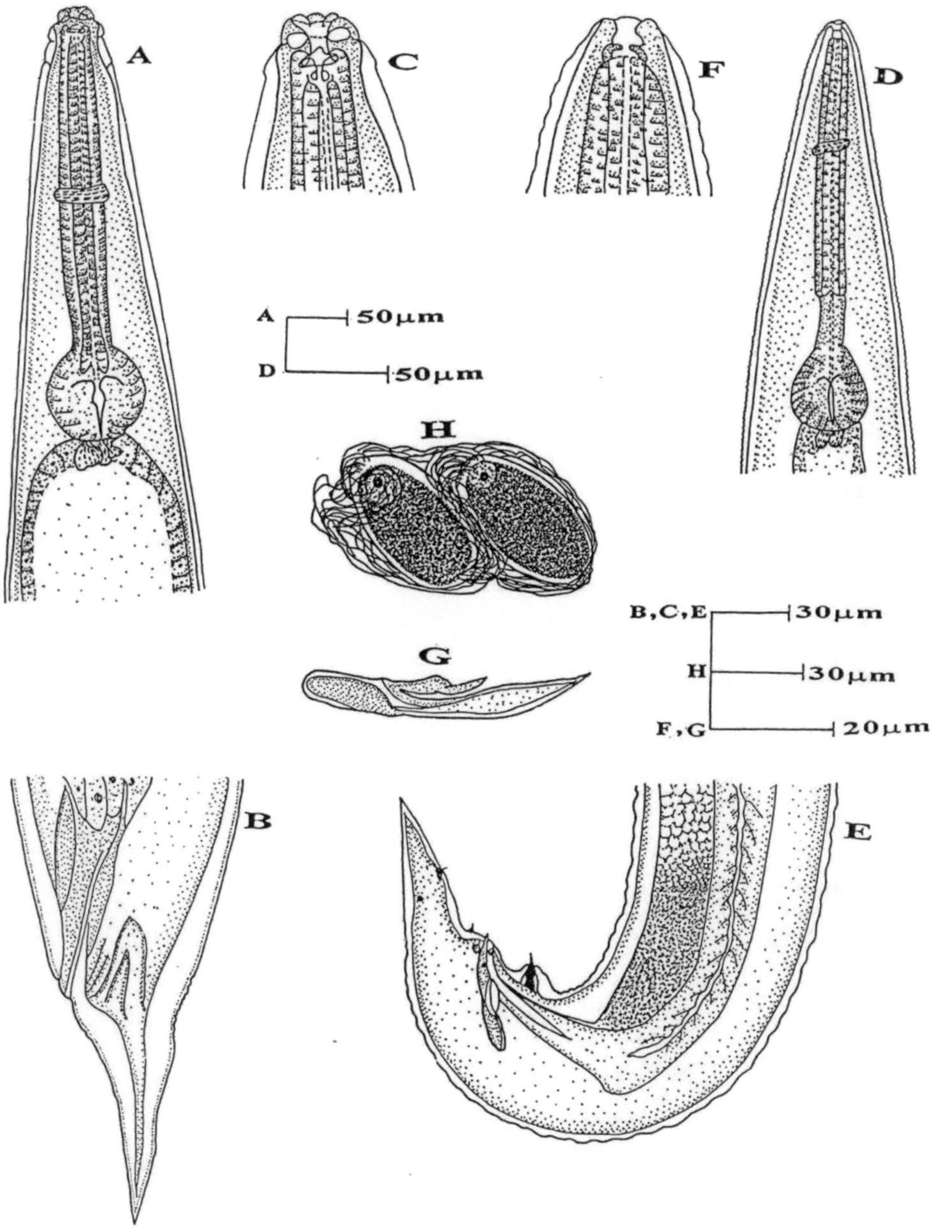

Fig. 16. *Binema ornata* Travassos, 1925: A-Female anterior end (lateral view), B-Female posterior end (lateral view), C-Female cephalic end (lateral view), D-Male anterior end (lateral view), E-Male posterior end (lateral view), F-Male cephalic end (lateral view), G-Spicule (lateral view), H-Eggs (Shah & Rizvi, 2004a).

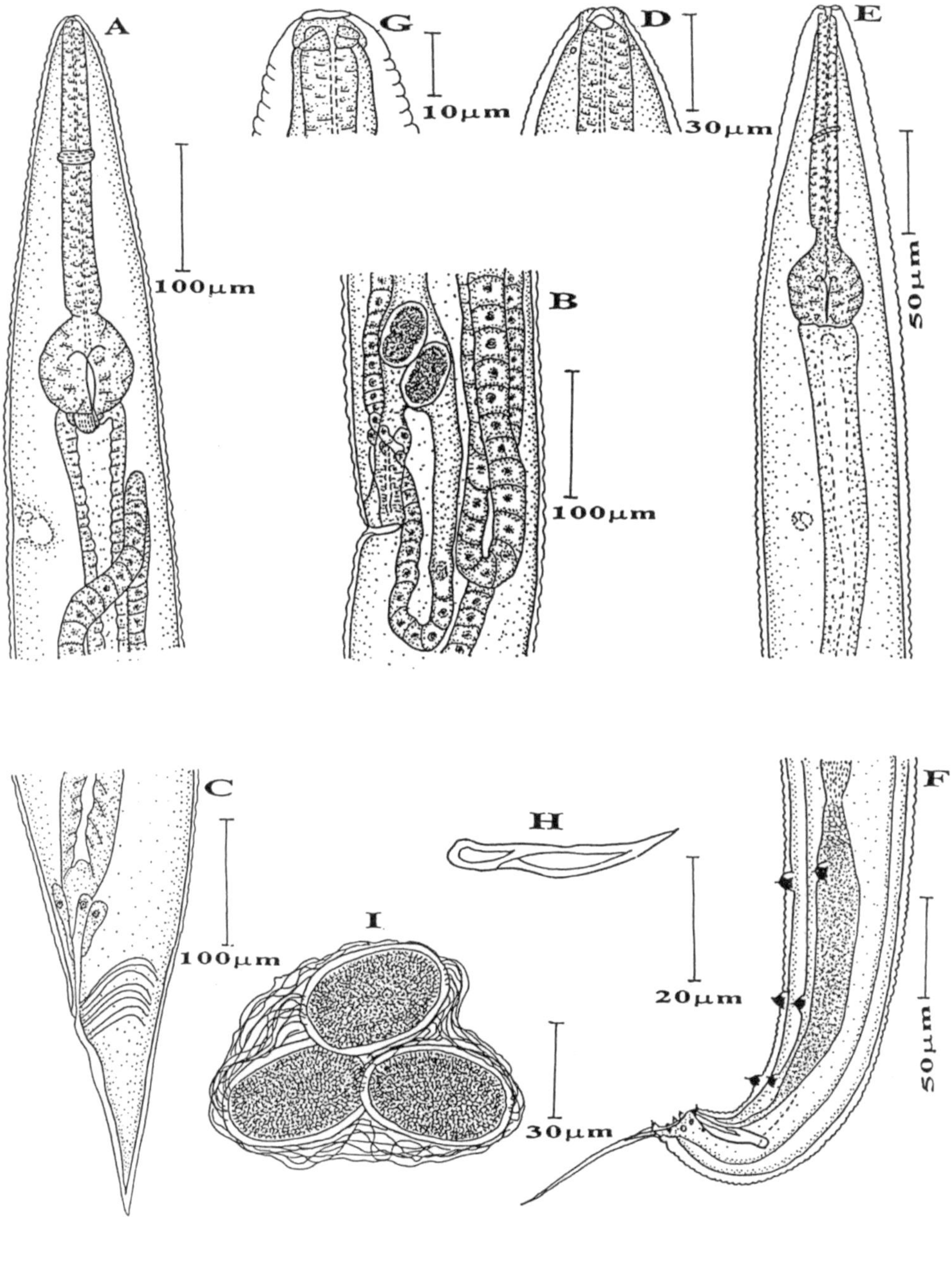

Fig. 17. *Binema korsakowi* Sergiev, 1923: A-Female anterior end (lateral view), B-Female vulval region (lateral view), C-Female posterior end (lateral view), D-Male cephalic end (lateral view), E-Male anterior end (lateral view), F-Male posterior end (lateral view), G-Female cephalic end (lateral view), H-Spicule (lateral view), I-Eggs (Shah & Rizvi, 2004a).

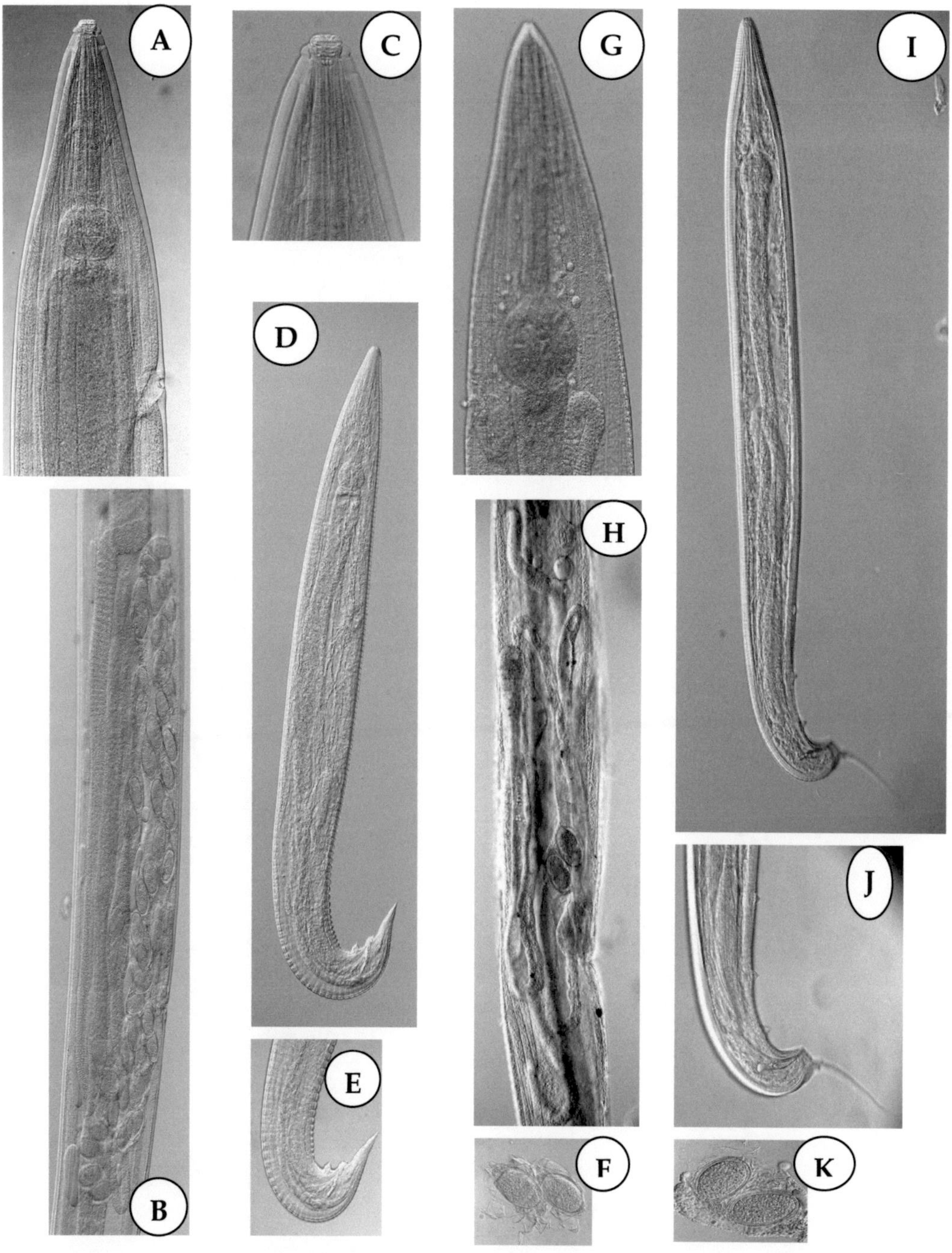

Fig. 18. Photomicrographs of *Binema ornata* Travassos, 1925 (A-F) and *Binema korsakowi* Sergiev, 1923 (G-K): A-Female anterior portion showing, excretory pore, B-Female gonads, C-Female cephalic structure, D-Entire male (lateral view), E-Male posterior end showing spicule and papillae, F-Eggs; G-Female excretory pore, H-Female gonads, I-Entire male (lateral view), J-Male posterior end showing spicule and papillae, K-Eggs (Shah & Rizvi, 2004a).

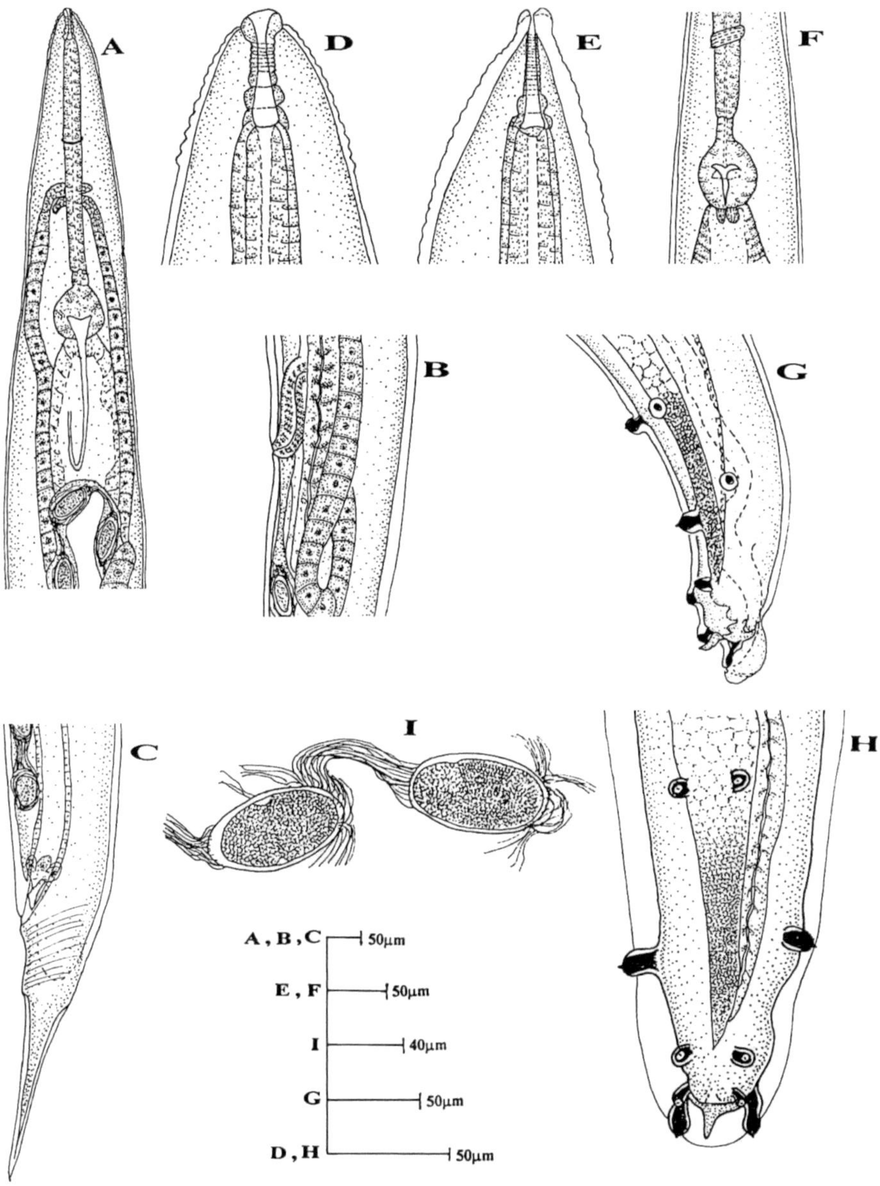

Fig. 19. *Binema mirzaia* Basir, 1942a: A-Female anterior end (lateral view), B-Female cephalic end (lateral view), C-Male cephalic end (lateral view), D-Male anterior end (lateral view), E-Female posterior end lateral view), F-Male posterior end (lateral view), G-Male posterior end (ventral view), H-Spicule, I-Eggs (Shah & Rizvi, 2004a).

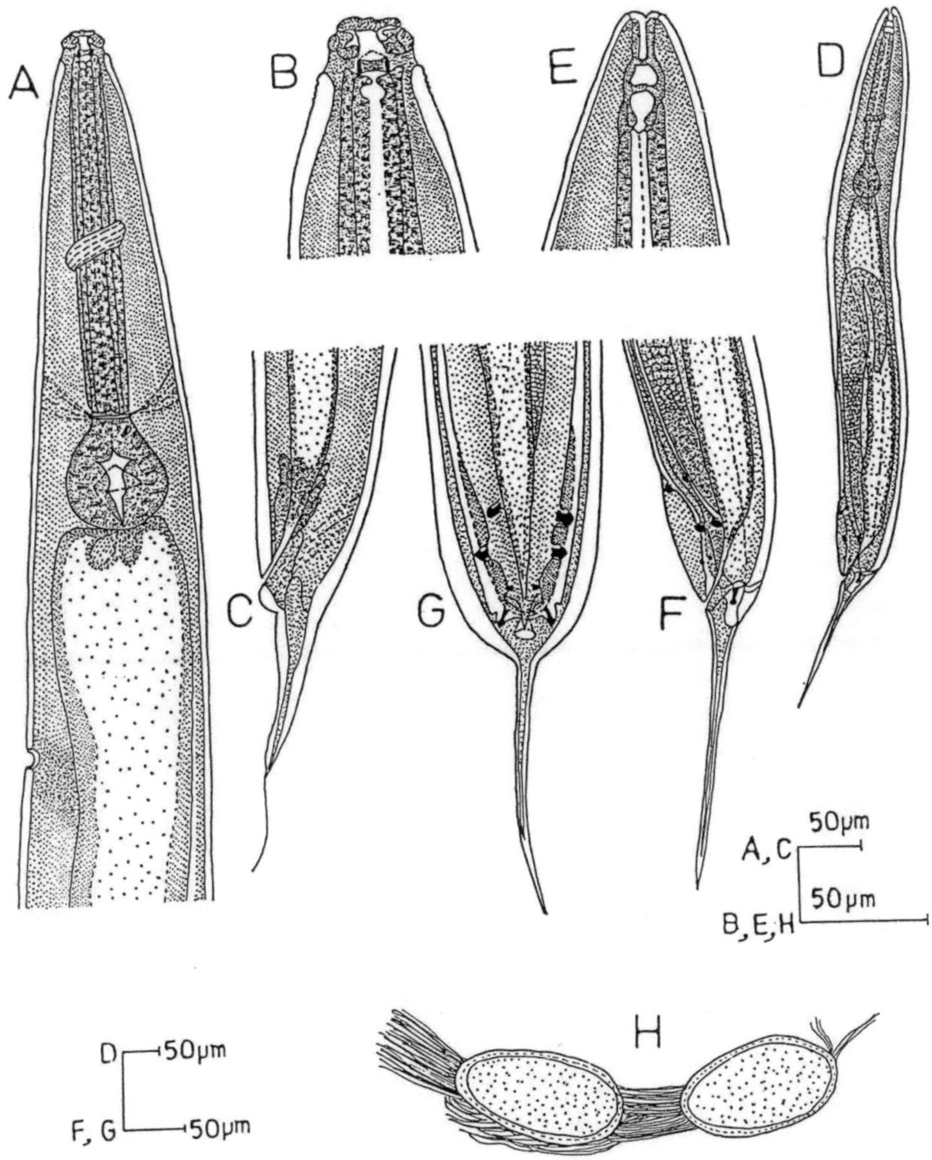

Fig. 20. *Binema anulinervus* Shah & Rizvi, 2004a: A-Female anterior end (lateral view), B-Female cephalic end (lateral view), C-Female posterior end (lateral view), D-Male entire (lateral view), E-Male cephalic end (lateral view), F-Male posterior end (lateral view), G-Male posterior end (ventral view), H-Eggs.

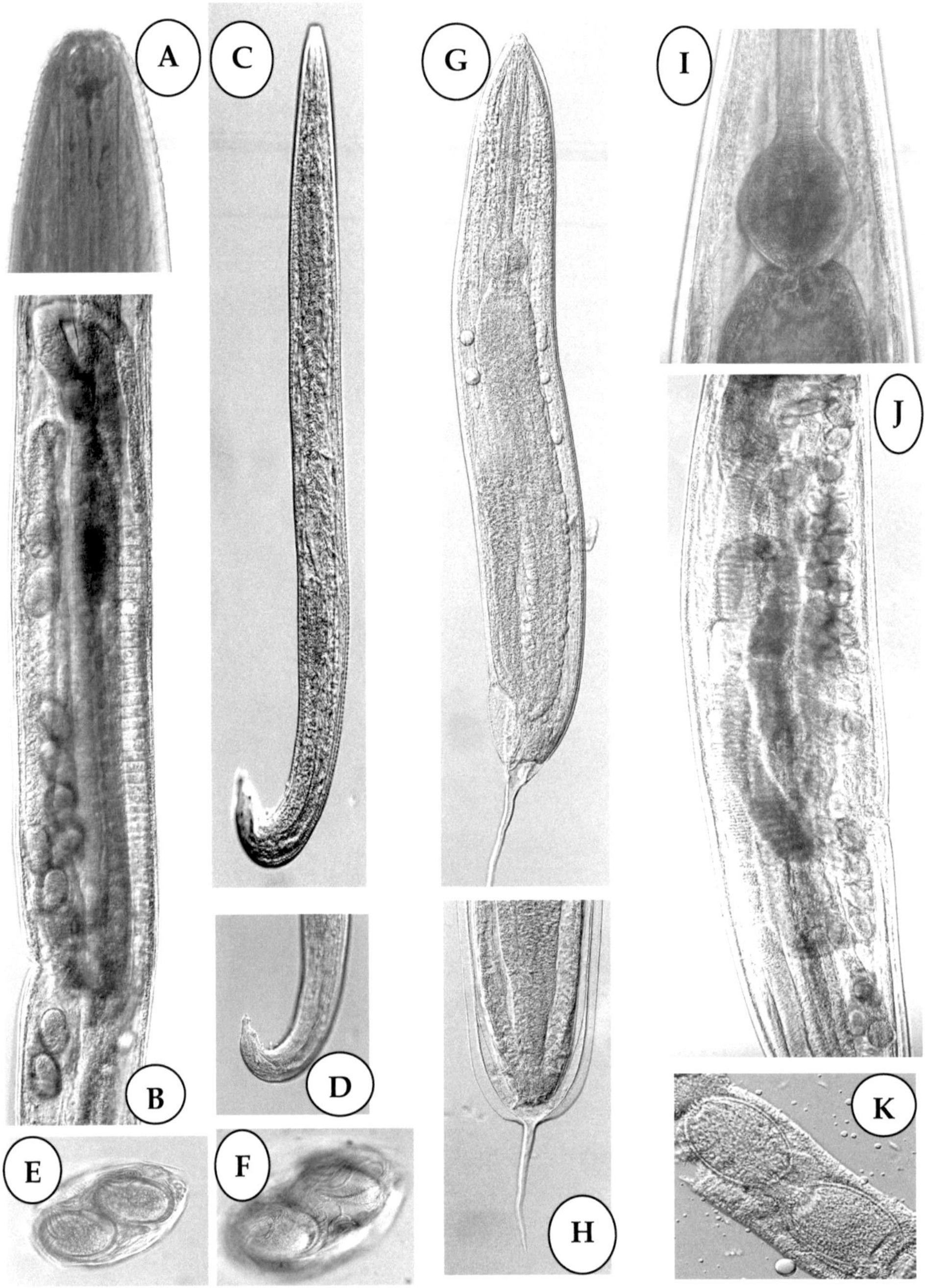

Fig. 21. Photomicrographs of *Binema mirzaia* Basir, 1942a (A-F) and *Binema anulinervus* Shah & Rizvi, 2004a (G-K): A-Female cephalic annulation, B-Female gonads, C-Entire male (Lateral view), D-Male posterior end showing spicule and papillae, E-Eggs (internal), F-Eggs (outer shell), G-Male entire (Lateral view), H-Male posterior end showing papillae (ventral view), Portion of female oesophagus showing ring like structure in the middle of Isthmus, J-Female gonads (Lateral view), K-Eggs.

7.3.6 Key to species of *Binema* Travassos, 1925

1. Female tail with flagellate caudal appendage...2
- Female tail without flagellate caudal appendage..3

2(1). Female length=2.423-3.273 mm, presence of a sub-ganglion at the middle of isthmus.. *B. anulinervus* Shah & Rizvi,2004a
- Female length = 6.98 mm, absence of a subganglion at the middle of the isthmus.... .... *B. pseudornatum* Leibersperger,1960

3(1). Buccal cavity present..4
- Buccal cavity absent.. *B. korsakowi* (Sergiev, 1923) Basir,1956

4(3). Lateral alae in male present..5
- Lateral alae in male absent..6

5(4). Annulation prominent only in cervical region and female tail=0.068-0.088mm....... .... *B. mirzaia* (Basir,1942a)Basir,1956
- Annulation absent in cervical region and female tail = 0.2-0.21 mm...................... ....*B. parva* Parveen & Jairajpuri,1985b

6(4). Male with five pairs of caudal papillae, buccal cavity with ornamentation............7
- Male with eight pairs of caudal papillae, buccal cavity without ornamentation........ ....*B. striatum* Rizvi &Jairajpuri,2000

7(6). Female buccal cavity with three sclerotized arches and male tail conical............... .... *B. bonaerensis* Camino &Reboredo,1999
- Female buccal cavity with projection; male tail forms a caudal spike..................... ....*B. ornata* Travassos,1925

7.4 Genus: *Chitwoodiella* Basir,1948b

7.4.1 Generic diagnosis

Female: Cephalic extremity formed by single lip cone. Buccal capsule long, tubular with striated cuticular wall, posterior part of which may or may not possess three cuticularised tooth like structures. Oesophageal corpus cylindrical. Prominent cardia with or without modification into a long tubular structure. Vulva between middle and posterior-third of body. Vagina short and directed anteriorly. Gonads amphididelphic. Blind ends of ovaries reflexed and reaching the oesophageal region. Eggs attached to one another in strings by polar filaments. Tail conical or subulate.

Male: Buccal capsule long tubular with striated cuticular wall, posterior part do not possess cuticularised tooth-like structures. Lateral alae present. Tail very short, truncated with caudal alae. Spicule absent. Caudal papillae five to six pairs. A median ventral, rod-like, bluntly pointed projection, juts out backwardly just behind the cloaca.

7.4.2 Species

Chitwoodiella longicaridia Shah, 2008 (Figs. 22 & 23); **Host :** *Gryllotalpa africana* Beauvois ; **Site :** Gut ; **Locality:** Imphal, Manipur, India

7.4.3 Key to species of *Chitwoodiella* Basir, 1948b

1. Cardia modified into a long tube..*C. longicardia* Shah,2008
- Cardia not modified into a long tube..2

2(1). Six pairs of caudal papillae in male; female buccal cavity with three tooth-like structures...*C. tridentata* Rizvi, Jairajpuri & Shah,1998

- Five pairs of caudal papillae in male; female buccal cavity without three tooth-like structure...*C. ovofilamenta* Basir (1948b, 1949)

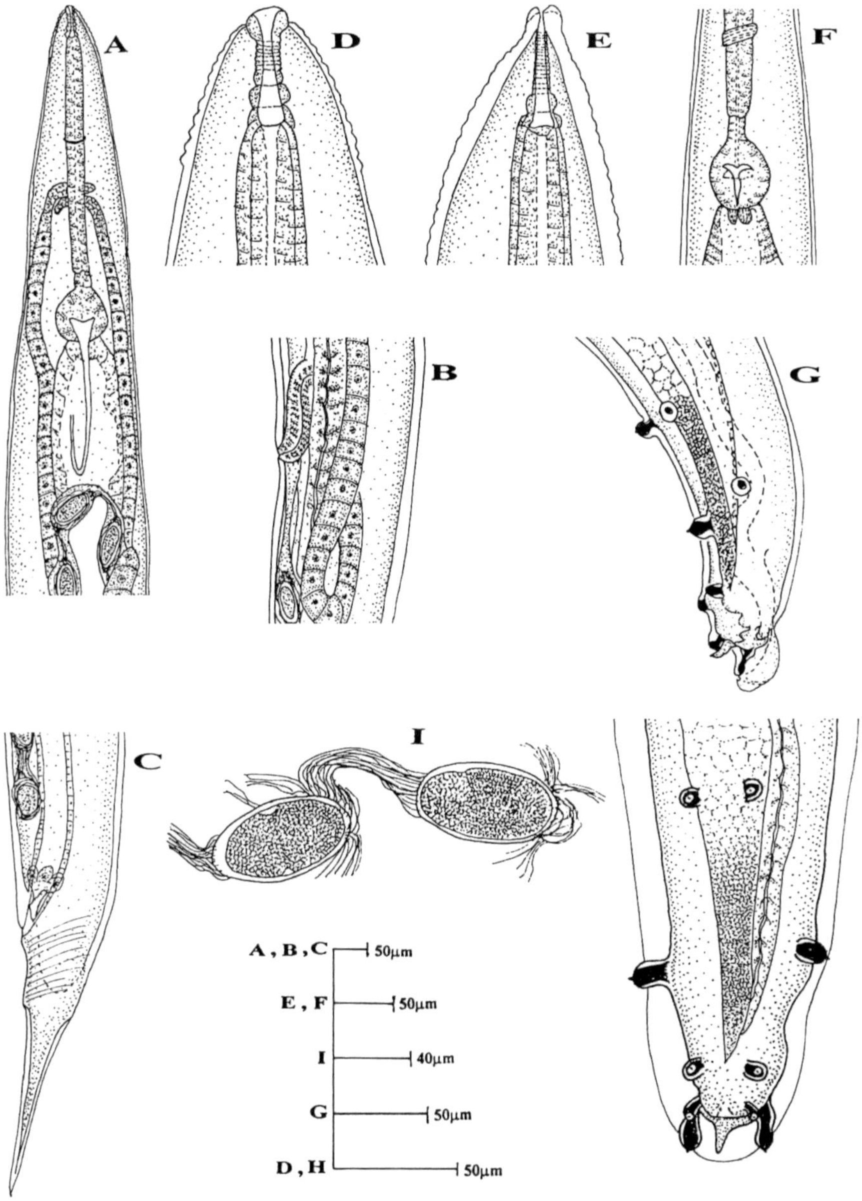

Fig. 22. *Chitwoodiella longicardia* Shah, 2008: A-Female anterior end, B-Female vulval region, C-Female posterior end (lateral view), D-Female cephalic end, E-Male cephalic end, F-Male oesophageal region, G- Male posterior end (lateral view under different focuses), H-Male posterior end (ventral view), I- Eggs.

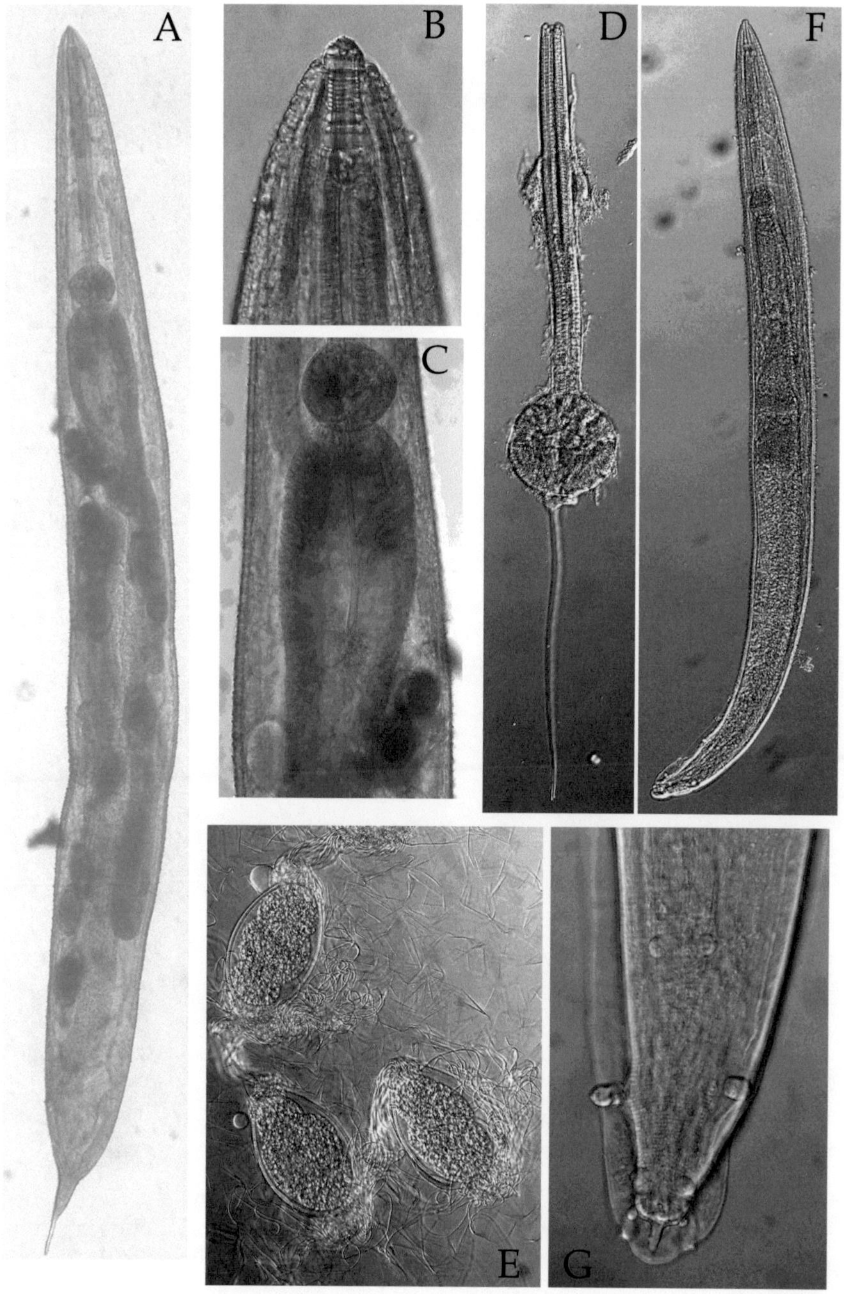

Fig. 23. Photomicrographs of *Chitwoodiella longicardia* Shah, 2008: A-Female entire (lateral view), B-Female anterior end showing prominent annulations in cervical region and in buccal cavity, C-Female oesophageal bulb and intestine showing modified cardia, D-Magnified and cut-open view of female oesophagus showing corpus, nerve ring, bulb and modified & elongated cardia, E-Eggs showing egg filaments joining one another, F-Male entire (lateral view), G-Male posterior end (ventral view).

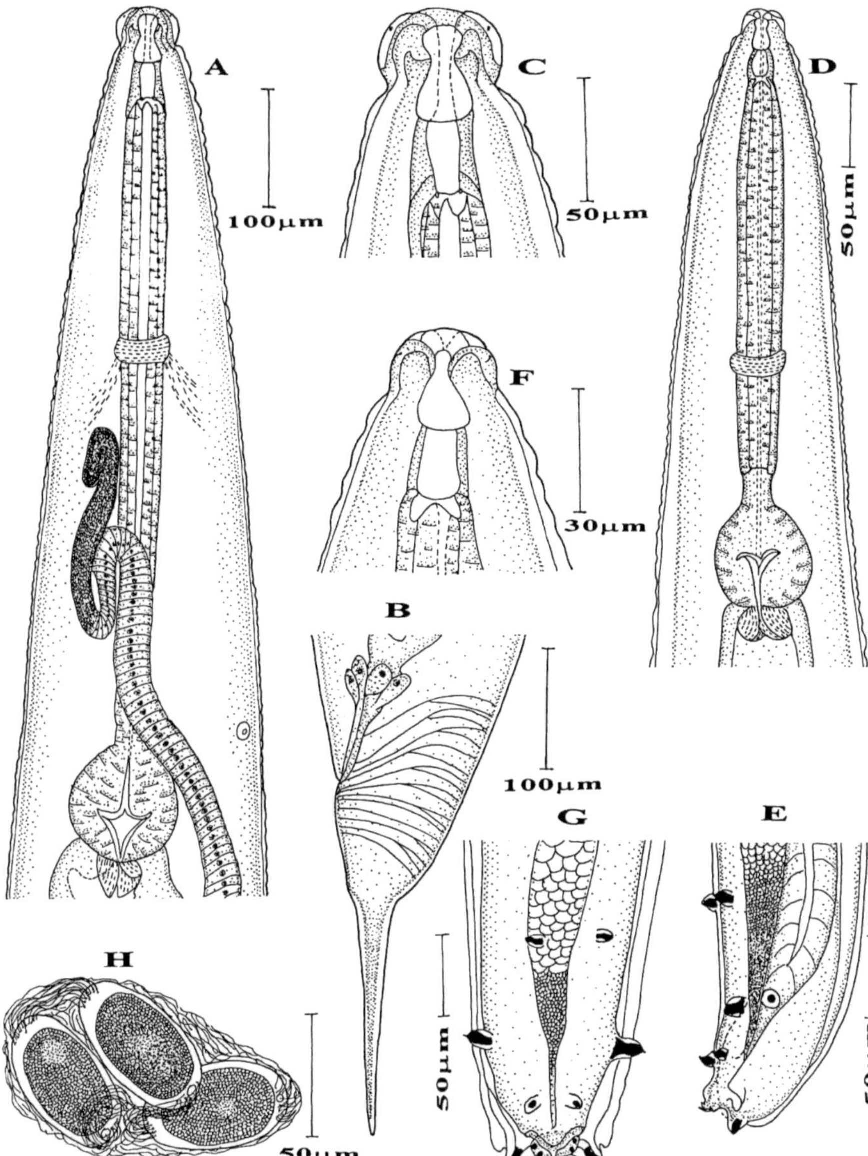

Fig. 24. *Mirzaiella asiatica* Basir, 1942: A-Female anterior end, B-Female posterior end (lateral view), C-Female cephalicd end, D-Male anterior end, E-Male posterior end (lateral view), F-Male cephalic end, G-Male posterior end (ventral view), H-Eggs (Shah, 2008).

7.5 Genus: *Mirzaiella* Basir, 1942a

7.5.1 Generic diagnosis

Cephalic extremity formed by prominent cephalic annule. Oral opening surrounded by three lips, one dorsal and two subventral. Buccal cavity long, tubular, formed by two distinct parts of almost equal length. Oesophageal corpus very long, widest at its anterior end, shaped like an inverted club, isthmus short and bulb spherical. Excretory pore anterior to the base of the oesophagus. Vulva near posterior-third of body. Vagina short, muscular and anteriorly directed. Amphidelphic. Eggs oval shaped, attached to one another by polar filaments, laid in mucus capsules, each capsule containing two-five eggs. Tail short, blunt or rounded or subulate, with or without spine-like appendage. Lateral alae absent in female. Gonads two, ovaries reflexed at both ends, the anterior one extends upto the middle of the corpus and the posterior one a little above the anus. Caudal extremity in male rounded. Caudal papillae four to seven pairs. Spicule absent. Pointed cuticularized accessory piece present immediately behind the anus.

7.5.2 Species

Mirzaiella asiatica Basir, 1942a (Fig. 24); Host: *Gryllotalpa africana* Beauvois; Site: Gut ;Locality: Imphal, Manipur, India

7.5.3 Key to species of *Mirzaiella* Basir, 1942a

1. Female tail with a distinct constriction in the middle.............*M. alii* Farooqui,1967
- Female tail without distinct constriction in the middle.......................................2
2(2). Three chitinous teeth at the base of the buccal cavity present in female..................
........................*M. indicus* (Singh & Singh, 1955) Adamson & Waerebeke,1992b
- Female buccal cavity without teeth...3
3(2). Spicule present in male...
......................*M. gryllotalpae* (Singh & Singh,1955) Adamson & Waerebeke,1992b
- Spicule absent in male...4
4(3). Caudal papillae five pairs, only caudal alae present..............*M. asiatica* Basir, 1942a
- Caudal papillae seven pairs, caudal alae extend upto midbody.................................
....*M. haroldi* Farooqui, 1968b

8. Acknowledgements

The authors are thankful to the Head, Department of Life Sciences, Manipur University for providing necessary laboratory facilities. The financial assistance provided by Ministry of Science and Technology, Department of Biotechnology, Govt. of India, New Delhi is also thankfully acknowledged by the first author.

9. References

Adamson, ML and Waerebeke, DV(1992a). Revision of the Thelastomatoidea, Oxyurida of Invertebrate host. 1. Thelastomatidae. *Systematic Parasitology* 21: 21-63.

Adamson, ML and Waerebeke, DV(1992b). Revision of the Thelastomatoidea, Oxyurida of Invertebrate hosts II. Travassosinematidae, Protrelloididae and Pseudonymidae. *Systematic Parasitology*, 21: 169-188.

Adamson, ML and Waerebeke, DV(1992c). Revision of the Thelastomatoidea, Oxyurida of Invertebrate host. III. Hystrignathidae. *Systematic Parasitology* 22: 111-130.

Adamson, ML (1984). L'haplodiploidie des Oxyurida. Incidence de ce phenomene dans le cycle evolutif. *Annales de Parasitologie Humaine et.Comparee* 59: 387- 413.

Adamson, ML and Nasher, AK(1987). *Hammerschmidtiella andersoni* sp. n. (Thelastomatidae: Oxyurida) from the diplopod, *Archispirostreptus tumuliporus* in Saudi Arabia with comments on the karyotype of *Hammerschmidtiella diesingi*. *Proceedings of the Helminthological Society of Washington* 54: 220-224.

Adamson, ML (1989). Evolutionary biology of the Oxyurida (Nematoda). Biofacies of a haplodiploid taxon. *Advances in Parasitology* 28: 175 - 228.

Adamson, ML and Buck, A (1990). Pinworms from water scavenger beetles (Coleoptera: Hydrophilidae) with a description of a new species *Zonothrix columbianus* sp. n. (Oxyurida: Pseudonymidae) from Western Canada. *Journal of Helminthological Society of Washington*, 57: 21-25.

Ali, SM and Farooqui, MN (1969). *Cordonicola blaberi* n.gen. n.sp. from the black roach *Blaberus* sp. and Cordonicolidae fam.nov. from Marathwada, India. *Rivista di Parassitologia* 30: 121 - 123.

Basir, MA (1941). Two new nematodes from an aquatic beetle. *Proceedings of the Indian Academy of Science* 13 (Section B), 163-167.

Basir, MA (1942a). Nematodes parasitic in *Gryllotalpa*. *Records of the Indian Museum* 44: 95-106.

Basir, MA (1942b). *Protrellina phylodromi* sp. nov., a new nematode parasite of the cockroach *Phyllodromia humbertiana* Sauss. *Current Science* (Bangalore) 11: 195 - 197.

Basir, MA (1948a). *Cameronia biovata* gen et. sp. nov. (Thelastomatidae) a new nematode parasite of the mole cricket, *Gryllotalpa africana* Beauv. *Canadian Journal of Research* 26: 201-203.

Basir, MA (1948b). *Chitwoodiella ovofilamenta* gen. et sp. nov. a nematode parasite of *Gryllotalpa*. *Canadian Journal of Research* 26: 4-7.

Basir, MA (1949). A description of the male of *Chitwoodiella ovofilamenta* Basir,1948 (Nematoda: Thelastomatidae). *Proceedings of the Helminthological Society of Washington* 16: 112-114.

Basir, MA (1956). Oxyuroid parasites of Arthropoda: A monographic study 1. Thelastomatidae 2. Oxyuridae. *Zoologica (Stuttgart)*, pp. 1-79, 13 plates

Biswas, PK and Chakravarty, GK (1963). The systematic studies of the zooparasitic nematodes. *Zeitschrift fur ParasitenKunde* 23: 411-428.

Camino, NB and Reboredo, GR (1999). *Binema bonaerensis* n. sp. (Oxyurida: Thelastomatidae) parasite of *Neocurtilla claraziana* Saussure (Orthoptera: Gryllotalpidae) in Argentina. *Memorias do Instituto Oswaldo* 94(3) : 311-313.

Camino, NB and Maiztegui, B (2002). A new species of Thelastomatidae (Nematoda) a parasite of *Neocurtilla clariaziana* Saussure (Orthoptera, Gryllotalpidae) in Argentina. *Memorias do Instituto Oswaldo Cruz, Rio de Janeiro*, 97(5) : 655-656.

Chitwood, BG (1930). A new nema parasitic in the intestine of *Fontaria*. *Journal of Parasitology* 16: 163-164.

Chitwood, BG (1932). A synopsis of nematodes parasitic in insects of the family Blattidae. *Zeitchrift fur Parasitenkunde* 5: 14-50.

Chitwood, BG (1933). A revised classification of Nematoda. *Journal of Parasitology*, 20, 131.

Chitwood, BG and Chitwood, MB (1934). Nematodes parasitic in Philippine cockroaches . *Phillipines Journal of Science* 52: 381 - 393. 3 plates.

Chakravarty, GK (1943). On the nematode *Indiana gryllotalpae* gen et sp.nov. from *Gryllotalpa* sp. *Current Science* 12: 257 - 258.

Cobb, NA (1920). One hundred new nemas (Type species of 100 new genera). *Contributions to the Science of Nematology. (Cobb) Baltimore, MD, USA,* Waverly Press, pp. 217-343.

Courtney, WD, Polley, D and Miller, VL (1955). TAF, an improved fixative in nematode technique. *Plant Disease Reporter* 39: 570-571.

Dale, PS (1964).*Tetleys pericopti* n.gen. et sp., a thelastomatid nematodes from the larvae of *Pericoptes truncatus* (Fab.)(Coleptera : Dynastinae). *N. Z. J. Sci.*,7: 589-595.

Dale, PS (1967). Nematodes associated with the pine bark beetle, *Hylastes ater*, in New Zealand. *New Zealand Journal of Science* 10: 222 - 234.

De Man, JG (1884). Die frei der reinen Erde und in sussen wasser lebenden nematoden niederlandischen fauna. *Eine Systematische Faunistische Monographie, Leiden*, pp.206.

Diesing, KM (1857). Sechzehn Arten von Nematoden. *Denkschr der Kaiserlichen Akademie der Wissenschaften Mathemitisch-Naturwissenschaftliche Classe* 13: 6-26.

Farooqui, MN (1967). On a known and some new species of insect nematodes. *Zoologischer Anzeiger* 176: 276-296.

Farooqui, MN (1968a). On a new species of *Cameronia* Basir, 1948 from *Gryllotalpa africana. Rivista di Parassitologia* 29: 269-272.

Farooqui, MN (1968b). On a new species of *Mirzaiella* Basir, 1942 from *Gryllotalpa africana. Rivista di Parassitologia,* 29(1) : 21-24.

Farooqui, MN (1970). Some known and new genera and species of the family Thelastomaidae Travassos, 1929. *Rivista di Parassitologia* 31: 195-214.

Fotedar, DN (1964). A new species of the nematode genus *Pseudonymus* Diesing, 1857 from an aquatic beetle in Kashmir. *Kashmir Science* 1(1-2), 73-75.

Galeb, O (1877). Sur l`anatomie et les migrations des Oxyurides, parasites des insectes du genera *Blatta. Comptes Rendus a l Academie des Sciences (Paris)* 85: 236-390.

Galeb, O (1878). Recherches sur les entozoaires des insects.Organization et development des oxyurides. *Archives de Zoologie Experimentale et Generale* 7: 283-389, 10 plates.

Gupta, NK and Kaur, J (1978). On some nematodes from Invertebrates in Northern India Part-I. *Revista Ibérica Parasitologia,* 38, 301-324.

Hammerschmidt, KE (1838). *Helminthologische Beitrage. Isis Von Oken* 5: 351-358.

Jex, AR, Schneider, MA, Rose, HA and Cribb, TH (2005). The Thelastomatoidea (Nematoda: Oxyurida) of two sympatric Panesthiinae(Insecta:Blattodea) from south-eastern Queensland, Australia: Taxonomy, species richness and host specificity. *Nematology* 7(4) : 543-575.

Kloss, GR (1958). Nematodeos parasitos de Hydrophilidae (Col.). *Atas de la Sociedade do Biologia de Rio de Janeiro* 2: 21-23.

Kloss, GR (1959a). Nematodes parasitos de baratas. *Atas de la Sociedade do Biologia de Rio de Janeiro* 3(5): 6 - 8.

Kloss, GR (1959b). Nematoides parasitos de Gryllotalpoidea (Orthoptera) la Nota Previa. *Atas de la Sociedade do Biologia de Rio de Janeiro* 3: 9 - 12.

Kloss, GR (1959c). Nematodes parasitos de Coleoptera Hydrophilidae. *Estudos Tecnicos Ministerio de Agricultura (Rio de Janeiro)* 13: 101 pp.

Kloss, GR(1960). Organizacao filogenetica dos nematoides parasitos intestinais dos artopodos (Nota previa). *Atas. Soc. Biol. Rio de J.*, 4: 51 - 55.

Kloss, GR (1961). Dois nematoides parasitos intestinais de especies selvagens de Blattaria. *Papeis Avulsos do Departmento de Zoologia* ,SaoPaulo 14: 243-47.

Kloss, GR (1966). Revisao dos Nematoides de Blattaria do Brasil. *Papeis Avulsos do Departmento de Zoologia, SaoPaulo* 18: 147-188.

Leibersperger, E (1960). *Die oxyuroidea de europaischen Arthropoden. Parasitologische Schriftenreihe* 11: 1-150.

Leidy, J (1849). New genera and species of entozoa. *Proceedings of the Academy of Natural Sciences of Philadelphia* 4: 225 - 233.

Leidy, J (1850). Description of some nematoid Entozoa infesting insects. *Proceedings of the Academy of Natural Sciences of Philadelphia* 5: 100-102.

Parveen, R and Jairajpuri, DS (1981). Two new species of insect nematodes of the family Thelastomatidae. *Rivista di Parassitologia* 42(2) : 261-266.

Parveen, R. and Jairajpuri, DS (1984). *Cameronia klossi* n. sp. (Nematoda: Thelastomtidae) from the mole cricket *Gryllotalpa africana* from Aligarh. *Revista Ibérica de Parasitologia* 44: 153-158.

Parveen, R. and Jairajpuri, DS (1985a). *Psilocephala nisari* sp.n. (Nematoda: Thelastomatide), a new nematode parasite of the mole cricket, *Gryllotalpa africana* from Aligarh, India. *Helminthologia* 22: 263-266.

Parveen, R. and Jairajpuri, DS (1985b). *Binema parva* n.sp., a parasitic nematode of the mole criket *Gryllotalpa africana. Rivista di Parassitologia* 46(3) : 347-349.

Rao, PN (1958). Studies on the nematode parasites of insects and other arthropods. *Arquivos do Museu Nacional, Rio de Janeiro* 46: 33-84.

Rao, PN and Rao, VJ(1965). A description of a new species of the nematode genus *Blattophila* Cobb, 1920 (Thelastomatidae). *Papeis Avulsos do Departmento de Zoologia, SaoPaolo* 18: 61-63.

Reboredo, GR and Camino, NB (2001). A new species of the genus *Cameronia* Basir (Oxyurida: Thelastomatidae) parasite of *Gryllodes laplatae* Sauss (Orthoptera : Gryllidae) in Argentina. *Boletín Chileno de Parasitología* 56: 42-44.

Rizvi, AN, Jairajpuri, DS and Shah, MM (1998). *Chitwoodiella tridentata* sp. n. (Travassosinematidae) from a mole cricket from India with SEM observations on *Leidynema appendiculatum* (Thelastomatidae). *International Journal of Nematology,* 8(1): 13-16.

Rizvi, AN and Jairajpuri, DS (2000). Studies on a new and two known species of Travassosinematidae (Oxyurida). *International Journal of Nematology* 10(1): 112-117.

Rizvi, AN and Jairajpuri DS (2002). Studies on a new and some known species of insect oxyurid nematodes. *Revista Ibérica de Parasitología* 62: 1-7.

Rizvi, AN, Jairajpuri, DS and Shah, MM (2002). *Gryllophila nihali* n. sp., *Protrellatus indicus* n. sp. (Oxyurida: Thelastomatoidea). *International Journal of Nematology* 12(1) : 29-34.

Sergiev, PG (1923). Two new nematodes from the intestine of *Gryllotalpa vulgaris*. Rapport de 21 [e] siance de la commission pour l'etude de la faune helminthologique de Russie 1923 (In Russian). *Trudy Gosundarstvennogo Instituta K Experimental noi Veterinarii* 1: 183-190.

Serrano Sanchez, A (1945). *Hammerschmidtiella neyrai* n.sp. en *Periplaneta orientalis* L in Granada. *Revista Ibérica de Parasitología, Tomo Extraordinario,* pp. 213-215.

Shah, MM and Rizvi, AN (2004a). Some studies on three known a new species of the genus *Binema* Travassos,1925 (Travassosinematidae: Thelastomatoidea) from Manipur, North-East India. *Parassitologia* 46: 317-326.

Shah, MM and Rizvi, AN (2004b). *Pseudonymus basiri* sp. n. and *Zonothrix alata* sp. n. (Pseudonymidae: Thelastomatoidea) from water beetle *Hydrophilus triangularis*. *International Journal of Nematology* 14(2): 229-235.

Shah, MM, Rizvi, AN and Jairajpuri, DS (2005). *Protrellus shamimi* n. sp. (Protrelloididae: Thelastomatoidea) from the cockroach *Periplaneta americana* from Manipur, North-East India. *Journal of Parasitic Diseases*, 29(1): 47-52.

Shah, MM (2007a). Two new species of *Cameronia* Basir, 1948 (Oxyurida, Thelastomatoidea, Thelastomatidae) from Manipur, North-East India. *Acta Parasitologica* 52(3):225-232.

Shah, MM (2007b). Some studies on insect parasitic nematodes (Oxyurida, Thelastomatoidea, Thelastomatidae) from Manipur, North-East India. *Acta Parasitologica* 52(4): 346-362.

Shah, MM (2008). A new species of Chitwoodiella Basir, 1948 with first report on Mirzaiella asiatica Basir, 1942 (Nematoda: Travassosinematidae) from Manipur, North-East India. *Acta Parasitologica* 53(2): 145-152.

Singh, KS and Singh, KP (1955). On some nematodes from invertebrates. *Records of the Indian Museum* 53: 37-51.

Singh, HS and Kaur, H (1988). On a new nematode *Hammerschmidtiella basiri* [Sic] n. sp. from *Periplaneta americana* Linn. *Indian Journal of Parasitology* 12: 187-189.

Skrjabin, KI, Schikhobalova, NP and Lagodovskaya, A (1966). Principles of nematology, edited by K.I.Skrjabin. Vol.XV. Oxyurata of Arthropoda, Part 4. *Moscow Izdatelstvo, Nauka,* pp.1-538.

Spiridonov, SE (1984). New oxyurid species from the intestine of *Rhinocricus* sp. *Trudy Zoologicheskogo Instituta* 126: 33-49.

Schwenk, JM (1926). Fauna parasitologica dos blattideos do Brasil. *Sciencia Medica (Rio de Janeiro)* 4: 491-504.

Todd, AC (1942). A new parasitic nematode from a water scavenger beetle. *Transactions of the American Microscopical Society* 61: 286-289.

Todd, AC (1944). On the development and hatching of the eggs of *Hammerschmidtiella diesingi* and *Leidynema appendiculatum*, nematodes of roaches. *Transactions of the American Microscopical Society* 63: 54-67.

Travassos, L (1920). Esboco de uma chave gerale dos nematodes parasitos. *Revista Vetirinarias Zootecnia* 10: 59 - 70.

Travassos, L (1925). Contribuicau ao conhecimento dos Nematodeos dos Arthropodes. *Sciencia Medica (Rio de Janeiro)* 3: 416-422.

Travassos, L (1929). Contribuicão preliminary a sistemática dos nematodeos dos artropodes. *Memorias do Instituto Oswaldo Cruz, Supl* 5: 19-25.

Travassos, L (1954). Contribuicao para o conhecimento dos nematodeos parasitos de coleopteros aquaticos. *Revista Brasiliera de Biologia* 14: 143-151.

Travassos, L and Kloss, GR (1958). Nematodeos de invertebrados, 14a Nota. *Atas de la Sociedade do Biologia de Rio de Janeiro* 2: 27-30.

Travassos, L and Kloss, GR (1960). Sur un curieux Nematoda. *Robertia leiperi* gen. at so.nov., parasite de l`intestin de diplopode. *Journal of Helminthology, R.T. Leiper Suppment,* 187-190 pp.

Von Gyory, A (1856). Uber *Oxyuris spirotheca* (nov. spec.). *Sitzungsberichte der Kaiserlichen Akademie der Wissenschaften Mathemitisch-Naturwissenschaftliche Classe* 21: 327-332.

Van Waerebeke, D (1969). Quelques nematodes parasites de blattes a Madagasker. *Annales de Parasitologie et Humaine et Comparee (Paris)* 44 : 761-776.

Van Waerebeke D (1978). Description de *Cephalobellus ovumglutinosus* n. sp. et de *Leidynema portentosae* n. sp.(Nematoda: Thelastomatidae), parasites intestinaux de blattes, et redifinition du genre *Leidynema* Schwenk, 1926 (in Travassos, 1929). *Revue de Nematology* 1(2) : 151-163.

Van Waerebeke, D and Remillet, M (1973). Deux especes malgaches de Thelastomatidae (Nematoda) appartenanta un genre nouvean, *Jaryella tsimbazazae* gen. et sp.nov. et *Jaryella ataenii* sp.nov. *Cahiers ORSTOM, Serie Biologie* 21: 239-250.

Zervos, S (1987a). *Protrellus dalei* n. sp., *Blatticola barryi* n. sp., and *Suifunema mackenziei* n. sp., thelastomatid nematodes from New Zealand cockroaches. *New Zealand Journal of Zoology* 14: 240-250.

Zervos, S (1987b). *Protrellus dixoni* n. sp. (Nematoda:Thelastomatidae) from the cockroach *Drymaplaneta variegata. New Zealand Journal of Zoology* 14: 251-256.